THE
PUZZLE
PEOPLE

THE PUZZLE PEOPLE

Memoirs of a Transplant
Surgeon

Thomas E. Starzl

University of Pittsburgh Press
Pittsburgh and London

Published by the University of Pittsburgh Press, Pittsburgh, Pa., 15260
Copyright © 1992, Thomas E. Starzl
Eurospan, London
Manufactured in the United States of America

Library of Congress Cataloging-in-Publication Data

Starzl, Thomas E. (Thomas Earl), 1926–
    The puzzle people : memoirs of a transplant surgeon/Thomas E. Starzl.
      p. cm.
    Includes index.
    ISBN 0-8229-3714-X
    1. Transplantation of organs, tissues, etc.—History.   2. Starzl, Thomas E. (Thomas
Earl), 1926–   . I. Title.
    [DNLM: 1. Starzl, Thomas E. (Thomas Earl), 1926–   .   2. Organ Transplantation—
history.   3. Organ Transplantation—personal narratives.   4. Surgery—personal narratives.   WZ 100 S796]
RD120.6.S73   1992
617.9'5'009—dc20
[B]
DNLM/DLC
for Library of Congress   92-455
                                                                              CIP

A CIP catalogue record for this book is available from the British Library.

Material in chapter 24 is reprinted with permission from *Dialysis and Transplantation* 16, no.
8, August 1987.

Contents

Figures

Photographs follow pages 140 and 236.

Preface

This book is about organ transplantation, or to be more accurate, about some of the people who made development of this field possible. My inclination to record these memoirs about events that shaped transplantation had feebly surfaced and been summarily rejected from time to time during the past few years. The impulse had become more insistent after I underwent two operations on my heart during the summer of 1990. It now seemed to me that what I had experienced might help someone else who feared along the way that their best efforts were leading nowhere. Or failing this, perhaps I could shed light on how advances occur in clinical medicine; what goes on in the middle of the night in laboratories and hospital corridors; what the interactions are between the involved physicians, scientists, and patients; and how the patients themselves inevitably emerge as the heroes.

The reader who wants documentation of the events in transplantation can find scientific trails in the memoirs of early workers in the field which recently were collected by Dr. Paul I. Terasaki of Los Angeles.[1] My contribution to Terasaki's book described and annotated the steps in transplantation of the last thirty-five years that involved me and others. These were the ingredients of formal history. It will be evident that most of the incidents to be described in this book comprised the rest of the story. They will be remembered with a smile or frown, or even a tear, by those who also were there.

Two people made the book possible. One was my wife, Joy, who was a heroine in its pages but a temporary widow during its writing, which required almost a year. The other was Mrs. Terry Mangan, whose own family paid the price for the laborious preparation of the manuscript. Accuracy and fairness were my foremost objectives; I therefore gave to the people mentioned in the book those portions involving them, or frequently the entire text.

My special thanks go to Dr. Francis (Franny) D. Moore of Harvard whose wise comments as sections came to him piecemeal could by themselves make an engaging separate volume. At first, my nonliterary background made difficult the organization of such a complex undertaking. Moore became an informal and painfully frank pen pal for four months during this critical early time. Otherwise, the project would have been abandoned.

Later, two other people became advocates of the book and saved it from abandonment. One was Dr. Luigi Fassati, a transplant surgeon in Milan who is himself the author of a popular novel. The other was A. Ralph (Jay) Dantry, owner of Jay's Book Stall, a bookstore which wins awards yearly for being Pittsburgh's best.

The ultimate fate of a manuscript depends on its editor. This book was blessed by falling into the skillful hands of a remarkable lady named Catherine Marshall whose care can be sensed on every page. If gold can be found by the reader, it was she who uncovered it. Where base metal is encountered, the fault lies with the author.

THE
PUZZLE
PEOPLE

1

The Puzzle People

At a meeting in Capri not long ago, I was asked by an Italian journalist, "Do you think that in the next decade a puzzle man with a heart, liver, and pancreas taken from other human beings might be feasible?" I answered, "There are already examples of puzzle men and women who have received a heart and kidney, a pancreas and kidney, a heart and lungs, liver and heart. Other and more complicated combinations will be forthcoming in the near future."

Later on, it occurred to me how incomplete and anatomic my answer had been. Every patient who went through the experience of receiving someone else's organ, whether one or many, was a puzzle. It was not just the acquisition of a new part or parts; the rest of the body had to change in many ways before the gift could be accepted. And this was only the beginning. It was necessary for the mind to see the world in a different way. How the physical and mental parts were put back together was not predictable. Many died. Some found the world a better and kinder place than they had ever known before. Others encountered a cruel swamp in which their vulnerability was turned against them in ways they could not have imagined.

That the journalist's question would be asked by a rational person was inconceivable when I was young. As I grew older, transplantation became a very large miracle, perhaps the least anticipated and potentially the most important one in the history of medicine. How the miracle came about is not so easy to understand as we might be led to believe in the histories written for or by physicians, in which someone's life can be summarized with a single phrase or by a number in a table.

When I began work in transplantation in 1958, the landscape was almost bare. There were no human organ recipients except for the few who had received kidneys in Boston from their identical twin donors. Three years later, in January 1961, when John F. Kennedy was inaugurated president of the United States, transplantation was still an esoteric exercise for a small number of dreamers in an even smaller number of surgical research laboratories. Few things seemed less realistic than the hope that successful transplantation of the kidney or any other life-supporting organ could be accomplished consistently in humans.

Yet, by the time Kennedy was assassinated, in November 1963, kidney transplantation was being used effectively to treat a slowly growing number of patients with kidney failure, and the first attempts had been made in humans to replace the liver. A new field in medicine was being born. Before the inflated expectations of that early time could be fulfilled, many more years would pass.

During those years, the patients were not the only puzzle people who were being forged. The surgeons and physicians also changed — not so rapidly, because their own lives were not at stake, but inexorably, because the lives of others were in their hands. Some were corroded or destroyed by the experience, some were sublimated, and none remained the same.

Most of the key professional figures of the early days of transplantation are still alive and some still practice medicine. Now they are working their way one by one to the side of the stage. Passage into the wings is done by steps, minuet style. One device to get there is with a conference at which past contributions and efforts are celebrated by one's friends and former foes. These have become frequent occasions lately; they resemble the tours from city to city made by aging baseball stars, some modest and some not, who are in their final season of play. The meetings are not designed to discover why these men and women did what they did. The secrets are within them, hidden beneath a pile of emotional stones which only they have a right or the knowledge to probe.

Somehow, the explanation of the riddle of striving must start in the earliest years. Because children sometimes see shapes and colors that escape the eye of learned men and women, it will be best in telling my own story to begin at the beginning.

2

Printer's Ink

After I learned to read, the definition of a gyroscope in the dictionary did little to explain the fascination of my favorite toy: "gyroscope . . . device consisting essentially of a spinning mass . . . which maintains its angular orientation with respect to inertial coordinates when not subjected to external torques."[1] I do not know anything more about gyroscopes now than when I was a child. My question then was how this mysterious object stayed upright. Its strength clearly came from rotary movement, and the movement required energy.

Staying upright in a small town in western Iowa should not need much energy. Our house at 205 Central Avenue, South West, in the town of LeMars, Iowa, was a railroad track away from downtown, two blocks from the Royal Movie Theater, and four blocks from the building that housed the semiweekly newspaper owned by my father, his sister Adele, and his brother Frank.

Frank left LeMars in 1922 before I was born on March 11, 1926, but his shadow lingered on, fed by complimentary hearsay in town and by proud family gossip at home. He had earned my father's undying disapprobation by legally changing his last name to Starzel because his journalist colleagues could not learn to spell and pronounce it correctly.[2] However, to a small boy, and even now, his qualities were heroic. A high school football star, he enrolled at Notre Dame where a crippling knee injury ended his athletic career in his freshman year. He transferred to the University of Iowa to study journalism and became managing editor of the Iowa City

Press-Citizen while he was still a senior. After several years of moving from paper to paper, he joined the Associated Press in 1929, and after a few years he became bureau chief for Ohio with an office in Columbus. In 1942 he was appointed traffic executive for the Associated Press worldwide. I never knew exactly where he was living, but always was vaguely aware that it was someplace exotic and apt to be in South America.

His ascendancy was completed in 1948 when he became the general manager (chief executive officer) of the Associated Press (AP) news agency with offices at Rockefeller Plaza in New York. He moved to 1 Forest Court in Larchmont. As chief executive officer he was responsible for both the administrative and journalistic conduct of the Associated Press. Burl Osborne, a young reporter from Spokane, Washington, who was recruited during Frank's tenure as CEO, subsequently developed renal failure, and on July 27, 1966, I performed a kidney transplantation on him. By 1977, Osborne had risen to the position of managing editor with the Associated Press, and in 1980 he joined the Dallas *Morning News* of which he now is the editor and publisher. I talk to him from time to time, and he never fails to dwell on his affection for my Uncle Frank who is now eighty-seven years old and living in Denver.

After Frank left LeMars he never came back for more than a few days. When he did, it always was a special occasion and usually a funeral. Tall and powerful, he exuded confidence and seemed to know everything. His memory was astonishing, and still is. He was blessed with a pleasant deep voice and an off-center smile. Burl Osborne told me that when Frank ran the Associated Press, he knew every employee in the organization and interviewed all new recruits before hiring them. I realized many years later that this reflected genuine kindness, not expediency. Frank and his wife, Sally, have a son, Bob, who practices law in San Francisco, and a daughter, now Sue Swanson, who lives in Denver.

Adele Starzl, my father's sister, died suddenly in 1944 at the age of thirty-seven after a short and not altogether happy life in spite of being beautiful and well educated. My father, the oldest of the three newspaper co-owners, spent one year at Northwestern University in Chicago—the only one who did not have a complete university education. I do not know why. It may have been because of the time he lost during his army service in World War I. More likely, the viability of the family newspaper depended upon the presence of at least one of these three talented children.

The paper originally had been bought in 1897 by my grandfather, John V. Starzl, who emigrated with his parents in 1874 at the age of six from what now is the Czechoslovakian-Austrian border. He was raised on farms in Iowa and South Dakota in a German-language household before moving for unknown reasons to Chicago where he purchased a pharmacy. It is not clear why he bought a newspaper and moved back to northwest Iowa where he had spent his first days in America as a farm boy herding cattle and sheep. The purchase probably was financed by his new wife's family.

The newspaper, called *Der Herold*, was one of the diminishing number of German-language papers in the United States. At the time it was well supported by a large local constituency of German-speaking immigrants in and around LeMars. It also had a substantial circulation list in continental Europe. The anti-Teutonic sentiments aroused by World War I, which eventually reached rage proportions, resulted in the closing of *Der Herold*, but my grandfather had acquired a second newspaper, an English-language paper called the LeMars *Globe Post*.

The Starzl family was particularly vulnerable to wartime community passions because my paternal grandmother, Margaret Theisen, also had a German lineage. This was traced to 1759 by her brother, Dr. Harold Theisen, who became a successful surgeon in Cleveland. Margaret, Harold, and several other children were born into a German-speaking household in Schleisingerville (changed to Slinger after World War I), a small town in Wisconsin about thirty miles from Milwaukee. She married John Starzl in 1897, in Chicago.

Margaret may not have been happy in the small town in Iowa. It is said that she was fond of traveling in Europe and going to exclusive resorts in America. I have no way of knowing the income necessary to support these activities and can only surmise that it was above average. My German grandparents lived in a beautifully appointed home with a better location than ours but only three or four blocks away.

I was encouraged not to go there toward the end of my grandmother's life when her behavior became so unconventional that she required periodic institutionalization. She died in 1937, five years after my grandfather died of complications of diabetes mellitus from which he had suffered for years. Both reached sixty-five. The LeMars *Globe Post* was left to their three children—my father (Rome), Uncle Frank, and Aunt Adele.

As I grew up, I gradually learned about the newspaper's troubled history. The best source of information lay in a large steamer trunk in the basement of our house. My older brother, John, my two younger sisters, Nancy and Marnie, and I were forbidden to open it. The fear of retribution was not enough to keep us out. Inside were stacks of magazines, almost all containing science fiction stories by R. F. Starzl, Rome Starzl, or Roman Frederick Starzl. Other published articles described hospital experiences and were signed Anna Laura Fitzgerald. This was my mother's maiden name. All had been written by my father.

Beneath the magazines was a layer of delicate Irish lace, and under this was a collection of newspaper clippings, dated 1918. They told about the trial for the crime of sedition (or treason) of my grandfather, John Starzl. The charge, brought by the government under the Alien and Sedition Act of 1906, was based on an editorial in the LeMars *Globe Post* criticizing the inhumane conditions under which soldiers were being transported to France after the United States entered the war in 1917.[3] During the trial in Sioux City, John Starzl, the ostensible author, was a perfect target for cross examination with his unmistakable German accent and imperfect grasp of the legal process. Also, he was burdened with a far greater handicap. He did not want it known that the real author was his son Rome (my future father), a soldier in an army officers' training school in Texas. This could not be concealed, however, and when it became known, my grandfather was acquitted. Later, the Alien and Sedition Act was declared unconstitutional.[4]

I wish that I could have known my real grandfather, the John Starzl whose family's youthful vision had brought them to these shores. By the time I met him, he had become aloof. Although we lived less than four blocks apart for the first six years of my life, I cannot remember a single conversation with him. It would have been nice to talk to him in German. This also had been my father's first language, in spite of his birth in America, but I was never taught. It was as if destruction of the language would remove the pain.

Those who knew John Starzl well always spoke of him with much more than affection. It was esteem. He may have remembered the yellow paint splashed on his house long ago in the middle of the night, or the days in the dock during the Sioux City sedition trial. It seemed to me that the "external torques" had been too strong and that the gyroscope had gone down. Now a mound of silence, bewildered also by the changes in the lady of his life, he waited patiently for what lay beyond. If I wanted to see my true grandfather, it had to be in the faces of his sons, Frank and Rome.

» «

More of their story was in the same steamer trunk that contained the clippings of the sedition trial. The trunk itself must have been seen as trash by someone who later lived in our house on Central Avenue. It disappeared along with the science fiction stories by my father, the enigmatic R. F. Starzl. Ten years after Rome died on April 8, 1976, my son Tom began a remarkably successful search for the missing magazines, which included some of the best known of their day. Most of R. F. Starzl's stories were about space exploration, describing in detail a technology that was not yet on anyone's drawing board but soon would be with rocket flight and lunar exploration. A strong and resourceful woman usually accompanied the hero as he dealt with environmental vicissitudes and well-armed, unfriendly life forms.

Science fiction in the late 1920s and early 1930s was just becoming popular. Ray Bradbury, one of the most successful of the next generation of writers, was an acquaintance of my father, but far more successful and persevering. Tom's investigations showed that the short stories and novelettes of R. F. Starzl began to appear in 1928, reached a peak in 1931, and were last seen in 1934 when he was thirty-five years old.

What R. F. Starzl, the author, left was a distinctive mark as the originator of a science fiction genre. He envisioned universes within universes down to microscopic size, each with its own sophisticated life organization. Into these unfamiliar environments he inserted humans, transmuted to the appropriate diminutive size and brought there by intention or by some scientific accident.

I have found that people do what they want to or find easy, and later explain why it was necessary. My father enjoyed writing and was good at it. But he also needed money, more than the miserly salary his parents paid him. His penalty may have been linked to his mother's disapproval of the Irish lady whom he married, my mother, and to the Great Depression which arrived before my third birthday. The need for money increased. After his father died, leaving him a portion of the paper, my father decided to become the sole owner of the *Globe Post* by buying up the stocks willed to his mother and to Frank and Adele. The science fiction stories provided capital. Late at night, I could hear the clatter of the typewriter. In the morning, he would go to work at the newspaper.

When the night noise finally stopped, I knew that the paper was his. Henceforth, he was to be an editor and publisher, involved in every phase of the business which, in addition to journalism, included a major printing shop. There was no task in the publication process which he did not do well, from the lowliest function of the "devil" who scavenged lead from the print shop, to typesetting, either by hand or with the sophisticated linotype machines. He was a superb photographer and built a darkroom on the second floor of the four-story plant to develop his own film.

I was expected to work at the *Globe Post* from the time I was twelve or thirteen years old, first as a paper carrier, but later doing all those tasks which my father had himself mastered. On the days of the *Globe Post* publication, Monday and Thursday, giant rolls of paper weighing nearly a thousand pounds were bulldozed into place to feed the presses. The devil (which was my job for a long time) and the strongest of the fledgling printers were assigned this undesirable task, which was made even more unpleasant by the frequent necessity to descend into the pit—the excavation below the roller presses into which oil and ink drained.

Being the boss's son did not confer special consideration and may have had the opposite effect. One Thursday morning, my considerably larger work partner, irate at being nearly crushed by a runaway paper roll, invited me into the pit to settle whether the mishap was his or my responsibility. We fought steadily in the slippery grime for almost two hours before the foreman came down to check on the delay. Amazed by what he found, he fired us. After being rehired a few hours later, my pit adversary and I became good friends.

I never have seen matched the manual dexterity of the printers, not just the virtuosos but practically all of them. If in the 1930s I wanted to teach a class of surgeons economy and precision of movement, the print shop of a small town in Iowa would have been a good place to start. The technology of printing had already changed in larger cities, and would soon in LeMars as well. But at that moment, the training ground still was there.

Handsetting words, letter by letter, made alphabet idolaters of the printers who did it. The printer foreman, Larry Kohlker, was a slender blonde man with a face of feminine beauty and an air of refinement difficult to reconcile with grimy hands, perpetually black fingernails, and muscular power. He worked for my father for more than twenty years, beginning when he left high school. They were like father and son. Years after I had left LeMars, he fell in love with my younger sister, Nancy, and she with him. The union would have been providential except that he already had a family. Larry was fired and Nancy returned to the university. Twenty-five years later, she died of cirrhosis of the liver. I have often wondered if there was any connection. Nancy, a lonely girl after our mother died in 1947, had not been a person to give her heart freely.

It is pointless to dwell on the successes of the *Globe Post*. The moral authority which the paper acquired was based not only on the integrity of its positions—whether one agreed with them or not—but also on the way these positions were stated. The *Globe Post* was regarded by many journalists as a close cousin of the *Emporia Gazette* (Kansas), the organ of William Allen White. My father reviewed every article with the care that is feasible only with small and exquisite things.

It did not seem to me then or later that this was enough for him. The science fiction, now behind him, had been a hollow exercise of imagination. The love of translating ideas into real structure led to his next passion, which could be seen in the steadily expanding dimensions of the machine shop in the basement of our house. He hoped that his inventions would be practical and relevant to his newspaper. One of these creations was a machine that transformed photographs into a metal "stamp" that allowed these photos to be printed in his newspaper. The standard process for this purpose was a complex one called photoengraving in which photographic images were etched by a selective acid digestion process on the metal plate eventually used for imprinting. The conventional preparation of the plates by a photoengraving plant in Sioux City was expensive and time-consuming.

My father wanted to prepare these plates electronically, using a photoelectric eye to scan the surface of the photos. His plan was to transmit these messages directly to a cutting tip which would engrave the impressions on the zinc plate. Now, the nightly noise of the typewriter was replaced with the sounds of the machine shop, its boundaries expanding like a deadly cancer, pushing my mother's laundry quarters ahead. Nearly ten years of effort came short of perfection. Photoelectric engraving eventually became a standard technique, but his own plates were not good enough to be used. He had succeeded in principle but the pictures were not sharp.

My father's instinct to invent and to build his own machines was unquenchable. The basement went through so many phases that it would be tedious to describe them. The embers must have glowed long after the flames went out. In 1953, almost ten years after I had left home, I was working in the Halsted laboratory at the Johns Hopkins Hospital in Baltimore. One of our objectives was to develop a heart-lung machine so that surgical operations could be performed inside the heart. In one of my letters to my father, I mentioned that the main sticking point was the inability to get oxygen into the blood without damaging the red blood cells.

A few weeks later, a large crate arrived from LeMars containing a farmer's cream can that had been converted to an oxygenator. The oxygen entry was via a jet which dispersed the gas directly into the blood. Beyond this was a defoaming chamber to remove the resulting oxygen bubbles before the blood was pumped back into the animal (or patient). I was embarrassed to see this cumbersome device, because our conviction was that the blood must *not* be exposed directly to oxygen. It was put in the corner and never tested.

Several years later a team at the University of Minnesota described the successful use of a bubble oxygenator. I went back to the laboratory, dusted off the cream can, and realized that its design was almost identical to the University of Minnesota apparatus. Sadly, I wondered if my unconscious contempt for his initiative had cheated my father of the achievement for which he yearned. The distinction was drawing sharper between those plain people like him—the skillful printers, the farmers among whom I had grown up—and the erudite class to whom I was increasingly exposed whose special language often concealed a gap in primitive knowledge.

Perhaps these impressions of thirty-five years ago were like the recognizable but blurred images of my father's flawed photoengravings and have become perfectly clear only now that my own twilight has arrived. I believe that I perceived, even as a child, a divided loyalty between my father, who was a constant and sometimes stern companion, and his famous and romantic brother, Frank, who was more of a concept at that time than a real person. Their divergent paths, both into journalism, had played out the genre of science fiction for which my father was himself remembered.

Frank Starzel had transported himself from the microcosm that was a small town in Iowa and returned only to visit or to bury those who stayed behind. My father, R. F. Starzl, stayed in that tiny universe within a universe but never was reconciled to its limitations. When my time came, I wanted to escape. The fear of failing and being forced to return, defeated and condemned to a lifetime of regret, made trivial all other fears, even that of death. Like a grim watchdog, this feeling stayed until the long course was run.

» «

How to have two such different role models as my father and my uncle, one close at hand and the other distant, without betraying either, remained unresolved for many years. Only when they were very old, with me not far behind, did I understand that they were reluctant spiritual twins with their own special disguises. These were friendly, proud, and abstemious men. Their personal and professional integrity was naked, making them immune to the temptations that lead to corruption. Because of this, I carried the vain illusion for many years that journalism was synonymous with a search for truth and was perhaps the most pure and virtuous of all professions.

Both men were straightforward to a fault and left no doubt of their opinions and positions. I was in my twenties before I spent much time with Frank, but in the next forty years, I saw him often in the most intimate of circumstances. I never saw him weep.

While he was physically intact, my father cried only once, late at night when we should have slept. The sobs came like thunder shocks from the bedroom where he was with my mother. It was in 1944 on the eve of my departure for the navy, but that was not the reason. He had just learned that she had cancer and could not live long. It was the first time I knew that he was not made of steel.

Raw steel unadorned causes unease, but steel joined with flowers is another matter. Our flower was Anna Loretta (Laura) Fitzgerald, daughter of Irish immigrants who moved in 1891 from a village called Clonbullogue in County Offaly to a farm a few miles from Newcastle, Nebraska. Almost exactly one hundred years later, a child named Colin McStay and his parents drove from their Dublin home and visited the oratory where my grandparents were married. Some years earlier, in October 1984 in Pittsburgh, I had operated on two-year-old Colin, the first Irish person to have a liver transplant. His mother wrote a best-selling book about this experience and then became curious about the grandparents of her son's surgeon.[5] Why had they left the comfort and security of Ireland for a hard life in the American great plains? Between Mrs. McStay's research and what I had learned as a child, it was possible to reconstruct the ancient event.

Poverty had not driven them. In Ireland, their families were landowners whose holdings were still intact and managed by direct descendants a century later. Opposition to the marriage was a possibility because they were cousins whose marriage required a special dispensation from the Catholic church. Another explanation may have been that Tom Fitzgerald's activities on behalf of Irish independence put his life in jeopardy. He was highly educated and departed his homeland carrying his books with him. Three of the sisters he left behind were Catholic nuns.

Thomas Patrick Fitzgerald's wife, my grandmother, was Catherine Ann Mangan, who lived nearby in Ireland. She was less educated than he but more practical. She bore him fourteen children. The first five were boys and all died at birth (Richard, Robert, James) or before the age of five (Thomas, John). I caused sorrow nearly one hundred years later when I asked my Aunt Margaret, one of the surviving sisters, for their names. She remembered where they were buried with perfect clarity. Nine girls followed, of whom three died, two at birth and one (Marcella) about three months later. One of the survivors was my mother.

Tom Fitzgerald was not as resigned to an agricultural life as my grandmother, although both lived to the age of seventy. He and his library became an information source for rural eastern Nebraska. He helped educate the six girls, who assisted in running the farm before they began to make their own way. All six became teachers, taking care of the one-room country schoolhouses that provided an education through the eighth grade for most children in that part of the country. After doing this for three years, my mother enrolled at St. Vincent's Hospital School of Nursing in Sioux City, Iowa, graduating in 1920. She worked as a surgical nurse until she married my father in November 1923 and moved another twenty-five miles from Sioux City to LeMars.

Her thoughts were never far from her family. On weekends, we often drove the one hundred miles to the Fitzgerald farm. Several of my early summers were spent there with her happy sisters, most of whom had children of their own. If I had a favorite aunt, it was the beautiful Margaret, who was married to a quiet farmer named Frank Weber who died in 1989. She is eighty-six years old and lives now in the small town of Ponca, Nebraska.

My father realized that my mother liked these visits because he saw how freely she laughed when she was there. For a long time, she did not feel welcome in LeMars. My father's mother had not approved of this marriage, possibly (I have been told) because of the lower social status reflexly given in those days to Irish immigrants.

In LeMars, a town of five thousand, the heavily Catholic population was divided along ethnic lines. The Germans, who tended to have more money, lived on the east side of town, worshiped at St.

Joseph's Catholic Church, and sent their children to its parochial school. The church was a magnificent but somber Gothic structure which to a small boy reeked of major retribution for small sins about which the confessional priests wanted too much detail for comfort. This was where Rome and Frank had their religious instructions.

Most of the Irish and other Catholics lived on the west side and went to the less opulent St. James' Church which was presided over by Father Cooper, an aging priest who spoke with a strong and pleasant brogue. Our house on Central Avenue was in a neutral zone between the two churches. The fact that the R. F. Starzl family went to the St. James' Church seemed to be a constant source of friction between my parents and my German grandmother. She held my mother responsible for the decision, which I believe was true. My mother was determined that her children would go to the public schools. The flower could turn to steel, and did so down the years on all matters of genuine principle. She was anything but an ornament. Needless to say, we were enrolled in the public elementary, junior, and senior high schools of LeMars.

It was a good decision. The administration of the public school system consisted of males who were distant figures. The working educational core was a collection of middle-aged and older women, almost all unmarried. Mention of their names—Miss Waddick, Miss Meade, Miss Thompson—made young boys and girls tremble. Miss (Mary) Waddick was the oldest and retired a few years after my exposure to her in the third grade. For those in LeMars, the departure of a great president of the United States was no more significant. This was my opinion also.

Miss Meade lived on Central Avenue in a small white wooden house, three or four blocks from my home. When I brought the *Globe Post* to her door on my delivery route, this was the one paper that must be in the perfect place. After a while, she married someone and had a baby. These were incomprehensible events. Later, the sight of a child in the yard made the incongruity complete. Icons did not do these things.

I caused Myrtle Thompson sorrow, but I also may have given her something valuable. With Miss Waddick and Miss Meade, there was an unmistakable bond of student-teacher affection and trust. Miss Thompson, who taught English and Latin in the junior high school, became convinced that I was cheating systematically in her eighth grade Latin class. Latin was a subject which interested me beyond all others at the time. Every night, I spent hours converting Caesar's conquest of Gaul to English. During class, I habitually sat in the most secluded seat in the back row from where I responded with studied diffidence when called on for translations. Frequently, this was followed by a search of my desk and books for the "pony" that Miss Thompson was convinced must be the explanation for my facile performances.

The conflict was made more complicated by the presence in the class of a very intelligent farm boy named James Deegan whose gentle and refined ways may have come partly from his suffering from a chronic illness. He had heart disease, which was said to have resulted from rheumatic fever much earlier. No one ever called him Jim. James sat quietly in the front row. He also rendered perfect translations when called upon and freely volunteered these when he was not. I liked him, but understood that he had been made into an opponent.

Miss Thompson warned me that a day of reckoning was coming. At the end of the year, she planned to give a standardized Latin examination that was used nationally. When the day came, she insisted that I sit in the front row, under her direct supervision. The test, which was like a slender book, had to be completed in two hours. After twenty-five or thirty minutes, I finished it and turned it in. Deegan and the others had barely started.

Later in the day, after she had graded the books, Miss Thompson sent for me. She sat behind her desk in the empty classroom and asked me to close the door, which I did, bracing for another accusation. I was twelve or thirteen years old at the time, but more than fifty years later, I remember exactly what she said and how: "Oh Tommie, I am so sorry." Then she put her head down and wept bitterly. Between sobs, she said that I had written a perfect examination. Deegan had only done well.

It was not a small crisis. Her thin shoulders heaving, she continued to cry uncontrollably, temporarily composing herself only to break down again. When I tried to take the blame, it made things worse. Alarmed by all of this, I went home and told my mother that I had done wrong. It had been a silly feud, fed by pride, in which I made no effort to explain anything along the way. Perhaps, I had taken a perverse pleasure in letting the conflict develop, knowing all along what the outcome would be.

My mother went to the school immediately. It was the only time she had ever done this or ever would. She did not do it for me. After that day, I loved Miss Thompson. For many years, she wrote to me, always aware of graduations, honors that came, and other major events. Later on, she moved to Sioux City. When the letters stopped, I knew that she must have died, and this was soon confirmed. What passed between her and my mother on that fateful day, no one will ever know. Wise women take these secrets to the grave.

The older women (and a few men) who gave stability to the educational system in western Iowa were a minority. Many others were fresh from college. In the last year of high school, I encountered incredulity again but it happened with a young woman and had an inconclusive outcome. One year out of the university and on her first job, this high school English teacher assigned to our senior class (1944) the task of composing an essay on war. I already had enlisted and was waiting assignment by the navy. For some reason, I could think of nothing to write as the due date neared.

Then one morning, I woke from a dream with an unusual sentence in my mind which became as fixed as Miss Thompson's anguished apology: "When his eyes opened, he saw a bright green leaf, turgid from the morning dew." It was the beginning of a description of a fatally wounded marine who regained consciousness to discover that his body was paralyzed. The story consisted of his dying thoughts that defined the horror of war and the justification for it under the circumstances of that period.

After I turned it in, the teacher asked me where the original article was, assuming that it had been plagiarized. She was a city girl and no amount of discussion could convince her that it had been written by someone like me. The result was a failing grade. I was learning lessons about life, at a time when I possessed no protective armor. I do not know what happened to my teacher. She was young and very beautiful. Someday, she may have become wise. I do not remember her name.

» «

World War II was the catapult out of the microcosm of LeMars, not only for me, in March 1944, but also for my brother John, who was one year older. In 1942, John left high school to work as a welder in a ship-building factory in Bremerton, Washington, and later joined the navy. Having been selected for officers' training school because of a high aptitude score, he turned in an unsatisfactory academic performance and was sent as a seaman on the North Atlantic convoys supplying arms to Europe. John was a peaceful person and a gifted trombone player whose greatest ambition it was to be a musician in a jazz band. This passion was seen as degenerate by our father, and disputes about it led to violent arguments which may have explained his premature departure to the shipyards. The irony was that John's musical skills had resulted from a family-imposed program of talent development that included all the children. I became a cornet player, good enough to go to national championship competitions in Omaha and Minneapolis. Except for family vacations in Minnesota and the Rocky Mountains, these were my only excursions outside the environs of LeMars until I joined the navy. The activities in music gave way to the higher priorities of playing on the high school football and basketball teams. With John it was different. He was a much better musician than I was, and music overwhelmed all other priorities put together.

How wise it is to force such strong currents of desire into a different direction is open to question. John's dreams of glory in music would never materialize. The day the music stopped may have been the day his spirit died, although it did not leave his body until 1985, in Dallas. During his naval duties, John met a young woman at the port of call in St. John, Newfoundland. After the war, they corresponded and in June 1947, they were married in St. James' Catholic Church, LeMars. The ceremony was repeated in my mother's sickroom a few days before she died. If it had not been for her well-known wish to see one of her children married, what proved to be a disastrous union of two people who did not love each other might never have occurred.

As it was, the magnet of the *Globe Post*, with its beguiling safety net, captured John after the war as it had our father the generation before. When the marriage failed after a decade, John left town and resurfaced in different western cities from time to time, sometimes with gaps of years between. Understanding what was happening to him was like trying to read a book with most of the words deleted. On the evening after the Cotton Bowl in Dallas on January 1, 1982, we had dinner together at the Anatole Hotel. We talked with what was a strange mixture of deep affection, respect, and personal solitude. He died not long after. I learned of his death after he had been cremated.

As with John before me, my high school diploma was mailed to an armed forces address. There were forty-seven in our class of 1944. Four were good friends and future physicians whose paths crossed intermittently in high places in the coming years. Each of the four is fond of saying that he was the least successful of the group. Warren Stamp became one of the leading orthopedic surgeons in the world. For twenty-five years he has been the chair of the Department of Orthopedic Surgery at the University of Virginia, Charlottesville.

Alvin (Bud) Mauer's father was a dentist. Bud became a professor of pediatrics at Indiana University and after that the director of the famed St. Jude's Cancer Hospital in Memphis. Ours was a Damon and Pythias relationship throughout grade and high school. I cannot count the camping trips and amusing incidents we shared before real life came down on us with the war clouds of 1944. I saw him after that only at medical meetings in a formal setting. It may have been just as well not to reminisce because later his father was killed by a speeding car and his younger brother, who had moved to Washington, D.C., died in his twenties of an acute virus infection.

Bobby Joynt, also the son of a dentist, served as a faculty neurologist at the University of Iowa before becoming the chair of neurosciences, dean, and finally chancellor at the University of Rochester School of Medicine. When my father had the first of a series of crippling strokes in December 1955, Bob saw him as a consultant and continued to do so with great tenderness whenever he visited LeMars for the next twenty years.

Three of these four future physicians were members of the high school football team, and the fourth, Bud Mauer, was the trainer. I played right end and Stamp was the backup at this position. Because he was so shortsighted, Bobby Joynt had trouble making his way down a well lit, wide corridor. We claimed that he was the only legally blind halfback in the state of Iowa. We should have added the most courageous.

The football team of 1943 was a very respectable one, but not good enough to be enshrined for its unique athletic prowess. What was more interesting was how four members of the squad went on to medical training, an unusual event in a high school that normally produced one future physician every five to ten years. There were retrospective inquiries about this which came to nothing because of the monotonous responses. Each of the four credited the other three for stimulating their interest, but took no credit of their own. It was not hard to deduce why this undersized team with its dearth of natural physical ability had won many games.

» «

My mother died of breast cancer on June 30, 1947. How essential she was in our family would be truly shown only by her leaving it. By this time, she was thought to be a saint, not only by us but by that diversity of ethnic populations which once had seen her as alien. When she was gone, there was no family anymore.

A few weeks before her death, I graduated from Westminster College in Fulton, Missouri, the school where I had been assigned for the academic component of officers' training school. When the war ended and I was discharged from the navy, I decided to return to the civilian comfort of the small college. Playing on the basketball team the first year caused so many missed classes that I quit the team for the 1946–47 season. The reward was an admission slip to the Northwestern University Medical School beginning September 1947. During 1946, Winston Churchill came to Fulton to deliver his famous "iron curtain" speech warning against the perils of communism. This was marked by historians as the opening of the Cold War.

Graduation in May 1947 was a sad affair because of the sense of loss at leaving this sheltered life, but especially because my mother was too sick to come. My father stayed at home with her. As soon as the ceremony was finished, I took the train home and went to her shaded room at our house.

She was short of breath because of the liquid that accumulated around her lungs faster than it could be taken off. Every afternoon her doctor came, inserted a needle in her chest, and sucked out several quarts of slightly bloody yellow fluid containing particles of tissue which I was told were bits of tumor that had spread from the breast cancer. My instructions in the event of pain or restlessness between these procedures was to give an injection of morphine into a thigh muscle or the buttock. The morphine tablet was to be dissolved in a tablespoon of tap water which needed to be heated over the kitchen stove before drawing it into the syringe.

Her last day of life was sunny. At midmorning while I was sitting in her room, she told me that she was suffocating. Rushing downstairs to the kitchen, I began to prepare the morphine, only to have the spoon fall from my trembling hands onto the floor. When I succeeded the second time and returned, she was taking her last breaths. She managed to take off her diamond ring, and with her last words she asked me to give it to my sister, Nancy.

I could not believe that she was dead. Mr. Sylvester Luken, who owned a furniture store next to the *Globe Post*, also was a mortician. When he came for the body, I refused to let him come up the narrow stairs and held him at bay like a Spartan at Thermopylae while a crowd gathered. I had known Mr. Luken all my life. He knew my mother well. Twenty-nine years later, when he took care of his friend, my father, in the same way, I apologized, and he forgave me.

I went to the funeral mass. Although I once had thought of being a priest, and had become a Latin scholar, this was the last time I went into a church for the next twenty-nine years. The next time was to honor my father. After that, it was a little easier on special occasions. For a long time, I wondered if my ineptitude in the kitchen had contributed to my mother's death. For several years, a horrible dream recurred in which a rose was attached to a light hanging from an electric wire that came from the ceiling. The rose would bleed until I woke up with fear and trembling. Finally, the dreams went away.

The family came apart. Dinner, which had been a formal and pleasant part of our routine, became a time of bitter recrimination. One person would accuse another of having been callous or at least not caring about our dead mother. Not wanting to work again at the *Globe Post*, I accepted a job on a construction gang for the rest of the summer. When I took the train for Chicago to begin medical school in early September 1947, I had no intention of coming back.

3

Medical School (1947–52)

Northwestern University Medical School is located at 303 East Chicago Avenue, two blocks from the concrete "beaches" which were accessible by crossing North Lake Shore Drive. These had been constructed years before to replace the natural sand of Lake Michigan. Going west, the city layers in September 1947 were as thin as onion skin, changing so fast that a fifteen-minute walk or a five-minute ride on the Chicago Avenue trolley could lay bare a transformation from grandeur to misery.

First came North Michigan Avenue and its expanse of fashionable shops, business centers, and professional offices. One block farther west was Rush Street with lights that either stared brazenly or blinked in the night, inviting those with a taste for expensive food or those with more lustful propensities to visit its restaurants, nightclubs, and burlesque parlors. These were teeming with shapely women and comely young men of about my age, which was twenty-one years.

By the time the Clark Street skid row was reached, four blocks farther on, the price of self-indulgence could be seen in the eyes and desperate faces of the bums who walked in the streets or covered themselves in the recesses of the storefronts whose movable steel grids kept them at arm's length at night.

Just to the left on Clark Street was a strip-show palace where medical students sometimes came late at night for relaxation, taking care to bring some money. Not paying the bills was rumored to invite corporal punishment by the bouncers, who were said to use the small baseball bats that could be seen neatly stacked in an umbrella stand just inside the entrance.

On the corner of Chicago Avenue and Clark Street was a large, flashing, red neon sign which read "Stop and Drink." Gone were the youthful faces and trim bodies of the Rush Street employees. Here, even the sad-eyed strippers looked as if they had entered purgatory, if not hell, a long time earlier. The next street west was LaSalle and after that Wells. At first, this seamy world was unrelated to my life as a medical student. Aided by the GI Bill of Rights, I lived in the luxury zone of the city during my freshman year. My room was on the fourteenth floor of Abbott Hall, a bubble overlooking Lake Michigan that provided everything for the student from bookstore to cafeteria.

During the first year, the greatest hurdle for me was gross anatomy. The diener, a man named Scotty, brought the cadavers up from a subterranean storage vault where they were kept in tanks. Each cadaver was shared by four students. Most of the cadavers were old, but some looked as though their lives had been arrested in full flight in their youth. What awful event had brought them here, now inanimate objects, to be taken apart piece by piece under the bright lights of the smelly dissecting room? The sickening odor of the preservation fluid permeated everything and left the laboratory in my clothes. My grades were high, but I finished the two-semester course with the feeling that I knew little about the human body and much less than that about the human spirit. My mother had been the first unclothed dead person I had seen in my life. Perhaps I was seeing her again.

Dissatisfied with my knowledge of anatomy, I bought a cadaver of my own four years later during my senior year. This was an Indian lady, not to be shared with other students. Late at night and on the weekends I learned her body lovingly as if she were an old and dear friend, making amateur drawings as portions of her came off. She slowly disappeared. When she was gone, she had bequeathed me a knowledge of anatomy that I would carry for all my life. Whoever she was, she had become to me the noblest of beings.

» «

After the freshman year, I moved inland near the Wells Street– Chicago Avenue junction, to the ghetto that received freely those who could not or did not want to go elsewhere. This was by choice and as a matter of principle. My father had come to Chicago to explain the loneliness of his life after twenty-four years of marriage. He had met and was seeing another Irish lady named Rita Kenelay who had spent her life on a farm near LeMars. He asked if I would object to his marrying again. I told him no, and that I would come to the wedding, but at the time I meant, "Yes, I object."

I have long since recognized how mean that inner voice was. History continued to repeat itself. Rita came to 205 Central Avenue S.W. in LeMars and faced the hostility that Anna Laura Fitzgerald had met. Only this time I was a conspirator, posted so far away that my resistance did not matter and probably was not perceived. From their marriage, I acquired a half sister, Cathy, who was born in April 1955. She lived at our family home after my father died until the neighborhood deteriorated.

I hardly know Cathy, but I do know that Rita is a great lady. She is seventy-three years old now and works every day at the LeMars *Sentinel*, which remained the only newspaper in town after the *Globe Post* burned to the ground on St. Patrick's Day, 1964. Without Rita, my father could not have lived to the age of seventy-six, or if he could have, he would not have wanted to.

That understanding came much later. All I knew in May 1948 was that I must be independent of my father. I obtained a temporary job at the Chicago *Tribune* as a proofreader. Before long, this function changed to copy reading, which involved converting information provided by reporters (particularly on medical stories and columns) into accounts that could be published.

More importantly, I found a second source of income as well as a place to live with a night and weekend job at an industrial surgeon's office in the ghetto at the junction of Chicago Avenue and Wells Street. What was entailed would not be legal today, but in 1948 about 10 percent of the medical students paid their way by providing care for employees who were injured or became ill at work.

During the day and for a few hours on Sunday, a physician named Dwight Gerhardt and a younger associate were available for these services. The medical students did the rest. I never understood why Dr. Gerhardt was in this place. He was very competent and taught me many things about wound care that were validated as correct by later experience. The modesty of his office blended perfectly into the shabby neighborhood. Patients had to pass through locked doors, after signaling their presence with buzzers. They ascended a flight of narrow stairs to reach the second floor where a small sign on the locked door read "Dr. Gerhardt, Industrial Surgeon." Missing the left turn-off would send the patient to the next level of the wooden building where strange people whom I seldom encountered occupied commune-style sleeping quarters.

The medical student tour of duty began at 6 P.M. and ended at 7 A.M. All night long the doorbell would ring. Whichever medical student was on call would take care of the problem, usually some kind of injury. Although we had finished only our first year, there were not many problems we could not handle, and I can remember only a few times when we asked Dr. Gerhardt to come in from his suburban home to help. I genuinely liked him. He paid us $100 a month which I split with another student named Phil Wiley. However, the greatest financial incentive was that we had a free place to stay. In the back of the office was a two-tier bunk bed and behind that a tiny kitchen with a gas stove.

This was my home for the next three years. After a year, my first partner, Phil Wiley, developed tuberculosis of the lung and left for two years of treatment at a sanatorium in New York. After he had lost weight and coughed up blood, I had made the diagnosis by taking a chest X-ray with a machine in the office. Wiley was one of those rare people who grasped complex issues instinctively, seemingly without effort. When he recovered from his lung infection, he finished medical school and practiced surgery in Traverse City, a resort town in northern Michigan. Following his departure, other students came and went but none could match him. His intelligence and aptitude had brought us through the first year of providing medical services despite the poverty of our training and knowledge.

It was not safe to descend into the streets at night, and I usually avoided this. One night I walked across Wells Street to a mailbox and saw what I thought was an animal being beaten by a burly man at the foot of a stairwell. When I intervened, I saw that it was a mentally retarded child. After a few minutes, her mother arrived

and sided with the man. A few moments later I heard a shot and felt
the bullet as it shaved the side of my head before it landed behind
me in the wooden wall of the building. I fled ignominiously and
reported the incident in the morning to Dr. Gerhardt. He laughed
and provided the advice, which by now was unnecessary, to mind
my own business.

» «

Nothing is more boring than medical school stories to those who
have not been there; even for those who have been, the tales are
pretty much the same. My time at Northwestern was five years
instead of the usual four. The reason for the extended duration was
a man named Horace W. Magoun, professor of neuroanatomy, who
taught his course during my sophomore year. His lectures were
supreme examples of clarity. This was because he wrote down
everything he was going to say and then memorized it so that it
sounded extemporaneous. There was substance as well as style in
these talks, each of which was more like an oration than a lecture.

By the spring of 1949, Magoun's research had made him one of
the world's leading students of nervous system function with a
particular interest in sleep and wakefulness. From his own teacher,
Stephen W. Ranson, he had learned techniques by which fine
electrodes could be directed to hidden parts of the brain from an
external frame attached to fixed points on the head. Magoun could
then study in animals what the effect was of stimulating or destroying the brain structures into which the electrodes were inserted.
His principal collaborator when I met him was Giuseppe Moruzzi,
a visiting professor from Pisa, Italy.

Before Magoun's work, the oversimplified view taught to students was that control of voluntary movement started almost
exclusively in the cortex, the surface layer of the brain, from which
the messages directing the body to move were transmitted to the
muscles of the arms, legs, and so forth. Magoun and an earlier
collaborator named Ruth Rhines already had shown how nerve cell
nests that were deeply buried far below the cortex helped to modify
and coordinate such voluntary motion. Their research helped to
explain how certain kinds of neurologic disorders, including strokes,
could immobilize victims without destroying their intellectual

function. Soon, my father was going to be an example of such a stroke although I had no way of predicting this.

The new question being asked by Moruzzi and Magoun in 1949, along with a psychologist named Don Lindsley, was how messages coming in the other direction from the outside world (pain, touch, light, and hearing) reached and affected the brain cortex. These sensations were known to start with nerve fibers posted like satellite discs at or near the surface of the body. From there, they begin their long journey to the brain, passing through relay stations (synapses) on the way. Like a well-organized pony express, each of the senses has its own special pathway which terminates at a relatively small strip of the brain cortex. For example, visual messages from the eyes end in the back of the brain near the protuberance which the reader can feel on his or her own head, whereas sound messages go to the brain at the temple areas on each side of the brain.

Magoun and Moruzzi suspected that there must be sensory pathways in addition to these well understood but limited ones. Beginning in the summer of 1949, I became the person who demonstrated the validity of this concept. Then twenty-three years old, I was looking for a day-time summer job to supplement my income from the night-time industrial surgeon duties. Magoun offered me a student scholarship. Within a few days, he showed me the technique for stimulating the deep brain structures and also how to record the responses at the brain cortex. Almost immediately, I changed the method around so that the deeply located needle tip could be used to record responses rather than to stimulate.

I have never understood why such a simple idea had not been exploited before. With my deep recording technique, the electrical record of responses to sensory stimuli could be tracked systematically throughout the deep recesses of the brain. All that was necessary was to provide a stimulus, as, for example, the noise of a toy cricket or a sudden light flash, and to see where the resulting electrical impulses were found. The amount of information that could be acquired was staggering.

It was like exploring the deep sea for the first time. I canceled my registration for the fall medical school term and continued to work with Magoun on what became known as the "extralemniscal sensory system." With this new concept of an alternative pathway for sensory stimuli, it was unnecessary to think of the brain's relation to the outside environment in the same limited way as before.

Magoun and I understood the importance of the discovery. We worked on its development full-time almost every day from early summer 1949 until he went to California a year later. At noon we walked to lunch at the Allerton Hotel cafeteria on Michigan Avenue, several blocks from the medical school. After a while, he timidly pointed out that my selections never changed, ended with a large custard, and always cost eighty-eight cents.

The food was only a source of energy; Magoun's conversations were magic. He taught me the true meaning of research as no one else could, or would ever try to. Not knowing the answer and wanting to get the conceptual picture right instead of being diverted into learning more and more about less and less was the framework for future research that he gave me. In 1950, Magoun left Northwestern to go to a new job at UCLA where he was founding chair of the Department of Anatomy at that now great medical school. I joined him there for five months in 1951 to complete my Ph.D. in neurophysiology.

Because Dr. Magoun's administrative duties before and after going to California were heavy, I did much of this later work alone, wrote the articles describing it, and took pride in its acceptance. It continues to be cited today.[1] But I knew that my contributions merely enriched the concept that Magoun had been delineating about brain structure and function. I wanted to do more. In addition, I knew by now that I wanted to take care of patients and to fulfill the ambition of becoming a surgeon that had been instilled in me as a child by my nurse mother. This seemed realistic. I had realized from performing the complex neurosurgical procedures required by our animal experiments that I would be competent, and possibly better than that.

The consequence of my decision to be a clinical doctor was that I returned from California to Northwestern in October 1951 to complete the senior year of medical school. Magoun had arranged for me to go instead to the Karolinska Institute in Stockholm for a fellowship with the Swedish neurophysiologist Ragnar Granit, who later was awarded a Nobel prize (1967). At the time, I believe Magoun thought that my decision to be a surgeon instead meant that both of us had failed. If so, I hope that he changed his mind. Ten years after I returned to Chicago, Magoun became dean of graduate studies at UCLA, one of several positions which he held with great distinction for almost three decades. He died of a stroke in March 1991 at the age of eighty-three.

» «

The Northwestern chapter of my life closed with another remarkable figure, the neurosurgeon Loyal Davis, who already had been chair of the Department of Surgery for sixteen years when I arrived and who remained in this post for another sixteen. Throughout most of this time he also was editor of *Surgery, Gynecology and Obstetrics*, the official journal of the American College of Surgeons. The fact that he functioned in these two powerful administrative positions in an intelligent and creative way was part of the explanation for his long tenure in both offices. His dominant personality was the rest.

I met Dr. Davis within the first few days after my arrival in Chicago. He always gave a lecture to the freshman class on the first Saturday morning of the academic year. If a pin dropped while he talked, he would find out where and why. In rapid order, he explained our duties and responsibilities, the suffering we would have to endure, and the monolithic purpose to which we had committed ourselves. When we left the room, the veterans, back in school after their wartime military service, remarked that this was going to be worse than the army.

Davis had himself been a colonel in the army, serving in England during World War II. It was rumored that his tenure was a stormy one. He bitterly fought what he thought were policy errors in military surgery and remembered specific tragic events which he recounted for the students. He had a particular interest in cases where the spinal cord was severed, causing permanent paralysis of the arms and legs. Some patients with less severe injuries were spared paralysis, only to have the spinal cord sheered off later during rough handling as they were evacuated or even in the course of subsequent hospital care. According to Nicholas Wetzel, one of

Davis's neurosurgical associates at Northwestern, this is what happened to General George Patton, who was initially intact after his fatal jeep accident. Someone flexed Patton's neck forcibly in order to allow him to smoke a cigarette, and Wetzel believes that the maneuver is what irreparably damaged Patton's spinal cord.

To prevent this complication, tongs similar to those used to pick up large blocks of ice were hooked into the sides of the head of some patients, and vertical traction was applied to the spine by hanging weights on an attached cord which was led through a pulley at the head of the bed. Davis told of a young soldier in North Africa whose neck had been broken in the same kind of accident as had occurred with Patton. In recounting this story, Davis described an astonishing mistake.

An inexperienced surgeon, taking care of the soldier and working from pictures in a book, had drilled a steel rod straight through the brain, creating a stirrup instead of tongs on which to pull. The patient was brain damaged for life by those charged to help him. The story was not told lightly. Davis was making the point of *primum non nocere* (first, do no harm). He asked the chances of violating this principle before every operation he personally performed.

The last three months of my senior medical school year were on Dr. Davis's neurosurgical service. This was not my choice, and in fact, I had made every effort to avoid the rotation. Neither Magoun nor Davis said so openly, but I believe that they had the cool disdain for each other that sometimes separates brilliant basic scientists and outstanding clinicians who are interested in the same organ system. Dr. Davis must have suspected that I had been made wary of him during my long stay in the other (Magoun's) camp.

For his part, Davis had an obvious interest in me because he knew of my work in neurophysiology, and I was not surprised to find the notification from the dean's office of an assignment to Passavant Hospital on Dr. Davis's busy service. I may have learned more about surgery from him than in any other three-month period in my life. Apart from that, a number of harrowing, and for the most part amusing, incidents occurred. It is strange how the humor has survived for forty years, along with deep affection for Loyal Davis, long after all else has faded.

A second student, older than I by eight or ten years, was Stuart Olson, a former saxophone player with the pioneer jazz artist, Stan Kenton. Olson, who was irrepressible as well as immensely likeable, directed his humor to Dr. Davis, who may have been half aware of this. Olson and I smoked, which was anathema to Dr. Davis if it was done in public. Having just lit up one day on the elevator, I sensed that Dr. Davis was outside when the door started to open on the next floor. I quickly dropped the forbidden cigarette and stepped on it. My instinct that Davis was close by was confirmed when he stepped inside, smelled the smoke, and demanded to know who was responsible. When we denied all knowledge, he asked to see what was under first one shoe (nothing, of course), and then the other shoe, under which lay the cigarette. He asked whose it was. After a pause, I told him, "You can have it, sir— I believe you saw it first." His associates were stupefied. After a moment's silence, he smiled, and after he left the elevator, I heard him laughing as he walked down the corridor.

The experience was revealing. To some people who did not know him well, Dr. Davis seemed like a hard and unyielding person. I never saw him that way again. Later on, he became an increasingly important person in my life until he died on August 19, 1982. By this time, his daughter, Nancy (Davis) Reagan, was mistress of the White House.

Like a bird sensing a change in season in early 1952, I prepared to move on. Dr. Davis wanted me to stay in Chicago and reacted angrily when I told him of my decision to go to the Johns Hopkins Hospital to begin a surgical internship. Six years passed before I returned to his department, but we wrote often and I visited him whenever I came to Chicago. Nearly thirty years later, a few days before he died, he called me in Pittsburgh about a woman who was in poor health in Mount Lebanon, a nearby suburb. They had been high school sweethearts in Galesburg, Illinois, more than sixty years before. He instructed me to call her family and to arrange for the best care possible. The message was brief because he was short of breath. I did exactly what he said. This was vintage Loyal Davis.

» «

In May 1952 I received an urgent summons from Richard Hale Young, dean of the school of medicine. He was waiting alone in his office, chain-smoking cigarettes. He was white-faced, agitated, and deeply angry. He blurted out that he had canceled my impending graduation. The reason was that some bound medical journals in the library on the subject of neuroanatomy had been defaced. Whoever did it had cut out articles from the books, using a scalpel or razor blade. The ruined books lay on his desk. For Young, who was a scholar, there could be no worse crime.

His investigators already had read my published papers in the related field of neurophysiology and had read my Ph.D. thesis to see if the missing articles were cited. Although they were not, I was the chief, and as far as I could tell, the only suspect. It appeared that I already had been convicted and that only the sentence was at issue.

It was a moment of supreme despair. A few years earlier, a faculty member named Leonarde Keeler at the Evanston campus at Northwestern had invented the polygraph (lie detector) and had opened a commercial service in an office on Rush Street. Later that day, I arranged to have the test. It was a humiliating experience because of the necessity to establish the reactivity of the subject about delicate matters such as sexual activities. By asking about these embarrassing things it was established that I easily could be made to sweat, that my heart rate would increase, and my blood pressure would soar. These changes also occur in a person who is lying. When asked if I knew anything about the book defacement, I answered no, with no change in the measurements. I had passed.

The report, which I paid for (about $200), was not accepted on face value when it was received by Dean Young. He told me that there were insufficient grounds to stop my graduation, but that he thought my knowledge of the nervous system had allowed me to fool the machine. More than fifteen years later, I received a letter from him with the solution to the mystery. Another medical student, by now a successful practitioner in the Midwest, had sent a large donation to the Northwestern library with a note to Young explaining that he was the person for whom they had been looking. He described the weight of his guilty conscience and his regret that suspicion had been directed elsewhere.

Not long after this, in 1969, I returned to Chicago to receive a cherished Merit Award from my old school. Dean Young was dying from cancer of the lung and had only a few months to live. We sat in his office together for the first time since that distant episode. He had difficulty talking because of his disease and had to rest between sentences. When he brought up the book incident, I remarked that he easily could have concealed the outcome. His response was that this would have been a monstrous crime compared to that of which he had accused me. He wanted only to be forgiven. This was easy. A few months later, he was dead. Afterward, I thought what a grand person he really was.

» «

My father came to the Northwestern graduation ceremonies in early June 1952 when I received my M.A., Ph.D., and M.D. degrees. Without fully understanding why, he believed more than I did that there would be some kind of larger purpose in my life. We talked often during these few days. Then he returned to his work in the small town in Iowa. Now twenty-six years old, I drove east to Baltimore. The word *transplantation* was not yet in my daily vocabulary, but I am confident that it was in his. Everything else was.

4

The Johns Hopkins Hospital

My interview for a surgical internship at the Johns Hopkins Hospital was arranged by Dr. Magoun and took place during my trip to Los Angeles in 1951 (see chapter 3). It was conducted by William P. Longmire, formerly a faculty surgeon at the Johns Hopkins Hospital and subsequently founding chair of the UCLA Department of Surgery. The starting date for the internship was July 1, 1952.

The heart (or perhaps today the soul) of the Johns Hopkins Hospital was the original infirmary at 5201 Broadway Avenue in East Baltimore. Just inside the front door was a giant statue of Christ, so tall that it reached up beyond the walkway on the second floor which gave access to sleeping rooms for interns and residents as well as some administrative offices. It was comforting to see the statue there when coming back late at night, or to look down on it from the third floor after climbing the stairs to my room.

The first person I met when I pushed open the front door was W. Dean Warren, an intern from two years before. He was on his way out, having decided after his first year of assistant residency to move to the University of Michigan for continuation of his surgical training. Ultimately, he completed his residency at Barnes Hospital, St. Louis. Warren's performance at Hopkins had been exemplary, and those in charge of the program liked him. I never found out why he had had enough.

The stated reason was financial. Whether he could have improved his subsequent record is doubtful. He became chair of the Department of Surgery at the University of Miami a dozen years later, and chair at Emory University School of Medicine in Atlanta after that. Before dying from cancer in 1989, he achieved recognition world-wide as the inventor of an operation known as the "Warren shunt." He was a profound student of liver disease and one of this century's greatest medical educators.

The second person, just inside, was George Zuidema. Zuidema grew up in Holland, Michigan, but was then a senior Hopkins student who had just completed an elective assignment at Harvard. He was covering one of the surgical services during the "bridge period" at the end of each June when an imperfect time fit between those leaving and those arriving created a shortage of personnel. George went back to Boston for his training at Massachusetts General Hospital, but returned to Hopkins in 1964 where he held the position of surgeon-in-chief for the next twenty years. Since 1984 he has been vice-provost for medical affairs at the University of Michigan.

These two men seemed perfectly normal, as did the next fifteen or twenty whom I met. Their appearance was deceptive. Almost all of them went on to preeminent positions. The talent pool at Hopkins in 1952 seemingly was without limits. Another good example was James V. Maloney, my roommate, an assistant resident who one year later became the chief resident. Maloney had an encyclopedic knowledge of heart function from research that he had started while in medical school at the University of Rochester and continued at the Harvard School of Public Health. Ascetic and deeply religious, he had the most remarkable intellect of the glitter-ing array of surgeons I have known during the last forty years. The fact that he prayed every night before going to bed made me envy his faith, and respect him more. Many years later, he became the second chair of surgery at UCLA, succeeding Bill Longmire.

As arduous as it had been, my Chicago life did not prepare me for the new challenge. The Hopkins intern was on duty twenty-four hours per day, every day of the year except for a one-week vacation. Apparently, some attrition was expected. The training program was "pyramidal" in that only two of the eighteen starting interns could be retained for a full six- (or seven-) year residency. Sur-prisingly, only a few, like Dean Warren, dropped out voluntarily.

The extras were culled, and most of these were deployed to other universities where they were eagerly received because of their generally high level of industry and ability.

It was a ruthless educational philosophy, one that permanently embittered a Harvard student who lived across the hall from me. This man went back to the Peter Bent Brigham Hospital in Boston and later established a fine academic reputation. Many others who were dropped also fared well and contributed to the growing Johns Hopkins aristocracy which became a powerful force in American academic surgery. It was a curious fact that these men always identified themselves as of Hopkins origin, no matter how short their stay in Baltimore. Perhaps this was understandable. The average level of technical surgery and the opportunity for clinical experience during that era at Hopkins were unparalleled.

It was a seller's market. The salary for the internship year was zero, and after this it was symbolic only. During my fourth and last year I reached the level of $36 per month. I had arrived in Baltimore with $500 in my pocket from a Borden Research Prize. Even without this advantage, conditions were workable for an unmarried house officer because the food was free and outstanding, and there always was a place to sleep if the time could be found. For some it was heaven, and for others hell. I found it to be purgatory. There were no women nor any black interns or residents during my four years there. The social climate was southern.

Alfred Blalock, the chair of surgery at Hopkins, was a gray-haired and revered figure whose every move and idiosyncrasy invited close study and often imitation. His variably kindly and merciless (usually the former) exposure of surgical principles and new ideas during interrogation of students and house officers in the "bull pen" of the Hurd Hall Auditorium was the teaching event of each week. His supporting cast was no less effective, made up mainly of higher-level residents and young faculty officers who recently had gone through the training program.

Henry T. Bahnson, who completed his chief residency in 1951, one year before I arrived, was the most respected of the group, not only because of his great skills and intelligence, but because of his zealous integrity and fairness in coming to judgment of other people. I learned much later that this stemmed from an unjust accusation directed at him during his childhood.

Bahnson had graduated first in his class at Harvard Medical School after being an all conference football tackle at Davidson College during his undergraduate years. His athletic skills, hand-eye coordination, and determination in the operating room could have been predicted from his football career. During the early 1950s, Bahnson published his epic work on the excision and repair of blow-outs in the main blood vessel carrying blood from the heart to all of the body (aneurysms). He already had made other notable contributions to surgery of other blood vessels and of the heart.

Bahnson's work and his precocious fame epitomized the excitement of the Hopkins environment in the early 1950s. Blalock, working with Helen Taussig and the same Longmire who had sent me to Baltimore, opened a new field when they carried out the first of their "blue-baby operations" in 1944. The institution became a crossroads for the new specialty of cardiac surgery. When I finished my internship and a chance came in July 1953 to go back to a research lab after an absence of nearly two years, I decided to study the cardiac conduction system. This system is a network of specialized muscle fibers which initiates and controls the rate of the heartbeat, although it normally is influenced by and subject to fine-tuning by the nervous system.

My project was to damage these fibers in dogs, thereby preventing them from conveying electrical messages from the two thin-walled upper heart chambers to the more muscular lower chambers (ventricles) which are the main blood pumps. Interruption of the fibers caused a condition called "heart block" and mimicked the situation in humans that frequently was caused accidentally during the heart operations that were being done in those early days without the assistance of heart-lung machines.

I devised an operation to cut the conduction fibers inside the dog heart during a brief period when one of the upper heart chambers was opened and cleaned of blood at the same time as blood returning to the heart was dammed up by clamping the incoming veins for the necessary three to five minutes. With successful cutting of the conduction fibers, the muscular lower heart chambers took up a new beat at about half the normal rate still seen in the naturally beating upper chambers. Then, it was possible to study both the resulting circulatory changes as well as the extent, which proved to be considerable, to which these could be brought to normal by electrically stimulating the slowed lower chambers back up to a normal heart rate.[1] Such stimulation therapy for patients with heart block promptly was introduced into the hospital.

While these experiments were going on, W. B. Kouwenhoven, retired former dean of the Johns Hopkins School of Engineering, was carrying out some different dog experiments down the hall which seemed crude by comparison. He and a surgical resident named James Jude caused heart stoppage in dogs by electrocution and other means. He then massaged the heart by external compression without opening the chest and without directly squeezing the heart with the hands as previously had been thought necessary. After prolonged periods of such treatment, Kouwenhoven was able to restore the heart to a normal beat by shocking it through the unopened chest wall. Before long, the method was tried successfully in patients. Almost overnight, external (closed chest) massage found its way to every emergency room and intensive care unit in the world. Kouwenhoven, who already had a long and distinguished career as a scientist and educator, had demonstrated the power of a simple and logical idea when it is steadfastly tested. All of his many other accomplishments were outweighed by what he did near the end of his life.

Another important research program was going forward at the same time. Hank Bahnson's preoccupation during my laboratory stint was the development of a heart-lung machine for open heart surgery. Because I was not schooled in physics, I was not as committed to this project or as helpful as I should have been. In late 1953, Bahnson organized a trip to Jefferson Medical College in Philadelphia for observation of the artificial heart-lung that had been developed by engineers at the IBM Corporation and by the surgeon John Gibbon. Gibbon already had used the apparatus to treat four patients by closing abnormal holes (septal defects) between their upper or lower heart chambers under direct vision.

Although three had died, one had left the hospital and it seemed clear that a revolution in cardiac surgery was close at hand.

A few months later, we flew to the University of Minnesota to learn what we could from C. Walton Lillehei, F. John Lewis, Richard Varco, and their associates. John Lewis's assistant in training was a young man with a crew cut and a wry sense of humor named Norman Shumway who was destined to be the father of heart transplantation. These men and their associates were attempting to do open heart surgery with three different methods.

Lewis's technique was similar to that used for my heart block operation in dogs except that the patient was cooled to increase the time when circulation to the heart and brain could be suspended. The second method of operating inside of the heart was with a heart-lung machine developed by two surgeons, Richard Dewall and Herbert Warden. It was the same in principle as the bubble oxygenator designed by my father (see chapter 2). The third and most controversial technique was called "cross circulation." In this procedure, Lillehei tapped the circulation from the large vessels of a healthy partner whose normal heart was strong enough to be put "on loan" to support the circulation needs of a sick patient while the patient's heart was opened and repaired.

From the observation dome of the human operating room, we witnessed a tragedy during an attempt at cross circulation. The healthy member of the connected pair was accidentally given a large amount of intravenous air from a bottle that had been internally pressurized to increase the rate of fluid infusion. No one had noticed when the bottle became empty of its solution. Moments later, the previously healthy cross-circulation partner who had been pumped full of air had a heart stoppage.

Although heart massage was successful, I learned later that the healthy patient had suffered permanent brain injury and ultimately died. It is impossible to convey in words the sense of grief and horror which pervaded the university hospital at the time of our departure. I remembered Dr. Davis's admonition *primum non nocere* (first, do no harm). The thought came again many times when we began to use living related donors eight years later for kidney transplantation.

» «

On November 27, 1954, near the end of the Halsted laboratory experience, I was married to Barbara June Brothers of Hartville, Ohio. We had met at Rehoboth Beach, Delaware, six months earlier. My father came to the wedding. He, and others, warned me of the perils of preoccupation with work. I paid too little attention to their advice. The best man was Hank Bahnson, in whose home I had been a constant nuisance and would be again.

The wedding was at the Brothers home, one of the fourteen or fifteen houses distributed around the periphery of the Congress Lake Country Club, midway between Canton and Akron. The owners of these estates, bearing names like Firestone (tires), Timken (roller bearings), and Moore (newspaper chain), created an atmosphere of affluence. Barbara's father, John Brothers, owned a chain of hardware stores centered in Canton.

The wedding was a major social event. My father became an instant celebrity when the golf course where guests' cars were parked was deluged with rain and turned into a mud pond. He organized and led wrecking crews to pull the stranded cars from the quagmire, becoming more encrusted with dirt each passing minute. As he effortlessly lifted the rear ends of cars from their ruts, I was almost ashamed to see how powerful he was in comparison to some of the bemused guests.

I was twenty-six years old at the time, but it still seemed to me that my father was invincible. From the time I was a child, we had had half-serious wrestling matches, testing each other's strength. He always won, but then at the last moment, arranged to lose. Now, we went through the ritual again. Although I was in good condition and thirty years younger, he still was stronger and had to contrive a last minute capitulation. It was the last time for this charade. The next time I saw him, thirteen months later, the left side of his body was paralyzed. Although his right side still was powerful when we wrestled again, it was I who pretended to lose.

After the wedding, Barbara and I drove to South Londonderry, Vermont, where we stayed at the Starlight Farm, a second home owned by my Uncle Frank. When the honeymoon was over, it was time to return to Baltimore—to the responsibilities of patient care and to a new way of domestic life in an apartment across the street from the emergency room instead of a hospital sleeping room.

» «

Eighteen months after returning to the clinical service, Barbara and I left Baltimore. My fit with the Hopkins system, which of necessity was a highly regimented one, was uneasy. I may have had a deep-seated resistance to the obsessive attention to detail and the formation of a reproducible decision-making process which are essential for responsible patient care. Only later was I to appreciate my lifetime debt to the program, including David Sabiston, one of the chief residents during my internship and a faculty officer during my last year, whom I imagined to be my greatest source of anxiety and internal conflict. Sabiston is a great educator who epitomized the philosophy of Hopkins surgical training in that era.

By the time I left, the pyramidal system had eliminated all but two of eighteen starting interns. Toward the end of my fourth year, only I and my friend Robert Gaertner were left. Bob, who was the second author on all the heart block papers, finished the chief residency but died of liver cirrhosis ten years later. In early spring 1956, I had a long conference with Dr. Blalock, who offered me a fifth—but explicitly not a sixth—year. Angry at what I construed to be an affront, I declined.

Within a few days, I had made my own arrangements to go to the University of Miami where a new medical school and surgical department had been founded recently. The chair at Miami was John J. Farrell, a name previously unknown to me. Behind the scenes, Dr. Blalock and Dr. Bahnson helped me to obtain this senior and chief residency, but I had not requested their assistance nor did I know of it until much later.

Thirty-five years have passed since I left Baltimore. I still cannot see clearly what this four years meant beyond knowing that it was the most formative period of my surgical life. In 1981 at the University of Pittsburgh, I rejoined two members of the legendary inner circle of the previous era, Hank Bahnson and Mark Ravitch. I found both to be as loyal to Hopkins as I was, but just as ambivalent in their retrospective assessment. When I was in Baltimore, I could sense the changes that had to come. Leadership in the field of cardiac surgery, which had started there, was slipping away and soon would be gone. I could not see what would replace it as a banner.

Surgical research, the original basis for the cardiac revolution, had slowed to a desultory and unsophisticated pace at Hopkins. Merely being able to operate well would not be good enough for the next generation. The talent pool was being exsanguinated as the rising stars were recruited elsewhere, and its replenishment was being inhibited by the de facto exclusion of a part of the population which possessed great vitality and creativity. Where were the women and the minorities?

The one black face that moved freely in and out of the surgical offices, but never to the bathrooms and doctors' dining room, belonged to Vivien Thomas. He was Dr. Blalock's personal laboratory technician, moving from Vanderbilt to Baltimore with Blalock in 1941. The master surgeons at Hopkins told tales of his natural skills and of his ingenuity in working out the blood vessel reconnections that were the basis of the blue-baby operation. When this procedure first was used in humans, it was reported that he stood behind Blalock in the operating room and gave suggestions and instructions. Then, like Matt Henson, the black man who went with Perry to the North Pole, he was denied the recognition that he had earned.

Dr. Blalock, a man of honor, took steps to right the wrong, and those whom Blalock had trained heaped honors on Vivien when he was old. Although Vivien never finished high school, he was given an honorary doctor of laws degree at the Johns Hopkins University in 1976. Today his oil portrait hangs in the lobby of the Blalock building, which was built in 1954 and later named for his chief.

These honors came late. When I knew Vivien in 1953, he drank heavily throughout the day and was a shadow of the heroic figure he must have been earlier. I saw him again in 1978 when I went back to Johns Hopkins to give the Reinhoff Lecture. He was dignified and dry. Justice had been done.

But all that was history yet to come. In the mid 1950s, Hopkins had one foot mired in the glorious past while the other groped for a stone in the torrent which would carry it over the flood. What was done in that great American institution to move into the new world in later years reflected its true fiber. However, this is not part of my story.

The four Hopkins years and the five that followed were the most turbulent and confusing ones of my life. I felt like a missile looking for a trajectory.

» «

There was another factor in my desire to leave Johns Hopkins which I was reluctant to discuss with anyone at that time or subsequently. After being financially independent for six years, I had had to accept money from my father in order to maintain an apartment and way of life for my new wife and subsequently for our first child. This need for subsidization became even more painful when, in December 1955, my father suffered his first stroke, which left him paralyzed on one side. Although he was able to return to work at his newspaper, he would never be the same again. I needed to find a place to complete my training where some kind of reasonable salary was paid. I never considered asking for help from my wife's wealthy family.

5

A Trip South

The job in Florida paid $300 per month—enough to live on without depending on regular support from my father, who still was recovering from his stroke of seven months earlier. I was not yet qualified on paper to practice surgery. Obtaining this credential was the reason to go to Miami. The starting date for the fifth-year residency was July 1, 1956. My wife, Barbara, and I drove down the east coast with our sixteen-month-old son, Timothy Wakefield Starzl, in the same car I had used for the trip to Los Angeles five years before (see chapter 3).

When we arrived, we had lunch at a restaurant overlooking the channel (Biscayne Bay) that separated Miami Beach and the mother city. They were two different worlds. Miami Beach was where the often dissolute rich made their last stand, soon to be invaded by an aged population which had been lured there by illusions of utopia, only to find hunger and despair. Those in Miami across the bay were more rustic in taste and behavior. They referred to Miami Beach as "rotten in paradise," perhaps with envy because they were not there themselves.

Jackson Memorial Hospital, our destination in Miami, was a rectangle of old and new buildings around an open yard which held a police facility. At an emergency room which was accessible by ascending a ramp from the court, injured prisoners were brought in wagons or squad cars to be booked, interrogated, or have their wounds or complaints taken care of.

Some of their injuries appeared to have occurred en route to the hospital. One night I walked in on a struggle that left one of those strong memories that never fades. A Spanish-speaking prisoner in a wagon refused to come out, possibly because he could not understand what was being asked of him. He fought furiously, using his arms and legs to hold himself in and to ward off the blows of five or six muscular officers who became more enraged, white-faced, and trembling with every passing moment. They pummeled him with their fists and night sticks. When he was limp and cried out no more, they removed him. It was not an isolated incident.

Was this gratuitous brutality or the justified use of legal force in what was a sea of crime and violence? Jackson Memorial Hospital had one of the busiest emergency rooms in the world, the number of cases exceeding by far that at Johns Hopkins. Within a few months, I had seen and operated on several patients with gunshot wounds of the largest vein in the body (the inferior vena cava) which drains blood from the legs, trunk, kidneys, and other tissues and organs. This kind of injury rarely had been reported in the medical literature, only seven examples with survival having been recorded up to that time. It was being seen routinely in Miami.[1] Night and day, the casualties came. Fear of being accused of exaggeration inhibits a guess of the number of operations that I performed during this two-year period. I once estimated two thousand.

My surgical training came not only at the beginning of open heart surgery, but also at the dawn of blood vessel surgery which, like many other advances in medicine, had been driven by the exigencies of war. Back at Hopkins, Hank Bahnson, a pioneer in vascular surgery, had established a bank where arteries and veins were stored after their removal from people who had died recently. These were kept in the refrigerator or in a vacuum tube after drying and were brought out as needed for blood vessel replacement. There was no such facility in Miami. I organized one with Dr. Francis Cooke, a Korean war veteran with field experience in vascular grafting. A report about this vessel bank was my first contribution to the literature of transplantation.[2]

I removed the blood vessels from the corpses in the hospital morgue, using a sterile surgical kit from the operating room. Nowhere have I seen such a parade of sorrow: drowned children;

raped and murdered women; blond, suntanned muscle-builders with neat bullet holes in their heads; and victims of automobile accidents. I dreaded the summons to the morgue, not wanting to know what had happened to the blood vessel donor, but realizing that this knowledge would be the price for providing the vessel graft to someone who needed it.

The worst sight was of a young man who had worked in a stone quarry. His job was to run an automated stone breaker that consisted of multiple hard instruments which gained momentum at the end of long chains or ropes in order to crack the stone targets. Apparently, he would amuse other workers by jumping into the pit where these instruments were swinging like balls on the ends of strings and then by dodging them. This day, he had miscalculated and was crippled by a first hit. By the time someone could turn off the machine, the other stone breakers had taken their turn as if infuriated by their unintended use for entertainment. Almost nothing was left of him.

Presiding as the founding chair of the Department of Surgery and chief of my surgical service at this new medical school was John J. Farrell, a man in his early forties who had been recruited from a junior staff position at Albany Medical College in New York. How this choice was made, and why, was a matter for speculation then and for years afterward.

The reason for perplexity was an absence in his case of the record of scholarship which usually is a condition for appointment to such a high academic post. He had published only one or two inconsequential articles in medical journals and did not belong to any of the important surgical organizations. These deficits are serious enough for a composed and wise individual, but they portend disaster for a volatile person with deep insecurities. To add to his woes, or perhaps because of them, Dr. Farrell drank to excess. Thus, the quality of patient care was unusually dependent on the people who were ostensibly in training but who actually were more competent than the man to whom they were responsible.

It is painful to write these thoughts even a third of a century later, and perhaps it is cruel because Dr. Farrell died in April 1983 of cancer of the throat and can not respond. In 1958, before I left for

Chicago, he asked me to stay on his faculty. After I was gone, he came to Chicago and tried to persuade me to come back. By this time, his faculty members had lodged a complaint against him with the American Association of University Professors (AAUP), charging him with academic misconduct. While the case played out publicly in the AAUP journal,[3] Dr. Farrell tried to enlist political support from the American College of Surgeons (ACS). I was interviewed in Chicago by two ACS officials, Dr. Loyal Davis of Northwestern and Dr. I. S. Ravdin of the University of Pennsylvania. I tried to say as little as possible. It was like watching a Eugene O'Neill tragedy in which the mismatch between the anti-hero and the environment was so great that disintegration and failure were inevitable. In 1961 he was removed from the surgery chairmanship.

In October 1965, after his career was ruined, I ran into Dr. Farrell at a meeting in Atlantic City. I was successful by then in ways to which he had aspired, and he spoke of his pride in having one of "his products" do well. I was located at the University of Colorado instead of at the University of Kentucky because of his unfriendly intervention at Kentucky (see chapter 7), but there was no reason to tell him that I knew this. It occurred to me how lonely and unhappy he must be, and what a nice man he might have been if his aims in life had been different and more attuned to his capabilities. After a long walk on the beach we shook hands, and I never saw him again.

This was later. In 1957, Dr. Farrell told me a lie which would make it impossible for me to consider working for him. During a volatile discussion I spoke with admiration of Dr. Blalock, my previous chief at Johns Hopkins. In response, Dr. Farrell said that before I came he had received a letter from Dr. Blalock which had deprecated me and that he, Farrell, had decided against Blalock's negative advice to accept me for the senior residency. His secretary, a kind woman, overheard the conversation. Realizing how deeply wounded I was, she came back to the office late that night, made a copy of Dr. Blalock's letter, and gave it to me. The content was the opposite of what Dr. Farrell had said.

Not long after, this secretary, who previously had been devoted to Dr. Farrell, quit her job. A promising group of young faculty officers were soon to follow, about a year after I had gone. These men and the positions to which they went included Robert Litwak (chief, thoracic surgery, Mount Sinai School of Medicine, New York), Frank Kurzweg (founding chair of surgery, Louisiana State Medical School, Shreveport), George Prout (chief, Division of Urology, Medical College of Virginia, Richmond; later, chief of urology, Massachusetts General Hospital, Boston), and Rufus Broadaway (private practice, Miami). John J. Foman was the only one who stayed. The stage was swept bare for the arrival in 1963 of the new chair, W. Dean Warren, the first person whom I had met at Johns Hopkins in 1956 (see chapter 4).

By the time Warren came, a few years later, the world had changed. During 1956–58 the restrooms and dining rooms still were segregated by the color of skin, and so were the hospital wards — as they had been at Johns Hopkins. The floor where black patients stayed was in an old part of Jackson Hospital, far from the operating rooms. This necessitated a long trip on a stretcher for those needing surgery. It also placed them far from the safety of an intensive care unit to which they might have to go if they needed to have emergency breathing (ventilator) support.

Intensive care as we know it today did not exist. For patients whose kidneys failed, there was nothing to do but wait and pray for a miracle which usually did not come. The musky odor caused by the body's growing chemical imbalance would fill the room as hope for spontaneous recovery slowly faded. There was dignity in the death watch. The patients knew what was happening but were not frightened. The poisons that would kill them descended like a gentle cloak on their consciousness, allowing sweet farewells before oblivion. There were no artificial kidneys in Miami, nor for that matter in most other centers.

One of my patients on the black ward was a young woman on whom I performed a chest operation, removing the diseased part of her left lung. After the operation, her kidneys stopped making urine. Seeing this beautiful and vital person edge toward eternity was a familiar experience. Then suddenly, she began to produce urine in quantities that became voluminous after a few days. We were overjoyed and could not refrain from a daily war dance when we came to her bed. I carelessly remarked that we would soon bath and swim in the urine as it swept us away. She misinterpreted what I said and wept. I can not remember being more ashamed of myself. Within five years, a revolution in the specialty of kidney disease would make a return from the shadows an expected outcome, no longer the cause for wild celebration.

Those planning public policy were aware that medicine was on the march and were concerned that there would be a shortage of physicians. As a result, new medical schools were founded at an unprecedented pace during the two decades after World War II. The University of Miami was one. Another was being constructed at the University of Florida at Gainesville in the northern part of the state. The founding dean was George Harrell who also would be responsible a few years later for the founding of the medical school at Penn State.

Knowing that I would not be willing to stay at the University of Miami, I had written to Dean Harrell and asked if I could see him about the possibility of finding a faculty position in surgery. He knew of my earlier research with the nervous system and heart physiology and agreed to talk to me. Another option that I wanted to explore was to go into private practice in the town of Sanford, near Gainesville, which was served by the Seminole Community Hospital. If private practice was to be my fate, I wanted to explore the possibility of being a volunteer faculty member at the University of Florida.

These inquiries came to nothing. However, on the way north in the flatlands of central Florida, my car broke down nearly twenty-five miles from the nearest town. After trying to flag a ride for an hour or so in the hot sun, a truck finally stopped which was driven by a middle-aged black man. He was very courteous, and for a while we talked about small things. Then he asked me to conceal myself, so that I could not be seen by passing cars. I was astonished until he mentioned that it had become commonplace for citizen vigilantes, enraged by seeing cohabitation of cars by mixed races, to draw up alongside and discharge a shotgun blast at the occupants. I did as he said.

When we reached town, he let me off a block from the gas station. I thanked him and tried to pay him something, which he refused.

By now, he will be very old, and even if he is still alive, it does not seem likely that he will read these words. But if by chance he does, I wonder if he will even recall his kind act so long ago. For me, it was one of those small things that grew a little every time it came back in memory until suddenly it was a mountain.

Many of the relics of the postbellum south were still standing. The need to care for all people gave to medicine its own special role in the social changes that were occurring. In October–December 1957, I took a three-month rotation in surgery at the Tampa General Hospital, which much later became the primary teaching hospital for another new medical school, at the University of South Florida. Here as in Miami, medical care was segregated. Many black patients were treated in a white frame building called the Clara Frye Memorial Hospital, several blocks down the street. Most of the patients were extremely sick, and despite the equipment and personnel limitations, complex operations were carried out there.

Late one afternoon, I was performing an operation called an "abdominoperineal resection" on an elderly black lady who had a large cancer a few inches above her anus. The first part of this operation is done from above, through an incision in the abdomen which allows the large intestine to be prepared for removal. The final part of the operation including removal of the anus and surrounding tissues is done from below with the patient lying on her back with legs spread apart and held up in stirrups.

At this stage it is necessary to join up the lower and upper fields of operation by separating the anus and rectum from the tailbone and spine at the back, and from the vagina and bladder at the front. This is the most dangerous and bloody part of the procedure. There was a thunderstorm outside, and just at this critical moment, the electrical system failed. I finished the operation successfully in the dark, aided by nurses who held pocket flashlights and the battery-powered special instruments which are used by specialists to examine the back of eyes. Always fascinated by the quaint architecture of this hospital, I tried to visit it a few years later. It had disappeared.

» «

If I had come to Miami in search of surgical competence, I achieved it automatically by caring for vast numbers of patients over the period of twenty-four months. In seeking a purpose beyond this, something at a subconscious level seemed to point to the liver. For centuries, the liver, an enormous and silent reddish-brown organ, had withheld many secrets of its own function. It also was hostile to surgeons. Those who tried to remove part of the liver, or to cut it for other reasons, placed their patients at risk of fatal bleeding. Almost half of the blood circulating in the body every minute passes through the liver. Part of this flow is arterial (delivered by the hepatic artery) and the rest is venous (delivered by the portal vein).

These two sources of the liver's blood supply can be distinguished by a casual observer in the operating room. When the hepatic artery or its branches are cut, blood spurts in a jet stream under high pressure. The bright red color of this arterial blood is due to oxygen which has just been taken up from the inspired air by its red blood cells during passage through the lungs. The blood is pumped by the heart directly to all of the body's tissues and organs.

In contrast, when the portal vein branches are cut in the operating room, they do not spurt because their blood contents are under low pressure. The blood is dark because so much of the oxygen has been left behind to nourish the pancreas, intestines, and stomach through which it already has passed by the time it reaches the liver. During the passage through the first organs, the portal venous blood picks up half-digested food from the intestines, insulin from the pancreas, and other special substances that are brought to the liver in high concentration from the organs being drained. The portal vein contributes about 75 percent of the liver blood flow compared to 25 percent from the artery.

Normally, the liver offers no resistance to the passage of the oxygen-poor but otherwise enriched portal blood. It takes up and uses many of the food products and special substances to which it has special access. However, the liver disease of cirrhosis—caused by alcohol, other toxins, or viruses—can block the blood passages within the liver through which the portal blood should pass. Like a river clogged with debris, the blocked portal blood seeks a way around the liver by alternative channels—other veins called collaterals which are normally small and carry little blood. These collateral veins in the human tend to be heavily concentrated at the

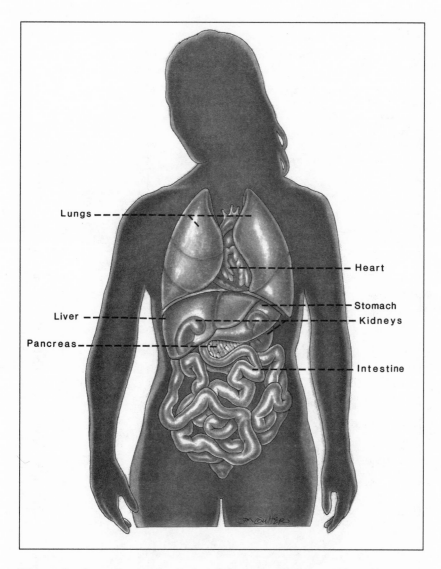

Figure 1. Location in the body of the commonly transplanted organs. Note that every normal person has two lungs and two kidneys. The kidneys are behind the liver on the right and behind the stomach on the left.

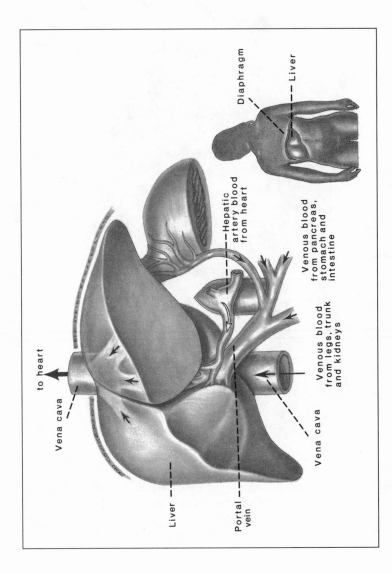

Figure 2. Normal blood supply of the liver. The vena cava runs behind, not through, the liver and therefore does not nourish it as do the portal vein and liver artery.

junction of the esophagus (gullet or upper food pipe) with the stomach. The now distended veins with their thin walls are unaccustomed to such a high flow and pressure. They may burst at any time. As when a dam breaks, blood rushes out of this point of least resistance.

The medical term for this complication is *bleeding esophageal varices*. A message from an emergency room containing these words implies a dire emergency. There is no more terrifying sight in medicine than an ashen and panic-stricken patient, bleeding internally into the esophagus and stomach and then vomiting his life's blood onto the floor before anything can be done to help. Many patients do not survive the first such incident.

The year before coming from Baltimore to Miami, I had helped Dr. Blalock treat a patient who had this complication of liver cirrhosis. The patient also suffered from sugar diabetes requiring insulin. Using a surgical operation called a "portacaval shunt," we relieved the high pressure of the distended veins by rerouting the portal vein flow around the liver, just as might be done by building a large bypass canal around an obstruction in a river. The operation was successful, leaving the liver to survive with artery blood alone. What caught my attention was the fact that this patient's sugar diabetes also was relieved. He no longer needed insulin to control his blood sugar.

I wondered if this had occurred because the natural insulin coming from the patient's pancreas into the portal vein was made more effective after the operation because it no longer had to pass through the liver and be changed there by some process. If this were true, the sugar diabetes might be fundamentally a liver disease instead of a disease of the pancreas as was commonly thought. Animal experiments that I designed to test this idea proved it to be without merit. However, the experiments led in less than two years to the first attempts at experimental liver transplantation.

Testing these ideas in Miami was not easy. Because there was no large animal facility, I set one up in an empty garage across from the emergency room of the Jackson Memorial Hospital around which the University of Miami medical school was organized. The garage was a large single room with a water supply and a centrally placed drain down which we washed the waste (feces and urine) that had been collected in the handmade metabolic cages deployed around the periphery. Supplies were borrowed (or impounded) from the clinical operating room at Jackson Memorial Hospital. I maintained this primitive laboratory with the aid of one of the junior surgical residents (William Meyer), who eventually joined his father in practice in Fort Myers, Florida.

My wife, Barbara, cared for the animals among many other highly supportive activities. We obtained dogs from the city pound, made them diabetic with a chemical called alloxan which poisons the insulin-producing cells (Beta cells) in the pancreas, and determined their insulin requirements after they became diabetic. After this, we performed an operation on the dogs similar to that used for the patient in Baltimore whose diabetes had gone away. To my dismay, the insulin requirements after the operation increased drastically in these dogs instead of decreasing as I had hoped. In addition, the animals became emaciated, lost their hair, and appeared to be confused. Some had bouts of unconsciousness or convulsions from which recovery usually was spontaneous.[4]

That the brain was being damaged by the portal vein bypass procedure was not new information. The operation of portacaval shunt which I had performed on the dogs was first described in 1877 by a twenty-nine-year-old Russian military surgeon named Nicholas Eck.[5] Although Eck failed to appreciate the harmful effects of this procedure, the operation of portacaval shunt came to be known as "Eck's fistula." Its harmful consequences were discovered sixty-three years before our Miami experiments by the forty-four-year-old Russian physiologist and psychologist, Ivan Petrovich Pavlov (Nobel prize, 1904). Pavlov's article on Eck's fistula in 1893 was one of the most powerful and incisive contributions ever made to knowledge of the liver (hepatology).[6] He called the nervous system symptoms of coma and convulsions "meat intoxication" because they could be caused or aggravated by a meat diet. He also noted that the livers in the animals after Eck's fistula were shrunken and contained abnormal amounts of fat.

Thus, aside from thoroughly demolishing my theory about favorably altering the diabetic state with Eck's fistula, our garage

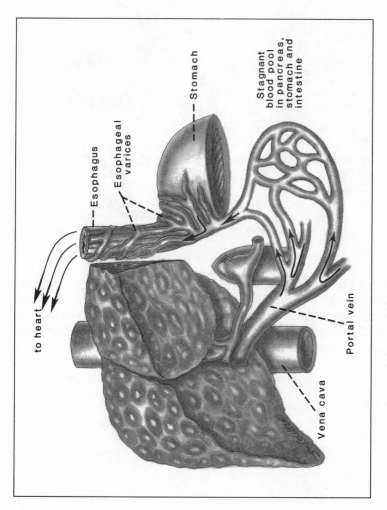

Figure 3. Varices formed when liver disease causes blockage of the portal vein blood, forcing this blood to find other ways back to the heart.

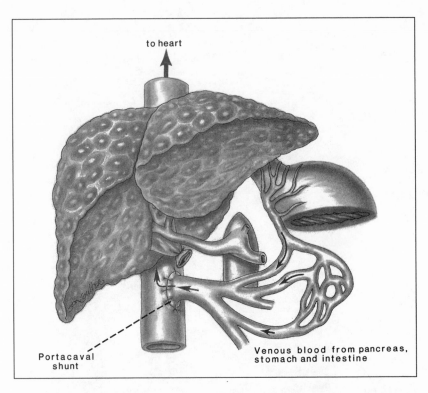

to heart

Portacaval
shunt

Venous blood from pancreas,
stomach and intestine

Figure 4. The surgical operation known as portacaval shunt reroutes the blocked venous blood returning from the abdominal organs around the obstructing liver. After the operation, the portal venous blood enters the vena cava and is carried behind the liver straight to the heart. This operation is also known as Eck's fistula.

experiments merely confirmed a well-known experimental phenomenon. Because I was too ignorant to be clever, these disappointments did not dampen my interest in the liver and the effect upon it of insulin. The questions about sugar and insulin metabolism raised by these still primitive thoughts and investigations during 1955–58 could not be answered without better models, including one of total removal of the liver (hepatectomy) in large animals. While still in Miami, I developed an improved method of hepatectomy in dogs who could live for twelve to twenty-four hours after this drastic operation.[7] It was a crucial step for the study of many metabolic problems, and my new technique of total hepatectomy quickly became the worldwide standard.

However, the most important consequence of the liver removal operation was the realization that a new liver could be installed (I thought easily) in the empty space from which the normal liver had been taken out. In fact, half of the operation of liver transplantation already had been perfected with the hepatectomy procedure. The other half would be to sew in a new liver. My two-year stay in Miami was nearing an end, and further work on this second half awaited my relocation in Chicago.

New ideas seldom have the simplicity of a switched on light bulb. Liver transplantation had never even been mentioned in the medical literature until 1955. In that year, a surgeon named C. Stuart Welch of Albany Medical College, New York, described the transplantation of a second (auxiliary) liver in dogs without disturbing the recipient's own liver.[8] This was not the liver replacement to which my own research led me, but there may have been a connection between Welch and my decision to go forward with liver transplantation.

John J. Farrell, the surgical chair at Miami, had himself come from Albany Medical College and was a protégé there of Welch, whom he idolized. It is hard for me to believe that Farrell did not know about and mention to me Welch's research on auxiliary liver transplantation. Furthermore, during my two years in Miami, while I was laying the groundwork for the alternative procedure of liver replacement, Welch visited Miami at least once. I met him.

To say more than this would require concocting an event and exchange of information which may have occurred but which I cannot recall. I wish that I could have this memory because, if I did, it would mean that much of what I achieved in the rest of my career could be traced back to the time I spent with John Farrell. Farrell was one of the few persons in my life for whom I had a genuinely low regard. I would like to believe that this was an unfair assessment.

6

A Fertile Vacuum

The summer of 1958 started as the most unpromising period of my life. The rationale for returning to Chicago after a six-year absence was questionable. Was this a reasoned decision or merely a clumsy effort to delay one? The ostensible purpose of this final year of training was to become fully qualified to do chest (thoracic) surgery, or more accurately, to obtain a certificate saying that I met this condition. In fact, I already was highly experienced in this field. The perception of some of those closest to me was that I was avoiding for one more year the final agony of growing up and going into private practice.

The truth was worse than anyone imagined. For the past six years, I had honed my surgical abilities. At the same time, I harbored anxieties which I was unable to discuss openly until more than three decades later, after I had stopped operating. I had an intense fear of failing the patients who had placed their health or life in my hands. Far from being relieved by each new layer of skill or experience, the anxieties grew worse. Even for simple operations, I would review books to be sure that no mistakes would be made or old lessons forgotten. Then, sick with apprehension, I would go to the operating room, almost unable to function until the case began.

Later in life, when I told close friends that I did not like to operate, they did not believe me or thought I was joking. Most surgeons whom I know have been able to protect themselves, either by rationalizing errors which they had committed or by promptly erasing the bad memories. I could not do this. Instead of blotting out the failures, I remembered these forever. With growing concern, I came to believe that I was not emotionally equipped to be a surgeon or to deal with its brutality. The incongruity was that I did not like doing the one thing for which I had become uniquely qualified. It was as if I had trained all of my life to become a violin virtuoso, only to discover that I loathed giving concerts or even playing privately.

What I have just written is not the revisionist musing of someone who has reached the age of sixty-five. I knew it all when I was thirty-two and understood the torment that lay ahead. But it was too late to change again. I had already forged a promising career in neurophysiology only to abandon it; I had dabbled for a year and a half in heart physiology, never to be heard from again. Surgery would have to be the end of the line. The further irony was that I was committed to a one-year fellowship in thoracic surgery, while already knowing that my main interests were below the chest, focused particularly on the liver. Was this latest interest going to be another passing fancy?

» «

F. John Lewis, the director of the Chest Surgery Division at Northwestern and my chief during the fellowship, was one of the brightest stars in the emerging new field of heart surgery when he came to Chicago in 1956 from the volatile environment of the University of Minnesota. Loyal Davis, the chair of surgery at Northwestern, was nearing retirement, and the tacit assumption was that Lewis, who was forty years old, soon would succeed him. Lewis was a fine surgeon and one of the most creative people whom I have ever met. "Witty" always was the first adjective used to describe him.

His innocent wit, which to me was irresistible, was not welcome to everyone. At conferences, he was able with a few words to puncture the pontifications of the more ponderous of his senior colleagues, invariably provoking laughter. The stiletto thrusts were remembered with a smile long after by his friends, and brooded over permanently by the victims. He was creating resistance. When Davis finally vacated the surgery chair in 1963, Lewis was passed over as the replacement, and in 1976 he retired prematurely to Santa

Barbara, California, where his life has been full. Now seventy-four, he recently wrote a book called *So Your Doctor Recommended Surgery*, which received good reviews. In medicine, he always will be remembered as the first person ever to operate inside the open human heart. His protégé at Minnesota, Norm Shumway (now at Stanford), became the father of heart transplantation. I was Lewis's protégé at Northwestern.

Although Lewis suffered no fools, it would be an oversimplification to say that his problems at Northwestern could be explained by his style. The institution was undergoing changes that were epidemic nationwide. Throughout its distinguished history, the clinical faculty of Northwestern had been practitioners who donated their time for the education of students in return for appointments at the "teaching hospitals" where they maintained their practices. Their motives were not necessarily altruistic.

An appointment at these hospitals (Passavant and Wesley in the case of Northwestern) brought prestige and access to a carriage trade of patients through inside referrals. Successful physicians and surgeons had little need for remuneration from the university, and for the most part they did not want it since this would imply an accounting of educational services rendered. These were closed hospitals that rarely allowed admitting privileges to outsiders who had not trained there and "did not know the system."

The volunteer system produced thousands of competent physicians and surgeons through the years, but it had disadvantages which caused its slow abandonment. Out of necessity for economic survival, most clinical faculty members pursued an individual practice as their first priority. Teaching and research occupied what time was left over. Only a few talented and highly motivated members could or would do consistently everything that was expected of them. More and more, universities were turning to full-time teaching faculty whose basic income was assured, and whose primary obligation was the advancement of medical science through research and education. Lewis was the first such appointment in a previously all-volunteer surgery department.

The recruitment of physicians and surgeons for whom the medical school provided a base salary was a policy change that created understandable political problems for the surgery chair, Loyal Davis, who was himself a volunteer. These concerned the extent to which the so-called full-time faculty members, who were viewed by many as tainted from university subsidization, should be encouraged or allowed to compete for private patients who needed conventional medical and surgical care. In defusing the situation, Dr. Davis made clear to Lewis—and to those like me who were answerable to Lewis—the desirability of developing a major and visible program in laboratory investigation. The result was an unparalleled opportunity to begin work in the seemingly esoteric areas that already had occupied my attention and would continue to do so for the rest of my life.

» «

Because Lewis's chest service was light, I began within a few days after my arrival on July 1, 1958, to try to sew in new livers in dogs whose own livers had been completely removed. These experimental operations were all carried out without an assistant at the Veterans Administration (VA) Research Hospital at 303 Huron Street. They were far more difficult and bloody than I had expected, and throughout the summer all the animals died during operation or within one or two days afterward.

Failure of the liver transplant experiments was a serious blow. The move to Chicago seemed more irrational with each passing day. While in Miami, Rebecca Ann, our second child, had arrived (January 1958), and now Barbara was seven months pregnant with our third and last child, Thomas Fitzgerald Starzl. Settling in for another year of hardship, we moved into the Town and Gardens (formerly Marshall Field) Apartments in the heart of the near North Side ghetto. Although I always had been healthy, I began to have bouts of abdominal pain, relieved by antacids. To my chagrin, a small duodenal ulcer was found with an X-ray examination. The antacid Gelucil became a constant and indispensable companion.

I began to suspect that this was what a misspent life looked like. Now thirty-two, I had become a perpetual student. When single, I was able to happily support myself in low style with night jobs, scholarships, and fellowships, depending on hospital support systems for food and simple lodgings. Now, I was an increasingly skilled financial liability, suspiciously viewed as such by part of my own family and that of my wife.

The time had come to stop dreaming and go into private practice. Passing general surgery board examinations was a prerequisite. I obtained these "boards" after taking the Part II oral examination in Philadelphia in August 1958. Even this step seemed symptomatic of the conflict between harsh reality and what I wanted to do. I could not afford to stay at a hotel the night before the examination and slept in a movie theater seat until the closing time at 3 A.M. The rest of the night I spent under a coat on a park bench near the University of Pennsylvania hospital, followed by an emergency shave before arriving for the tests.

Two of the examiners were Charles Kirby, a young thoracic surgeon from the University of Pennsylvania, and James D. Rives from Louisiana State University. Kirby recognized my name from my publications on heart block from Johns Hopkins and spent his examination time discussing this work instead of asking questions. When Kirby died suddenly in January 1964, from a myocardial infarction before he was forty, I felt a deep personal loss because of his kindness during our encounter.

Rives was dogged in his interrogation. I had no idea of the outcome of the all-day ordeal until late in the afternoon. I had gone to an enclosure in the bathroom because of abdominal pain, when Dr. Rives and some of the others came in and continued the discussion of candidates which they had started in their executive session. I realized from their remarks that I had placed first in the group. More than a year later, the acquisition of competency certificates finally came to an end when I also passed the thoracic surgery boards in October 1959.

Passing both of these specialty boards was important, but not a relief for my financial concerns. What I did not understand was that a change in fortune had been engineered by Loyal Davis, the department chair, and by Lewis. Both had become interested in what I was doing in the laboratory, realizing that it was unusual and potentially important. They advised me to apply for grant support from the National Institutes of Health (NIH), the federal agency which had become the chief source of research funds after World War II.

Compared with today, grantsmanship in 1958 was a primitive and ingenuous exercise. I sent a four-page grant application to the NIH requesting funds of about $30,000 a year for five years to support studies on both insulin metabolism and transplantation. All of the request was honored, and the money began to arrive in 1959.

More institutional support was coming. One afternoon in the late summer or early autumn of 1958, Dr. John A. D. Cooper, associate dean of the medical school, came to the laboratory of the VA Research Hospital where I was performing an experimental liver transplantation. He asked me if I wanted to be Northwestern's candidate for a Markle Scholarship. He explained that each medical university in North America could nominate one individual. I was supported by the same dean, Richard Young, who seven years earlier had considered disqualifying me from graduation from medical school (see chapter 3).

From the list of about eighty candidates from Canada and the United States, four or five would be chosen from smaller subgroups of about twenty during three- to four-day retreats in Colorado Springs, Williamsburg, and other similar resort centers—for a total of about twenty-five. The judges at these beauty contests were distinguished jurists, businessmen, educators, and representatives from other professions who were looking for qualities beyond those which could be read in a career summary.

The objective of the scholarships was to induce promising young physicians and basic scientists to stay in medical university work as opposed to more remunerative careers in private practice. Nomination by a university implied a long-term commitment by the sponsoring institution. Reciprocally, a lifetime pledge to university work was asked of the nominee. It was to this end of the bargain that Dr. Cooper directed most of his remarks when he first talked to me. I was expected to outline briefly a focused program of research and development that would have depth and a potential for longevity.

Having an appropriate plan of research was considered critical. It should not be something as trivial as a highly focused proposal that might be completed in two or three years. Equally unacceptable would be something unrealistic or manifestly unattainable. I suspected that liver transplantation might be seen this way because there were no clues about how to effectively control rejection, the mysterious process that destroyed transplanted organs.

My Markle selection group of about twenty candidates convened at the Broadmoor Hotel in Colorado Springs, February 2–5, 1959. On the way, I flew to Sioux City and drove the twenty-five miles to LeMars to talk to my father and obtain his blessing. Although he was still managing the newspaper, his *joie de vivre* had been eroded by his first stroke in 1955, which had left him paralyzed on one side and with a speech defect. He advised me to follow my own path, but he warned me not to aspire to too much. For much of his later life, he was tormented by the slowlyunfolding sad fate of my older brother, John, whose unfulfilled youthful dreams and ambitions led him to a life of reclusive and itinerant misery. I knew that my father's hesitation came more from love than from doubt.

The Markle interviews were an anticlimax. The four selected from our group, including me, fared no better in later years than those passed over, but in my case the purpose of the Markle Scholarship was uniquely served. The academic compass was in place, and I was committed to a lifetime of teaching and research. As it turned out, the subject of liver transplantation hardly came up at the interviews. When it did, I noted with amusement that the committee saw no reason at all why this could not be accomplished. They were far more concerned with our views on literature, music, social issues, and penal reform, and what we thought were the qualifications for leadership.

» «

On July 1, 1959, I became the second full-time member of the Northwestern surgery faculty, preceded only by John Lewis. My rank was associate in surgery with a salary of $12,000 per year including $6,000 provided by the Markle Scholarship. In order to avoid the same political problems encountered by Lewis, Loyal Davis made no arrangements for me to have hospital privileges where I could see private patients. I was a designated "dog surgeon" or "rat doctor."

Now completely free from patient responsibilities for the first time in four and one-half years, I was able to work in the laboratory all day every day. With grant money in hand, it was possible to transfer the projects from the VA laboratory to the more commodious surgical research unit on the fourteenth floor of the university (Montgomery Ward) building at 303 East Chicago Avenue. My office on the seventh floor was next to that of John Lewis, and beyond that was where Loyal Davis carried out his administrative duties.

Also on July 1, 1959, three members were recruited to what now became a liver transplant "team." Two were talented senior medical students named Robert Lazarus and Robert Johnson. The third and most important was Harry A. Kaupp, Jr., one of two third-year surgical residents who had been assigned by Lewis and Davis to a "lab year." My project and a second one directed by an established private surgeon each would have the services of a resident. Neither of the available residents was particularly anxious to join me on my first day as a junior faculty member. The choice was made by a coin flip. When Harry Kaupp lost, I gained a great friend and tireless worker. Within a few weeks, he and I were able to have dogs live through the operation of liver transplantation (liver replacement) on a regular basis.

The secrets were simple. First, we learned how to preserve the transplanted liver during its removal and while it was being sewed into the recipient. It was common knowledge that refrigeration was a means of preservation, although this usually was of food, not tissue grafts. At first, cooling the livers was accomplished by immersing the anesthetized donor dog in an ice bath, just as John Lewis prepared his patients for open heart operations. We soon learned that the liver could be cooled most easily by running a cold, salt water solution into it through its portal vein while the rest of its blood supply was interrupted. The same method, with very little change except for the solution used, is used today to preserve the human livers given to patients. The dog livers removed under these conditions and kept cold could be expected to function if they were sewed in within two hours.

The second key principle was to maintain the recipient's blood circulation in as normal a state as possible while the dog's own liver was being removed and while the new liver was being sewed in. During this period, it is necessary to temporarily clamp the two great veins (portal vein and inferior vena cava) that carry blood coming back to the heart (via the liver) from all of the body below the chest. In dogs, the effect of simultaneously obstructing the portal vein and inferior vena cava is devastating and usually leads to death within a few minutes or hours. With each beat of the heart, the organs of the lower half of the body become more stuffed with blood that continues to be pumped in but has no way to get back to the starting point.

We solved the problem of vein blockage by using plastic bypass tubes which we inserted into these two venous systems below the obstruction sites, took outside the body, and reinserted into one of the large veins in the neck. Envision a siphon from an overloaded gasoline tank to an empty one which feeds the same engine (the heart) and you will have a reasonable idea of what was done.[1]

Once we had standardized a system to siphon blood from the lower to the upper part of the body during the period of great vein obstruction, the operation became a more reasonable one. It still was necessary to reconnect the main blood vessels supplying the transplanted liver and to reconstruct the duct that takes away its excreted bile. These were sophisticated steps, but they were potentially within the grasp of trained surgeons.

After the operation, the dogs usually were normal for almost a week before they began to reject their livers. By the end of the summer of 1959, we were confident that this operation was not only feasible, but could someday be applied for the treatment of human disease. Armed with this conviction, Harry Kaupp and I left by car in the last week of September for the annual convention of the American College of Surgeons in Atlantic City.

» «

On the way east, we made a side trip to Morgantown, West Virginia. Dr. Kenneth Penrod and Dr. Calvin Sleeth, the founding vice-president and dean respectively of the new University of West Virginia Medical School, had invited me to visit their campus, which still was under construction. They were looking for junior faculty officers, and I believe that I was known to one of them who had been in Gainesville when I visited there from Miami two years earlier.

My career summary was unimpressive. In spite of this and although I was only two months out of my surgical training, I announced to Penrod and Sleeth that my interest was only in being the chair of the department. Nothing less would do. I am still embarrassed by this, but the surprising outcome several months later was that both men came to Chicago and spent a day and an evening with me and Barbara. I suspect that they were morbidly curious about my boldness.

We were too short of money to dine out or even to afford a main course item at home. We ate a rabbit that paid the supreme price after being smuggled out of the lab. The interlude with Penrod and Sleeth was pleasant, but in the following March, the chair was offered to Bernard Zimmerman of the University of Minnesota, who accepted. I was left with nostalgia about the beautiful lights on the suspension bridge over the Monongahela River, the coal jewelry which was being sold in the Morgantown trinket shops, and the lost chance to live in a small town.

After our visit to Morgantown, Kaupp and I continued on to Atlantic City. One of the two reasons for this long trip was to comment on a paper about liver transplantation in dogs which was scheduled to be given by a member of the Peter Bent Brigham Hospital surgery team headed by Francis D. Moore. While I was still at the Chicago VA Hospital, I had heard of the Boston efforts from Fred Preston, the chief of surgery there. Kaupp and I were anxious not only to learn what they were doing in Boston but to announce what we had achieved to what we envisioned wouldbe a large and appreciative audience. Our grandiose expectations were not met.

The anticipated amphitheater was more like a small classroom. Furthermore, it was not full. Two or three dozen restless or bored people seemed more interested in moving on to the next presentation than in hearing the liver transplant paper. The Brigham group had started on their project at the same time as I had, in the summer of 1958. They had encountered similar problems, including a high failure rate during operation, and they had arrived at the same general conclusions as we had. After their formal talk, I gave a discussion which I remember as faltering because of my inexperience in public speaking. The unexpectedly long survival of one of our animals was the main point and was undoubtedly overdone in the tradition of surgical braggadocio that characterizes our specialty. If this evoked as much as a stifled yawn, I did not see it. Neither the Boston manuscript nor my discussion of it was published.

The Atlantic City meeting could have distorted a reasonable person's sense of proportion. A second reason for going was to show a movie for an evening session called the Symposium on Spectacular Problems in Surgery. About one year earlier, while doing the fellowship in chest surgery, I had seen an elderly patient at the VA Hospital with an obstruction of the large blood vessel (abdominal aorta) that carries all of the blood being pumped down from the heart to the lower trunk and legs. Like a long cork, a hardened cylinder of clot and connective tissue occupied the channel through which the blood normally passes, and this extended like a giant inverted Y down into both groins. Going upward, portions of this corklike material passed out into the arteries supplying both kidneys, all of the bowel, and the stomach, pancreas, and liver. At a fourteen-hour operation, I removed the corklike material from the aorta and its many involved branches and restored a normal blood supply to the legs and each of the organs.

An Austrian photographer named Fred Hartman, who was head of the VA Medical Art and Photography Department, made a movie of the long operating room siege and edited it down to ten or twelve minutes. This was one of the most complex vascular (blood vessel) reconstructions that had ever been done, and even in 1991 it would rank high on such a list.[2] The Spectacular Problems in Surgery Symposium was a very popular event at these yearly meetings, and in preparation I memorized my narration, which I delivered live from the podium. Several thousand people were in the packed audience. The movie was a smash hit and made such a strong impression that I still am asked about it from time to time by people who were there.

Yet, I knew that this was an inherently inconsequential contribution, and that its meaning was trivial when compared to the paper and discussion on liver transplantation which almost no one had heard.

7

Substance or Stunts?

The work on liver transplantation by the Northwestern and Harvard teams resurfaced at the annual meeting of the American Surgical Association (ASA), held at White Sulphur Springs, West Virginia, on April 5, 1960. The ASA is not the oldest learned surgical society in America, but it is the most prestigious. Those who cannot gain membership call it the most pretentious. How precious admission to the inner circle is can be surmised by the active membership ceiling of 350 for the North American continent. All of the surgeons whom I have mentioned in this book already were members in 1960 or were soon to be, with the exception of John Farrell. I was an invited guest of Loyal Davis's.

Only thirty to thirty-five papers are selected for presentation at the annual meetings from a submitted list many times this large. Usually, the selections represent a field (or subject) that is well worked out, or ready to be brought into more general use. Transplantation has been an exception over the last two decades in that many of the steps in this discipline became well known for the first time at the ASA annual meetings long before they were ready for use in humans or even considered for it. So it was with liver transplantation and the presentation of the animal studies using this procedure.

The Boston results were given in 1960 by the Harvard team leader, Francis D. Moore, and published the following autumn in the *Annals of Surgery*. I discussed Moore's paper, based on our own investigations which were published at the same time as Moore's but in *Surgery, Gynecology, and Obstetrics*, the equally prestigious journal of the American College of Surgeons.[1]

The spotlight was on Moore this day. In 1960 and at all subsequent times, Franny Moore was a figure of remarkable grace whose knowledge of surgery and biology was so overwhelming as to intimidate anyone who disagreed with him or even appeared on the same platform. In 1948, at the age of thirty-four, he had moved from the nearby Massachusetts General Hospital to become the Moseley Professor of Surgery at Harvard and surgeon-in-chief at the Peter Bent Brigham Hospital, Boston. During the nine preceding years, Moore had advanced from his graduation at Harvard Medical College through an internship, residency, and staff position at the Massachusetts General Hospital. At the Brigham, he became the successor to Elliot Cutler, a pioneer heart surgeon, who in turn had succeeded Harvey Cushing, the father of neurosurgery.

It was not usual forty-three years ago for a surgeon who had strong links with one of these Harvard hospitals to assume a leadership position at the other. Although both were minions of the Harvard medical school system, these hospitals had their separate heritage, governance, and autonomy. They competed for resources, and most of all, they competed for glory. Those who trained at the Massachusetts General Hospital prided themselves above all on their ability to care for patients at the very highest level of surgical operating room competence. The image they projected was in part a product of the large size of the hospital (nearly 1,000 beds), the volume and variety of the patients seen there, and its long and distinguished history. In contrast, the smaller Brigham (284 beds) was only thirty-five years old when Moore arrived in 1948, its founding surgical chair having been Harvey Cushing. Those who worked there in surgery were scholars who with justification saw themselves as working beyond the envelope of conventional care.

Moore, the crossover, was a wunderkind, a phenomenon. He occupied his two new positions for the next twenty-eight years. His accomplishments in science and surgery mushroomed on such a grand scale that they could be imagined to be fictional were they not so easily verifiable. He presided over the early trials of kidney transplantation at the Brigham while abstaining from authorship on any of these reports. He was best known for his studies of body water and mineral composition as these were affected by injuries, operations, and diseases. This was his greatest legacy, one that already has influenced the practice of surgeons by the tens of thousands.

Moore's contributions to liver transplantation were made over a six-year period. His early investigations in dogs began in July 1958 when he was forty-five years old, and now, in 1960, he was reporting on thirty-one liver transplant experiments. Seven of these animals lived for more than four days, with a maximum of twelve days before death from rejection. From these seven animals he had pieced together a very complete picture of the postoperative course after liver replacement in the dog. There was no attempt to prevent rejection because the means were not yet available.

The first person to discuss Moore's paper was Stephen E. Hedberg, one of Moore's Brigham protégés who was serving his military obligation at the Walter Reed Hospital in Washington. Hedberg's comments were not directly relevant to the liver, but they stand out in my mind because I came to know him later under other circumstances. He returned to Harvard and became a well-respected liver surgeon at the Massachusetts General Hospital with special expertise in a technique for preventing or stopping the bleeding from the enlarged and thin-walled veins in the esophagus of patients with serious liver disease (see chapter 5). The method consisted of looking down the esophagus with a hollow tube which had a light at the end, finding the bleeding vein, and injecting it through a long needle with an irritating fluid that caused the vessel to shrivel up.

Years later, one of Hedberg's patients, who had liver disease caused by a virus, vomited blood on him, infecting him with the same disease and eventually causing the same complication of esophageal bleeding. He told me of this in a quiet and earnest conversation which we had in the spring of 1984 after a surgical conference in Miami where we had served together on the same program. He said that he was going to need a liver transplant before long. He wanted to put this off to make some personal arrangements. A short time later, one of his friends called to tell me that he had deteriorated rather suddenly and died.

My discussion of Moore's paper came next. What I said reflected my respect for the always gracious Dr. Moore and nervousness at saying anything at a meeting of such importance and formality. My approach had been and would continue to be strongly influenced by my original interest in the effect of portal blood (and insulin) on the liver. In more than eighty transplant experiments, I had systematically tested different ways of restoring the transplanted liver's blood supply. We showed that livers which were given a normal portal venous inflow performed better than those which were not. But the important achievement for the moment was that we had eighteen dogs with survival greater than four days, with one animal living for twenty and one-half days. I realized that we were ahead of the Boston team.

Before the 1960 ASA meeting, I had met very few of the celebrated surgeons whose names were familiar because of their professional contributions and writings. After three days, and the exposure caused by my discussion, I was no longer anonymous. In the lobby of the Greenbrier Hotel, two friendly young men whose faces I recognized introduced themselves. One was David Hume, a former Harvard surgeon who now was in Richmond. With him was Richard Egdahl, also of Richmond but in later years to be the surgical chair, dean of medicine, and director of the Boston University Medical Center. With them was one of their friends, John Mannick, who would soon join Hume in Richmond and much later (1978) succeed Franny Moore as surgeon-in-chief at the Brigham. In 1989, Mannick was elected president of the American Surgical Association.

They expressed interest in my work, but what they may not have appreciated was that I was far more intrigued with theirs. Just before Moore's presentation, Hume, Egdahl, a third surgeon named Charles Zukoski, and three other colleagues had given a paper on kidney transplantation in dogs.[2] Their work provided a remarkable insight into the difficulties to be overcome if any whole organ transplantation procedure was to have clinical value. Hume had tried to prevent kidney rejection by damaging the immune system of the recipient with X-rays.

The injury caused by exposure to X-rays had been known for more than a half century. A wealth of detailed research had been stimulated by the atomic bombings at Hiroshima and Nagasaki, which had left thousands of immunologically crippled victims. Their exposure to irradiation had stripped away their natural defenses against germs in the environment and had exposed them to the additional threat of cancer caused by tissue damage from the X-rays. Many of the survivors died later of infections and malignant tumors, in much the same way as after the Chernobyl incident in the USSR. This was a new field with many pathways, one of which had been identified as early as 1953 to lead potentially to transplantation. As it turned out, this was a blind alley, and it seemed to me that Hume's paper (which Moore discussed) had shown this.

When Hume's dogs were given more than 1,000 rads (the units of X-ray therapy) to the body, rejection of the kidneys could be prevented, but the animals all died of overwhelming infection. With less than this irradiation dose, survival was possible but the grafts were rejected. There was no margin of safety. Their findings did not surprise me. I had already tried to depress the immune system with X-ray therapy before liver transplantation. The results were so poor that a journal could not be found to publish them until two years later.[3] Irradiation of liver grafts had no beneficial effect, and irradiation of the recipient was overtly harmful.

As we continued to talk, Hume told me confidentially that he and two of his coworkers (Charlie Zukoski and H. M. Lee) were experimenting with a new drug called 6-mercaptopurine as a substitute for X-ray therapy. Six weeks earlier they had sent an abstract with their encouraging results to the surgical forum committee of the American College of Surgeons, to be considered for the meeting in San Francisco the following October. This was the first of many phone or personal conversations which I had with Hume, of which the last was at the American Surgical Association meeting at the Century Plaza Hotel, Los Angeles, in April 1973. This was a few weeks before he was killed in the crash of an airplane that he was flying. The thousands who attended his funeral expressed the mass bereavement that is reserved for kings and heroes.

A year after his death, a celebration in his memory was held in Richmond. By this time the apotheosis that follows the loss of great men was nearly complete. Most who spoke of Hume in glowing terms were largely paying tribute to themselves as they recalled warmly their exploits together. No matter, the silhouette was there of a truly remarkable intelligence and personality of which admirers and "friendly enemies" were still wary long after he was gone.

Hume always reminded me of a human buzz saw, constantly advancing but with such precision and beauty of motion that it was a masochistic thrill to realize that the cutting pathway was directed straight to you. When giving a lecture, he spoke rapidly without notes and covered more ground in a few minutes than anyone whom I have met. He was of medium height with a stocky build. Presiding over this marvelous physical apparatus was a handsome, close-cropped head. He had the whitest teeth I have ever seen, which were often displayed because he laughed at the slightest provocation, whether sad or happy. Few people passed through the veneer and were allowed to see behind. His was a strange combination of fire and ice.

Like Franny Moore, who was five years older, Hume had a strong Harvard background, but a discontinuous one. His father was a Canadian university professor (Toronto) and his mother was a concert pianist. He was raised in Muskegon, Michigan, where he was an average student according to Moore's eulogy of 1974, which also mentioned his irresistible attractiveness to women.[4] In spite of an indifferent high school record, he was admitted to the Harvard premedical curriculum and graduated in 1941. He was unable to obtain admission to the Harvard Medical College and went instead to the University of Chicago where he graduated in December 1943. Then he returned to Boston on January 1, 1944, to be trained in surgery at the Peter Bent Brigham Hospital during the next four and one-half years, with six months off for duty in the U.S. Navy.

One of the other four interns beginning at the Brigham with Hume on the bitterly cold day in January 1944 was Joseph E. Murray, whose contributions to kidney transplantation would lead him to Stockholm as the recipient of a Nobel prize in December 1990. From the eulogies given after Hume's death by Murray, John Merrill, J. Hartwell Harrison, and Franny Moore, the interlocking and indispensable roles of Hume and Murray in the early days of the Brigham kidney transplant program could be reconstructed.[5]

Hume was acknowledged by all four to have been the originator, and Harrison, his greatest admirer, called him the "father of renal transplantation." However, his research interests were split between investigations of the nervous system control of hormones and kidney transplantation until he left Harvard in 1956 to become the Stuart McGuire Professor and chair of the Department of Surgery at the Medical College of Virginia (now Virginia Commonwealth University). A second tour of duty in the navy during 1953–55 had precluded his participation in the first identical twin kidney transplantation which was the primary justification for Murray's Nobel prize thirty-six years later. Hume returned to transplantation after he moved to Virginia.

When Franny Moore transferred from the Massachusetts General Hospital in 1948 to take over the surgical leadership of the Brigham, his greatest inherited asset was the young star, David Hume, who also was his most nagging administrative liability. For an outsider to conclude that they did not like each other would belie the substantive support they gave to each other, as well as the flowery verbal bouquets they exchanged publicly, spiced with phrases of gentle faint praise. Of the two, I came to know Hume best, but both men came in and out of my life in the years ahead.

They were both maestros, but their interpretation of the score was different. Each would have to conduct his own symphony. The stage for Moore was already set when he arrived at the prestigious Brigham in 1948, with all the principal transplant players tuning their instruments. For the rest of his career, and long after his retirement, he would extoll and promote the achievements of the group and its individuals, fiercely defending all those who worked at his adopted Harvard hospital to which he gave his ideas and devoted the rest of his life. His heart belonged to all of Harvard, not just one part.

Hume left this place of privilege to go to a barren stage in the south where he overcame the resistance to his Yankee ways, piece by piece created his own ensemble, and captured his new city of Richmond. Both men far exceeded reasonable expectations and became legends.

» «

Six months after our encounters in April 1960, Moore, Hume, and I met again in San Francisco. I already had gone beyond simple liver transplantation and was scheduled to give a paper at the same surgical forum where the 6-mercaptopurine referred to by Hume was to be discussed. With our new operation, other organs were transplanted with the liver.[6] Instead of facing its new recipient environment alone, the liver was accompanied by the stomach, intestines, and pancreas of the donor. These were all organs whose blood outflow emptied into the portal vein before the portal vein passed through and nourished the liver. Thus, the transplanted liver could bring with it its own supply of insulin, food, and the other substances which are important for its health and which a few years hence would be called "hepatotrophic factors." The procedure was called "multivisceral" (many organs) transplantation.

Like the simpler operation of liver transplantation, there was no apparent clinical application of multivisceral transplantation since rejection could not be prevented. However, I had two objectives. One was to see if the liver as a component of this huge multiple organ graft would be rejected with the same intensity and speed as we already had established with the liver alone. Only five animals survived the difficult operation, but in each one, it looked as if rejection of the individual organs was less than would be expected if the organs had been transplanted by themselves.

Because the large grafts contained lymph nodes, spleen, and other elements which are part of the normal immune system, the second question was whether the multivisceral graft would "turn the tables" and try to reject the host. The answer was yes. Donald Brock, a young staff pathologist at the Chicago VA Hospital, found cells throughout the recipient dog's own tissues which he thought from their appearance (but could not prove) had come out of the graft with harmful intentions. For example, there was evidence under the microscope that the recipients' own lungs were being damaged by this counterattack by cells from the multivisceral graft. It would be another thirteen years before the extent of this problem, called "graft versus host disease" (GVHD), would be worked out in rats by the Massachusetts General Hospital surgeons G. J. Monchik and Paul Russell.

Because the work had been completed the preceding April, my interest in the multivisceral project was growing cold by the time of my presentation on October 12, 1960. It was put into the deep freeze by the discussion that followed. William P. Longmire of UCLA deflated any illusions I might have had about the importance of the contribution. He asked wryly if, rather than performing this complex operation, it might be easier to simply anesthetize the dog and have a laboratory assistant carry the animal from one table to another. The ripple of laughter from the audience completed my humiliation. Longmire had been one of the early workers in transplantation, and he was one of the most respected. He was implying what I already knew, that any such research was merely a technical exercise so long as we had no means of controlling rejection.

As far as I was concerned, X-ray therapy as an antirejection measure never would be practical. The faint hope that remained was the 6-mercaptopurine treatment which was described by Charlie Zukoski (with Hume) as weakening and delaying rejection.[7] Zukoski's results, along with those from skin graft experiments in rats and the independent observations by a young English surgeon named Roy Calne in dogs undergoing kidney transplantation provided hope where there had been none before.[8] However, the hope was dim because only a small minority of the dog kidney recipients could be kept alive for as long as one month, and none had truly long survival.

The early and late deaths of these animals either were caused by too little treatment, which allowed rejection to break through, or too much drug treatment, which caused fatal infections. In principle, the dilemma was similar to X-ray therapy, although the possibility remained of a narrow margin of therapeutic safety. It was also obvious that liver transplantation was much too complicated an operation to use for studies of immunosuppression. The road to the liver would have to lead through the kidney.

Knowing that Joe Murray's Brigham research team was interested in antirejection drugs in Franny Moore's surgical laboratory, I approached Moore as we walked down the street after one of the forum sessions. I asked him if he could accept me for a research fellowship in Boston, effective immediately if possible. The fact that I was a Markle Scholar gave me a small financial hedge since these funds ($6,000 a year for five years) could be transferred between universities. I had not discussed the matter with anyone, not even my wife or Loyal Davis, because leaving Northwestern had not occurred to me until that day.

I can remember how firm Moore was, but also how kind, as he denied my request. I know that Moore remembers the incident because two or three years later he told Bill Waddell, my new chair at the University of Colorado, about it and added that my move from Chicago to Denver had been one of the more successful transplantations in history up to the present time. I became (and still am) indebted to Moore for his decision which, because it was negative, moved me onto an entirely new level of development and responsibility.

Fourteen months later, I left Chicago to be an associate professor of surgery at Colorado. On March 27, 1962, three months after arriving, I performed the first human kidney transplantation at Denver on a patient who is still alive twenty-nine years later. Eleven months after that, on March 1, 1963, we made the first attempt at human liver replacement. As I had thought in San Francisco, the road to the liver would lead through the kidney, but I would have to find a pathway myself by becoming involved in the renal field.

» «

Deciding to leave Chicago in the space of a day in San Francisco was easier than actually doing it. I had no place to go nor any prospects because I had not been planning to go. For most of the first year after joining the faculty in July 1959, I had done no clinical work, and only recently had I been given attending surgeon duties on Charity Ward 56 at the Cook County Hospital. For the political reasons described in chapter 6, Loyal Davis did not want me to compete for private patients at the fashionable near North Side hospitals, Passavant and Wesley. I could not admit patients to these hospitals except on Davis's neurosurgical service, which was an inappropriate location for them.

I had moved our family from our ghetto flat to a large apartment at 3220 North Sheridan Road in a respectable neighborhood near

Lincoln Park and close to Lake Michigan. However, with a low fixed income and no means of supplementing it from practice, we were falling farther into debt. Worse yet, my clinical skills were being eroded slowly by disuse. The daily operations in the laboratory could not substitute for contact with patients.

Beginning a few months before the San Francisco meeting, I found an alternative solution at the Lutheran Deaconess Hospital, a small and very old hospital run by sisters of a Lutheran religious order at 1138 North Leavitt Street. It was two miles from where we lived. As so often happens, the solution became worse than the problem. My private practice grew uncontrollably as soon as it became known that I would take difficult or unusual cases. Most of the patients were referred from other surgeons who either had created complications already or foresaw them. Most of the surgery at first was in the abdomen, but soon I developed referrals for lung or esophageal surgery to this hospital—which never previously had accommodated chest cases. More organization was necessary, at first to make special care possible and later to make it efficient. I had no office hours and only saw patients who were in the hospital or who were visiting the offices of other physicians or surgeons where I also could provide follow-up care.

Life had become a round-the-clock nightmare. I made a special arrangement with the Lutheran sisters that allowed me to operate early in the morning beginning at 6:00 or 6:30 A.M., complete a major case, and arrive in the experimental laboratory at Northwestern University or on the clinical ward at the Cook County Hospital by 9:00 or 10:00 in the morning. Work there usually lasted long past dinner time so that evening rounds or examination of patients to be operated on the following day put off returning home even more. Knowing that fatigue was my enemy, I learned to fall asleep in strange places by closing my eyes tightly and imagining a tapestry of bright colors or a maze of glittering lights. When these began to turn and spin, sleep was close behind. It was like self-hypnosis. I was always wide awake or sound asleep, never in between.

The final blow came in late 1960 when a decision was made to close the Lutheran Deaconess Hospital and to slowly transfer its

functions to the new Lutheran General Hospital in the suburb of
Park Ridge, about twenty miles away. Now, to fulfill my patient
and research commitments, I left home at 4 A.M., drove one
hundred or more miles a day, and on lucky days returned home in
time to hear the Star Spangled Banner at 2 A.M. after the last
television movie finished. I already had used up thirty-five years
and did not see how I could make it to forty. By becoming a
commercial surgeon, I had freed myself from debt for the first time
in more than ten years. But the time and energy to accomplish this
had been stolen from the research program which was the justification in my mind for being in university life.

Eventually, a way off the treadmill was found for me by a surgeon
named Ben Eiseman who was the founding chair of the Department
of Surgery at the new medical school of the University of Kentucky,
which enrolled its first class in 1960. Before going to Lexington,
Eiseman had been professor of surgery at the University of Colorado and chief of surgery at the Denver VA Hospital. By his efforts,
he had made this hospital one of the crown jewels of the VA system
and a professional touchstone for many young academic surgeons.
The United States as well as foreign countries are dotted with
surgical professors who came there, spent their time with Eiseman,
and passed on. The direction almost always was up.

Besides being multitalented, with harmless passions for skiing,
mountain climbing, and military affairs (he is an admiral), Eiseman
was a talent scout. He made it his business to know who was
available in university surgery, why they wanted to move, and what
were their strengths and weaknesses. I learned of him first through
the surgical literature when I published a research report with
conclusions opposite to those which he had reached. Instead of
being angry, he wrote me a courteous letter asking for more
information.

Later, I met him. When he found that I wanted to move, he
invited me to come to Kentucky and join a young faculty roster that
was packed with talent. I agreed, but the appointment was effectively blocked by my earlier chair at Miami, John Farrell. Farrell
had previously served an internship at the St. Joseph's Hospital in
Lexington. During that time he had made friends with a local

neurosurgeon who had risen to be a member of the board of trustees at the university. What conversation transpired between Farrell and this trustee I do not know, but the result was opposition to my appointment.

Shortly thereafter, Eiseman was passing through Denver on a ski trip and met William R. Waddell, who had recently been recruited from the Massachusetts General Hospital to be the new chair of surgery at the University of Colorado Medical School. Waddell asked Eiseman who he thought would be a good candidate to take over the position as director of surgery at the Denver VA Hospital, the position that Eiseman had vacated to go to Kentucky. Eiseman recommended me. Before long, Waddell called me and arranged for an interview in Chicago.

If fate had been cruelly capricious until this time, it now made amends. The brilliant roster of surgeons gathered in Kentucky did not stay. Besieged with administrative problems, Ben Eiseman would return to the University of Colorado in 1966 to serve under Waddell's chairmanship and later mine. It is doubtful that the transplantation program that evolved almost overnight in Denver could have survived or even have been started in the smaller Kentucky school, which was undergoing its own particular brand of birth pangs. Ben Eiseman still has an I.O.U. out on me for putting me together with Bill Waddell.

8

The Rocky Mountains

By moving west from Boston, Bill Waddell was coming back toward his desert roots, a process that he completed when he retired from the University of Colorado in 1982 and moved to Silver City, New Mexico. Now seventy-two years old, he still sees patients. Once a week, he drives 200 miles to Tucson where he teaches medical students and residents at the University of Arizona. They see in him the wisdom of the ages. I met him there in January 1991. Like a piece of fine leather, he looked the same as thirty years before. His life is peaceful now, and he reflected back with modest pride. What he had done was no less than the friends of his young days, Franny Moore and Dave Hume.

The tranquility was hard earned. Like Hume in Richmond, Waddell found chaos when he arrived in Denver in the summer of 1961. In the 1950s, the Department of Surgery had been one of the most honored and productive in the country under the guidance of Henry Swan, a world leader in cardiac surgery, and Ben Eiseman, his VA chief. Now there was scorched earth. Swan had been deposed when he was in his early fifties and Eiseman had gone to Kentucky. The preeminence in heart surgery which Colorado had enjoyed for almost a decade was lost overnight. Worse yet, the machinery to train students and surgeons was teetering. Local critics of the university were fond of saying that the Department of Surgery had a hidden self-destruct button which activated every ten years or so, forcing a new start to be made, or allowing one, depending on the point of view.

The location of the button did not seem particularly mysterious to me. In principle, the problem was a variation of the one faced by Northwestern (see chapter 6), and for that matter by all medical universities of the time. This was the change from a trade-school approach to medical education, in which practicing community physicians volunteered their time, to a full-time plan with salaried faculty. Under the volunteer system, the non-paid faculty occupied the highest titular ranks and dominated the administrative policies of the teaching hospitals.

The educational hub of the University of Colorado School of Medicine was the Colorado General Hospital, located across the street from my headquarters at the VA. I worked at both places. A third institution, the Denver General Hospital, one and one-half miles to the west, had severed its historically important connection to the university during the kind of transition from a volunteer to a full-time salaried faculty that had torn Northwestern apart. The only differences were that Colorado was farther along and the wounds were deeper.

The implementor of the change was an outstanding dean (and later vice-president) named Robert J. Glaser who sincerely believed in the full-time system. Between 1955 and 1962, he recruited a new crop of young clinical chairmen (there were almost no women to be seen) from other universities. They took over from the town physicians and surgeons who had walked the corridors and filled the operating rooms of Colorado General Hospital since the founding of the school in the middle of the nineteenth century. Much of the other previous community support was withdrawn, not without bitterness, and a classical "town-gown war" ensued. Those already there in the old system, of whom Swan was one, could elect to become full time. Swan did so, but did not fit in with the new arrivals. As it existed when Waddell arrived in July 1961, followed by me in December, the Colorado medical school was the purest example of the full-time system in the United States.

The school was fiscally underprivileged. My appointment was "free" since my $18,000 salary was covered by a seven-eighths appointment at the VA Hospital plus most of the $6,000 per year Markle stipend which I brought with me. University policy did not allow faculty appointees to supplement their incomes from private practice. All such monies went into a dean's fund over which the department and its chair had no control and very little influence.

This administrative arrangement was essential for the school's survival. The reason was that the expenses of medical education, like those of health care itself, were skyrocketing with the postwar explosion in medical science. Income was needed to maintain the schools, and the single best source was the money from fees generated by the clinical faculty. It became more and more important for this money to come back into a central reservoir or dean's fund, which later would be called by its critics a "hog trough." From this reservoir, salaries were paid to those who contributed and to those who did not. Some of the race horses in the money-generating clinical disciplines quickly complained that they were being used as drays to pull the economic milk wagon.

The full-time system was an ideal way to support the basic scientists who could not practice medicine. The disadvantage was that it spawned a growing clinical faculty, some of whose members had no incentive to see patients in preference to pursuing career-advancing research or even a nonindustrious personal life style. This practical reality now created new pressures within the university. One way to activate the loafers was to re-create private practice incentives within the walls of the university itself. Eventually, intramural political struggles over the extent of these incentive plans, control of the dean's fund, and disposition of other economic resources wracked the University of Colorado and ruined the soil from which grew the transplant and other creative efforts of the 1960s. Fortunately, there was a golden period before this occurred.

The curious thing was that Bill Waddell did not believe in the strict full-time system. He came from a remunerative practice at the Massachusetts General Hospital, and just as I did, he accepted a large reduction in personal income from private practice in order to come to Colorado. He had promised his friend, Dean Bob Glaser, that he would not try to overturn the full-time system, and he kept his word long after they had grown apart. Waddell kept his disapprobation to himself, except to ask me to support him when there were intradepartmental revolts, which I did.

Later, I maintained departmental discipline while I was chair and he helped me. When cynical half-way reforms were imposed by economic necessity as a university policy in the late 1970s, it was one of the reasons that I left after nineteen years, but not the main one. Embittered by what he believed to have been bondage to an administrative system in which he did not believe, Waddell went home to New Mexico not long after I left for Pittsburgh in 1980. It was like the parting of brothers.

It is not for me to say why anyone might seek, or even accept reluctantly, an administrative position which requires decisions that can control or distort the lives of others. If I interview someone for such a post, I make two inquiries. One question is if the candidate has an important concept to be advanced or sustained. People who have an intellectual objective dream large and build castles. The second question concerns the candidate's preoccupation with the details of administrative control which he or she might acquire. Those who are morbidly concerned about such matters will defend castles and try to conquer more instead of building new ones because their instinct is the acquisition of power, not the promotion of ideas. Waddell was a pure example of the first category. He came to Colorado to teach and do research and probably did not even read the fine print about what tools he would have to do this.

» «

Neither did I. Beginning in December 1961, my principal administrative position in Denver was chief of surgery at the Denver VA Hospital. Because of its teaching activities, this hospital was crucial to the educational vitality of the school. When Bill Waddell came to Chicago to interview me, we had none of the discussions about salary, space, rank, fringe benefits, and other issues which today tend to sour relationships before the first day on the job. There were no requirements to see private patients nor any incentive plan to induce private practice activity. I never signed a contract during my nineteen years in Colorado, including the last eight years when I was the surgical chair. We bought a house one mile from the hospital for $32,000. It would be a perfect environment for work.

Waddell wanted transplantation to be the imprint of his new

department. Our mutual goal, and especially mine, was to bring liver transplantation to clinical use. However, we agreed that nothing like this could be tried until kidney transplantation was made to work. Waddell knew my opinion, and agreed with it, that an attempt to prevent rejection with any single agent or drug would do no more than add to the dismal record of repetitive failure which had been compiled to date in kidney trials elsewhere.

As a first step to the development of a clinical transplant program, I set out to relocate the Northwestern transplant laboratory to the Denver VA animal facility, which was essentially unused following the mass exodus of the surgical faculty the preceding year. The efforts were hampered by seizure of these laboratories by investigators from the Department of Medicine. Nothing was left for us except a small operating room with a kennel across the hall that could accommodate thirty or forty dogs.

What we aspired to seemed at first like lunacy to some of the people from the existing Colorado faculty whom we recruited to the transplant team in January 1962. Waddell had no experience in transplantation, but his long stay in Boston had exposed him to the much publicized kidney transplants at the Peter Bent Brigham Hospital. More than his critics, he realized how little actually had been accomplished elsewhere that would sustain any hope of achieving our objectives. The prospects in the field were largely illusory, based to an extraordinary extent on an operation at the Brigham, two days before Christmas, 1954, when Joseph Murray first transplanted a kidney from an identical twin donor.

This was the first example of successful transplantation of a vital whole organ, and it led to Murray's selection for the Nobel prize in 1990. However, this success depended on the perfect tissue match that can be obtained only with identical twins. Under these circumstances, rejection does not occur. Further progress in all other situations would require effectively weakening the recipient's immune system in treatment that is called "immunosuppression."

If a single figure were to be identified as the genesis of the concept of immunosuppression for purposes of transplantation, there could be no other candidate than Sir Peter Medawar, the English immunologist. Medawar's appreciation in 1944 and 1945 that rejection was an immune reaction—following recognition by the immune system that a graft is "foreign" and must be destroyed—made inevitable almost all the research done later. If rejection was an immune event, what could be more logical than to try to protect grafts by altering the immune system? By 1951, Medawar's group showed that natural hormones of the adrenal gland or synthetic chemicals with the same action (often referred to as corticosteroids or steroids) weakened immunologic defenses and delayed skin graft rejection in animals.

Total body X-ray was another way of weakening the immune system of a kidney recipient. On January 24, 1959, Murray and his associates at the Brigham broke through the immune barrier for the first time in humans when they successfully transplanted a kidney from a fraternal (nonidentical) twin to his irradiated brother. Five months later, the feat was duplicated by the Paris team of Jean Hamburger. Both of these patients lived for twenty-six years.

Thus, by the end of 1959, kidney transplantation had gone beyond identical twin transplantation, but only to the level of the fraternal twin. Using recipient irradiation, eleven attempts in Boston to use donors other than fraternal twins resulted in death of the recipients within zero to twenty-eight days—in two cases before transplantation could be done. In all eleven, infection played an overwhelming role in the fatal outcome.

Across the Atlantic during 1960 and 1961, more encouraging results using irradiation were reported by two groups in Paris, one led by Jean Hamburger, the physician who had participated in the first kidney transplantation from a living related donor nearly a decade earlier. Hamburger's team had prolonged survival of two of five recipients of kidneys from blood relatives (one a first cousin) more distant than fraternal twins. The kidney from the first cousin functioned for fifteen years, and when it failed, retransplantation was performed with a sister donor. The patient, who was eighteen years old, became first a physician and later a member of the national parliament. Now forty-eight years old, he is the longest living non-identical twin recipient in the world.

In addition to irradiation, Hamburger clearly understood the value of steroids, which he frequently used in his patients although the dosages were not well documented in his reports. In addition, he was systematically attempting for the first time to "tissue match" the donors and recipients. His surgical team had a clear understanding of organ preservation as exemplified by the fact that they cooled the transplants after these kidneys had been removed from the donor and while they were being sutured into the recipient.

During this same period, the other French team, headed by René Küss, also made a supreme contribution. In 1951, Küss had perfected and performed the renal transplant operation which was used subsequently in the historic twin cases in Boston and remains the standard kidney transplant procedure today. Without immunosuppression, all of these early patients died. Then, in 1960 and 1961, Küss performed his operation again in six patients who were treated initially with total body irradiation, followed later with unstipulated amounts of steroids and the new drug 6-mercaptopurine.

Three of Küss's six patients lived for a long time, although they eventually died after five, seventeen, and eighteen months. The two longest survivors were the first in the world to have protracted function of a nonrelated kidney transplant. This was an enormous accomplishment, far superseding anything previously achieved anywhere. Küss had introduced the concept of "cocktail" or multiple agent therapy. His recipient of June 22, 1960, became the first long-surviving transplant recipient to be given 6-mercaptopurine. The use of 6-mercaptopurine was particularly significant because it had become clear that irradiation for transplant purposes was too dangerous to be practical. This drug and its derivative azathioprine were central to the next stage of transplantation. These agents inhibit the metabolism and multiplication of the cells (lymphocytes) responsible for rejection.

» «

The parent 6-mercaptopurine compounds were synthesized in 1952 at the Burroughs Wellcome Company in Tuckahoe, New York, by Dr. George Hitchings and Gertrude Elion (Nobel laureates in 1988). Hitchings and Elion were looking for agents to treat leukemia, the special kind of cancer that affects white blood cells. In 1959, Drs. Robert Schwartz and William Dameshek of Tufts

University, Boston, demonstrated in a nontransplant experiment that 6-mercaptopurine inhibited the normal immune response in rats.

In London on September 7, 1959, the same team reported to the seventh European Congress of Haematology that this drug prolonged skin graft survival in proportion to the dose given. The work was submitted to the *Journal of Clinical Investigation*, but because of a delay in the review process, it was not published until June 1960. In the meanwhile, similar observations in rats were made by the team of Robert Good at the University of Minnesota and reported in December 1959 in a rapid-publication journal. Surgeons were quick to follow these leads by extending the experiments to kidney transplantation in dogs (see chapter 7).

Appreciation of the potential importance of these discoveries was what had prompted my decision to transfer to Colorado. In the meanwhile, Roy Calne had migrated from England to Murray's laboratory at the Peter Bent Brigham Hospital where he worked for fifteen months, beginning in July 1960. Like me, he was seeking a better environment to pursue the research he had started. Calne and Murray were studying azathioprine, a drug derived from 6-mercaptopurine, which still had only the code name BW 57-322. Later, its trade name was Imuran.

By the end of 1961, it was well worked out what 6-mercaptopurine and Imuran could and could not do. These drugs definitely delayed and reduced the rejection of skin or kidney grafts in experimental animals, leading to their systematic evaluation in clinical trials by Murray at the Brigham. However, prolonged survival of the kidney grafts was an uncommon achievement, either in animals or in humans. Of the first ten kidney recipients treated with these drugs at the Peter Bent Brigham Hospital from April 1960 through November 1962, eight died after zero to twenty-eight days, one lived for one hundred sixty days, and one whose transplantation was in April 1962 lived for eighteen months.

The trials were so unsuccessful that it was widely thought that the immunosuppression necessary to prevent rejection would almost always lead to immunologic invalidism and lethal infections. The results were uncomfortably similar to the early ones with total body irradiation. Thus, by the time I arrived in Denver in December 1961, the reason for having made this precipitous move had largely vanished. Transplantation appeared to be going nowhere. Or so it seemed to the pessimists who were in the majority.

Because of this gloomy picture, we did not see how we could hope to proceed with organ transplantation except under the most special circumstances. To avoid a false start, we would follow the tracks of Joe Murray and John Merrill and begin with an identical twin kidney transplant case. On March 27, 1962, at the Denver VA Hospital, our transplantation plans went forward when we performed the kidney transplantation on an identical twin recipient who had been cared for at a private Denver clinic. The attending physician held the patient in Denver until my arrival, instead of sending him to Boston as he originally planned.

Robert Brittain, my chief resident at the VA, did the donor operation under the watchful eye of Bill Waddell. Oliver Stonington, the chief of the Division of Urology, helped drain the connecting tube (ureter) of the kidney to the bladder. I did not have much experience with this part of the operation and had asked him if he would make me his student which he did. Both the donor and recipient teams had practiced the operation many times on cadavers in the morgue, and by the time of its performance there was little reason for anxiety. The result was perfect.

The good news was sent at once to LeMars, Iowa. It was just in time because tragedy was to strike there again. On the way west from Chicago in December 1961, I had seen my father. Except for looking older and more tired, he was much the same as he had been since the stroke of 1955. The one-sided paralysis annoyed him, and he cried easily. Now, on July 23, 1962, he had another stroke which completely paralyzed the other side. When I saw him next, his body was of no more use than an inanimate kitchen bowl containing and nourishing his brain with a blood pump. Except for the bright eyes which filled with tears. I would have to hurry if he was to know the end of *my* story. *His* story also could be told only through me, but that would be a long time in the future. I put the duty off for almost thirty years.

» «

It would have been difficult to find an easier first case, not only because of the identical twin donor, but also because this patient was given his new kidney before the old one had failed completely. This meant that he never needed treatment on the artificial kidney. The artificial kidney, an invention of the Dutch physician, Wilhelm Kolff, had been brought to America in 1949 and developed further at the Peter Bent Brigham Hospital by George Thorn, John Merrill, and Carl Walters. It was used for a long time only to tide patients over during an acute but reversible bout of kidney failure until the kidneys could recover and produce urine again.

In these patients, the surgical crosscuts to insert the plastic tubes from the machine into the blood vessels would start at the wrists, moving upward every few inches until the armpits were reached. When the arms were used up, the crosscuts would start at the feet and move to the groin. Once the leg vessels were exhausted, the string had played out and death would follow. Each crosscut could be used only two or three times. But this changed in 1960 when the University of Washington nephrologist, Belding Scribner, working with a young surgeon named David Dillard, introduced a new technique. By using "Scribner shunts," each crosscut could provide a set of vessels that might be usable three times a week for many months or years.

Blood vessel access for dialysis was not the only problem for patients with kidney failure. In 1961 and 1962, there were very few artificial kidneys available for chronic treatment. The problem was dramatically publicized in *Life* magazine, November 9, 1962, by pictures of a tribunal in Seattle deliberating which six patients among many candidates should be selected for entry into the only artificial kidney unit in the world designed for chronic care.

Joseph Holmes, the chief of nephrology (kidney disease) at the University of Colorado, had the equipment and the skill and experience to use it. He was a true pioneer in the artificial kidney field. Approaching sixty, he became the oldest member of the transplantation team. Chronically fatigued by overwork and lung disease which he "treated" by constantly smoking cigarettes, he fought to treat or hold back the tide of desperate patients who flocked to Colorado General Hospital. Not far behind them came an avalanche of remonstrances from administrators, complaining that his dialysis unit was consuming 10 percent of the entire hospital budget, which was true. Unanswered mail surrounded him in his tiny office as he sat smoking in the middle.

A child named Royal Jones came to see Joe Holmes a few weeks after the public announcement of the identical twin transplantation. It might have been appropriate for Royal to have a less regal name. Instead of power, fate delivered to him a crown of thorns. By the time he was twelve years old he had the marks of crucifixion on his arms and legs, where the cuts for connection to the artificial kidney machine could be seen. As for transplantation, his arrival was too early, because our team was not ready to treat him and would not be for another half year.

Holmes agreed to try to hold him on dialysis, and the countdown began. The sight of this brave and wretched little black boy dragging himself down the hallways of the Colorado General Hospital was enough to mobilize an army, and this was exactly what happened. The VA transplant research laboratory for which we had been slowly acquiring equipment sprang into action. Provisions were made for X-ray therapy, and surgical teams were assembled. Money was released by the VA and funds from the NIH grant that had been transferred from Chicago for liver transplant research were diverted.

Important new laboratory personal were recruited. A gifted technician named Ralph Huntley already had arrived from Marquette University, Milwaukee. In July, he was joined by Paul Taylor, whose contributions continued for the next twenty-nine years. Ruben Brochner, an Argentine neurosurgeon who was waiting for issuance of his Colorado state physician license, and Huntley set up a data system which had safeguards to prevent entry alterations or the unauthorized use of dogs.

The anesthesia machines were refurbished. Because Ben Eiseman had left skilled surgical technicians headed by a well-educated biologist named Fred Stoll, it was possible within a few weeks to perform eight or ten dog kidney transplantations in a day — or twice this number if necessary. A supply of Imuran, which was receiving its first trials at the Peter Bent Brigham Hospital, was obtained from George Hitchings of the Burroughs Wellcome pharmaceutical company.

Royal's mother was going to be his donor. Our dilemma was deciding how to treat him. We wanted particularly to see if total body X-ray therapy could be improved in view of the promising human results reported by the French teams of René Küss and Jean Hamburger. However, a disquieting effect was seen in dogs that received total body irradiation at the same levels planned for Royal Jones. Many of the transplanted kidneys quickly became enormously swollen and cyanotic (blue), seemingly worse than in untreated animals. Only an occasional animal had prolonged survival.

The best results were with Imuran. Some of these dog recipients lived on for years, long after discontinuance of the therapy. It was shown in these animals that steroid (prednisone) therapy could reverse rejection but caused death from its own side effects, of which ulceration and bleeding from the stomach and intestine were the most common. By the end of the 1962 summer we had concluded that survival for one hundred days after kidney transplantation could be achieved in no more than one of four mongrel dogs. There had been no time to test all the treatment combinations.

What to do with this incomplete information was the perplexing question. To abandon Royal was unthinkable in view of the deep commitment already made to him and his mother. We did not believe he could live much longer the way he was; dialysis was becoming more difficult daily. The possibility of failure and discreditation of the university, the program, and individuals of the transplantation team did not weigh heavily enough for anyone in the group to mention it.

The transplantation went forward on November 24, 1962, with combination treatment by irradiation, Imuran, and prednisone. To protect Royal from infection, he was kept in one of the Colorado General Hospital operating rooms for a month afterward. A few weeks following this, he returned to school. The transplant lasted until 1968 and then was replaced with a second one. Years later, the second graft also failed. Royal is still alive and awaiting his third kidney nearly thirty years after the original operation. The grandeur of his name did not bring him a royal kingdom, but it was better than no kingdom at all.

The success could have been a fluke. Within the next twelve weeks, three more kidney transplantations were performed. Two of these patients also still are alive, both with their original transplant from a brother or sister. The third patient died of an infection 113 days after receipt of an "unrelated kidney" donated by his wife. After the transplantation, he formed a large blood clot in one of his leg veins that migrated to his lungs, where it blocked the passage of blood through the heart. At an emergency operation, the clot was removed through a chest incision by Thomas Marchioro, the assistant chief of surgery at the VA Hospital. The patient never fully recovered but his new kidney functioned well until the end.

Using the drug combination of Imuran and prednisone, the first barrier had been passed with unexpected ease. This was an enormous achievement and a vital step in making kidney transplantation a practical means of treating patients. However, an even more significant consequence for us was that the stage was set for liver transplantation. It never would go this smoothly again.

9

The Failed Liver
Transplant Trials

Bennie Solis was a tiny spot in the universe, and a flawed one at that. The son of poor Spanish American parents, he was born with biliary atresia, a condition for which there was no medical or surgical treatment, nor any hope of divine intervention. His liver was incomplete. Its cells still could fulfil their sophisticated duties to the rest of the body, such as building and breaking down proteins, sugars, and fats. But his liver lacked the tubular duct system that normally collects the bile produced by the liver as part of its function of eliminating the body's waste products.

These ducts begin as tiny structures deep within the liver and join with other ducts as they work their way out. By the time the ducts reach the outside and can be seen at the undersurface of the liver, they have coalesced into a single structure called the common duct which resembles a hollow noodle. The common duct drains bile from all of the liver, carrying it to the intestine where it can be disposed of. The arrangement is like a super highway which is the culmination of millions of progressively larger feeder roads carrying cargo to a common destination.

When the duct is blocked or lacking, as in biliary atresia, the bile products of the liver cells can not be discharged and must find another way out. They pass into the blood stream, and soon their pigment can be seen in the yellow color of the patient's skin and by the lemon or orange hue of the normally white part of the eyes. This is jaundice. Driven by the body's needs, the liver cells continue to produce the bile until the blocked bile eventually damages them and erodes their many other vital functions.

In response to the damage, the liver tries to repair itself by laying down connective tissue—the first stage in scarring. The scarring then separates collections of liver cells into islands which lose their harmonious relationship to each other. In addition, the flow of portal vein blood that nourishes the liver is at first impeded and eventually blocked (see chapter 5). Thus frustrated, the obstructed portal blood seeks other avenues by which to return to the heart, with the consequent development of the dangerous thin-walled esophageal veins called varices which may rupture and bleed. The liver grinds down and with it the total body machinery dependent on the liver, which is the energy factory for other tissues and organs. That this occurs slowly contributes to the tragedy.

Reflecting on this evolution of events in the early 1960s, Willis Potts, a pioneer pediatric surgeon in Chicago, described biliary atresia as the blackest chapter in pediatrics. The victims of the disease seem normal at first, and they remain that way long enough to come into their new families, be loved, and leave those images which have no time to be created by the hapless stillborn infants or babies who die just after birth. The children with biliary atresia have personalities. In some cases, their slow transformation to physical pariahs only increases the affection which they receive. Their spindly and easily broken limbs often grow in the wrong direction off globular bodies that are increasingly bloated by enlargement of the liver and spleen, and by the accumulation of free fluid in the abdominal cavity (ascites). When death finally comes, it usually is from coma caused by the liver failure, or bleeding caused by the portal vein blockage combined with the inability of the failed liver to make clotting factors.

This was to be Bennie's fate. The day he was born, he began his slow walk to Calvary and was almost there when we saw him in February 1963 with C. Henry Kempe, chair of the Department of Pediatrics. Kempe was one of those chairs who elected to remain with Dean Glaser during the transition to the full-time system at Colorado. His special scientific field was infectious disease. He had become available for recruitment to Colorado from the University of California when he refused as a matter of principle to sign the "loyalty oath" that became a condition for employment at his institution during the anti-communist fervor of the early 1950s. Having escaped as a child from the holocaust of Europe, he would not help re-create the same thing here. He had no trouble distinguishing right from wrong.

Kempe was already a public figure in Colorado for another reason. During his career he had observed children in hospital emergency rooms and wards who had injuries that could not be explained easily by domestic accidents, as was claimed by those who brought them in. He identified the possibility that these babies and children had been tortured or maimed in bursts of anger or passion by parents or other guardians. The findings were characteristic. X-rays showed multiple bone fractures at different stages of healing, from which the time of the abusive incidents could be reconstructed. The marks left from fear and emotional repression of the children were harder to uncover.

Kempe coined the term *battered child syndrome*. He had discovered a dreadful social secret about childhood abuse and had exposed it. Later, he came to understand the extent of sexual abuse of children within families and founded a center for these victims (almost all girls) near the medical center. This was no ordinary pediatrician. He was a true defender of children.

Without hesitation, Kempe supported our proposal to attempt a transplantation for Bennie. His support, then and later, never wavered. What he saw as rectitude was not affected by failure in more than half of the cases over the next seventeen years. He protected the liver transplant program and helped take care of the patients, asking no recognition for what he did. When I came to the University of Pittsburgh in 1980, he reached another decision point.

Officials at the Children's Hospital of Pittsburgh, including the chair of the Department of Pediatrics, were uneasy about allowing an operation to be performed which still was classed as experimental. They called Kempe. Now invalided by heart disease, he reiterated his original position, and pointed out that the longest survival in Colorado was more than ten years after liver transplantation.

Paul Gaffney (hospital director) and William Donaldson (chief of surgery) decided to go forward with liver transplantation in Pittsburgh. Kempe died in Hawaii in early 1984 and was mourned for many reasons, of which most could be traced to his compassion and integrity.

Bennie's donor was another child who died during an open heart operation. In looking back, one can ask why Bennie, who himself was on life support with a ventilator, should not have donated a heart to the other child instead of receiving his liver. The question did not come up, and could not for almost five more years when the first heart transplantation was performed by Christiaan Barnard in Cape Town. Instead, the donor, who already was on a heart-lung machine, was cooled and maintained with an artificial circulation. The donor family gave permission for removal of the liver.

By this time, we had performed nearly two hundred liver transplantations in dogs, counting the original work in Chicago and that in the Denver VA laboratory. The effectiveness of Imuran-steroid therapy was considered established from the first human kidney cases. We viewed the principal hurdle to be the operation itself, which would be vastly more difficult than kidney transplantation.

However, nothing we had done in advance could have prepared us for the enormity of the task. Several hours were required just to make the incision and enter the abdomen. Every piece of tissue that was cut contained the small veins under high pressure that had resulted from obstruction of the portal vein by the diseased liver. Inside the abdomen, Bennie's liver was encased in scar tissue left over from operations performed shortly after his birth. His intestine and stomach were stuck to the liver in this mass of bloody scar. To make things worse, Bennie's blood would not clot. Several of the chemical and other factors which are necessary for this process were barely detectable.

He bled to death as we worked desperately to stop the hemorrhage. The operation could not be completed. Bennie was only three years old and had not enjoyed a trouble-free day in his life. Now, his wound was closed and he was wrapped in a plain white sheet after being washed off by a weeping nurse. They took him away from this place of sanitized hope to the cold and unhygienic morgue, where an autopsy did not add to our understanding of our failure. The surgeons stayed in the operating room for a long time after, sitting on the low stools around the periphery, looking at the ground and saying nothing. The orderlies came and began to mop the floor. It was necessary to prepare for the next case.

It was not the last time I would see this scene, both in my dreams and in reality. I never heard anyone who was there describe this as "the Solis case," or the first human liver transplantation. If they mentioned it at all, it was always just about Bennie.

» «

Bennie's operation was on March 1, 1963. During April, two more kidney transplantations were performed. Of the six kidney transplant recipients treated so far, five were alive, and four of the six were destined to survive for the next quarter century. Now that the kidney series was started, efforts in the research laboratories had turned back to the more difficult operation of liver transplantation. The main lesson that had been learned from trying to treat Bennie Solis was that the defective blood clotting that is characteristic of serious liver disease would have to be controlled. A German coagulation expert named Kurt von Kaulla who was working in the Department of Surgery was recruited to the team.

Von Kaulla identified the missing links in the clotting chain during liver replacement and how these might be corrected. It was clear that however seriously disturbed clotting was at the outset, it usually became even worse once the liver transplantation was started. In addition to a further decline in the already low clotting factors, a new sinister influence during operation was the development of an event called *fibrinolysis*. In some way, the operation itself caused the entry into the blood of substances called fibrinolysins which dissolved clots that already had formed. A burst of these fibrinolysins would turn circulating blood into a thin fluid which resembled red ink.

If this state did not spontaneously reverse, or could not be eliminated with a drug called epsilon aminocaproic acid (EACA), there was no hope of stopping the bleeding. No matter what else was done, the one absolute requirement for restoration of clotting was the use of a liver graft that functioned promptly and well. Von Kaulla recommended strategies to stop fibrinolysis, including treatment with EACA and infusions of specific clotting substances that could be obtained from the blood bank after their separation from donated whole blood.

In 1963, Denver did not have the high visibility to the national media that it later enjoyed, or labored under. Very little was known publicly about our trials of kidney transplantation, and the failed first attempt at liver transplantation went unnoticed by the press. At a professional level, Bill Waddell was in contact with Joe Murray and his other friends at the Brigham in Boston. Dave Hume called me often from Richmond. Through frequent phone calls I shared with Hume whatever information we were learning on a day-to-day basis, and learned from him in return. Both Murray and Hume were interested only in the kidney cases.

The existence of the Colorado kidney transplantation program was not widely known even within the medical profession until Bill Waddell announced it while discussing a paper given by Hume in 1963 at the American Surgical Association in Phoenix. Now it was made clear that a third active kidney transplant center in the United States had been added to those at the Peter Bent Brigham Hospital and the Medical College of Virginia.

I was at the ASA meeting at the invitation of Waddell, who was a member. That evening, guests as well as members were invited to a fiesta on the outskirts of the city. On the transit bus was an empty seat next to a stocky, square-jawed man with short sandy hair in which iron streaks were just appearing. I sat down beside him. He was Willard Goodwin, one of the world's foremost urologists. He did not know me, but after a few moments conversation, he realized that I was the person to whom Bill Waddell had referred in his discussion of Dave Hume's paper. We talked about transplantation and the Colorado kidney series, about which Goodwin had heard rumors only. Several years earlier, Goodwin had attempted several kidney transplantations at UCLA. From these cases, a number of important observations had been made which were of great help to later workers. The death of all his recipients had discouraged him and caused him to stop clinical trials.

The chance encounter introduced me to one of the most open-hearted and generous people whom I have ever met. These qualities, added to Goodwin's accomplishments in transplantation, gave him a special role in the new phase of transplantation, which already had begun in Colorado but was not yet recognized elsewhere. Until that night in Phoenix, I had no connection with the still small kidney transplant fraternity except for my conversations with Dave Hume. Goodwin told me of an impending meeting on renal transplantation in Washington, D.C., scheduled for September at the National Research Council. He said that he would arrange invitations for me and for Bill Waddell, which he did.

A few days later, Goodwin came to Colorado. I learned later that his habit was to glean information from these informal visits and report back to the UCLA transplant group, which included Paul Terasaki, a pioneer tissue typer. More than twenty-seven years later, in November 1990, a urologist named Jacques Poisson of Nice, France, gave me a yellowed copy of a six-page, single-spaced, intramural letter from Goodwin which Jacques had saved from his fellowship days in Los Angeles. Dated May 11, 1963, the in-house document started:

Dear Friends: On May 5 and 6, I visited Denver to learn what I could of the homotransplantation effort of the group there (Tom Starzl, William Waddell, Tom Marchioro, Oliver Stonington, and about a dozen others). The visit was most impressive to me, and I should like to share some of my impressions with you.

When I arrived on the evening of May 5, I went to the Veterans Hospital where I visited the completion of what must surely be the world's first technically successful homotransplantation of the human liver. The recipient, a patient of Dr. Waddell's, was a man with a primary hepatoma [liver cancer] involving the whole liver. He had had two explorations, 7 days and 1 day before the transplant. He was a non-veteran admitted to the VA Hospital in order to receive the transplant from a VA patient dying there of a brain tumor. The surgical team was waiting alerted for 48 hours, one of the drawbacks of cadaver donor transplantation.

When the white donor (the recipient was Afro-American) finally died, Dr. Marchioro and his team promptly introduced a catheter via the femoral vessel [main artery to the legs] and began perfusion (up into the aorta) at a slow rate with a heart-lung machine that was primed with

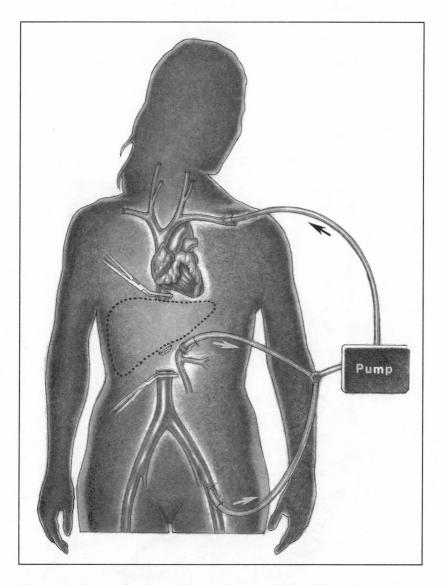

Figure 5. External tubing delivers obstructed blood from the lower to the upper half of the body while the natural liver is being removed and replaced. For humans, this system is pump-driven, as shown by the rectangular box.

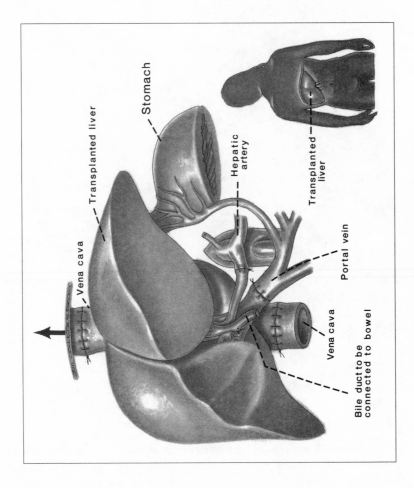

Figure 6. The transplanted liver in place.

refrigerated oxygenated glucose solution plus procaine. Later they opened the chest and also perfused the lower aorta and abdominal organs from above.

Preparation of the sterile donor liver took about 2 hours. Approximately another 2 hours were spent in transplanting the liver, performing all the necessary anastomoses [blood vessel connections]. When I saw the homotransplant in place, it had a good color and looked like a normal liver. A cholecystectomy was done [gall bladder was removed] and the gall bladder bed bled in a healthy normal way. A T-tube was placed in the common duct below the anastomosis and shortly thereafter, it began to drain clear bile. The above surgical procedures were done . . . with great skill and careful speed. . . . Starzl had tried this some weeks or months ago in a child with congenital atresia of the bile ducts. The procedure failed because the recipient bled to death under their eyes. There was lack of blood clotting. Because of this awesome previous education, they were prepared in the present case, and gave large amounts of human fibrinogen [a clot-promoting blood product] intravenously during the operation.

The next day, I saw and talked with the patient. His new liver was making large amounts of clear bile and he seemed to be in good immediate postoperative condition. It seemed to me that the patient was in better shape than the surgeons on the day after this monumental effort.

The rest of Goodwin's letter was concerned with the kidney recipients, many of whom he interviewed. As it turned out, the recipients to whom he talked are still alive, including Royal Jones and a young man who was having severe postoperative psychiatric problems. In his note about the latter recipient, Goodwin reported that "his donor brother was always bigger and better and handsomer and the better athlete, etc. The recipient was resigned to die and does not quite know how to cope with his new found life with his brother's kidney. He may not be up to it . . . we should really try again to get the psychiatrists interested in this problem. They could have a field day!" It is sad to relate that the donor later committed suicide whereas the recipient is still alive with perfect function of his original kidney graft more than twenty-eight years later.

Goodwin went on:

The Denver team has either 8 or 9 successful kidney transplants (2 or 3 since dead). . . . Another patient I was privileged to see is a 35 year old male who had come from Virginia to the Denver VA because he was told that the Denver and Los Angeles VA Hospitals were 'centers' for kidney transplantation. Denver was closer than Los Angeles, but somehow he got past Richmond and Hume. He received a kidney from his 32 year old sister in January, 1963. Before that, he had dialysis in Virginia (at the VA Hospital), and in Denver in preparation for the transplant. He appeared to be in excellent health. He had a moon face and ruddy cheeks. He confessed to an interest in sex and erections but evaded the question of whether or not he had intercourse (he is a bachelor). He apparently is presently a ward of the VA, and is being rehabilitated. I think that he takes Imuran and prednisone and I believe that he formerly had chronic glomerulonephritis [his original kidney disease]. He was a truck driver.

This patient also is still living with his graft, which is the longest surviving non-twin kidney transplant in the world.

A cadaver organ procurement program was a necessary condition for the Denver program and particularly interested Goodwin. Brain death and the concept of the heart-beating cadaver were five years away. Consequently, all donors were without a heartbeat and circulation for five to thirty minutes before an artificial circulation could be restored using a heart-lung machine.[1] Goodwin had not heard of this method and described

an intelligent program to harvest cadaveric organs (especially kidneys) for homotransplantation. . . . A very low pressure system is used with low rates of perfusion (aortic) so that the blood inflow (to the pump) matches the output. They feel that this is valuable and useful and have had some good animal experimental data to support them. . . .

A visit to their dog lab at the VA Hospital was most impressive. It is a well run, active place, air conditioned, and clean. They have plenty of technical help. They keep superb records on their animals, similar to regular hospital charts. They have one doctor in full time charge of records alone. They have a number of excellent kidney transplant experiments going on to test the value if any of splenectomy, thymectomy, etc. They also have an active program with liver transplants.

Near the end of Goodwin's memo was a comment about the interactions within any multidisciplinary group, showing his grasp of human behavior: "One of the interesting human aspects of this work, not only in Denver but everywhere, is how much each participant wants to be a part of the team and how each of us speaks so readily of '*our* experience,' while privately considering it '*my* experience.' Everyone with whom I speak is eager and ready to give credit where due, and at the same time wants to ensure his own niche and his own credit."

Reading his report nearly twenty-eight years later, I wondered if Goodwin might have set new standards in journalism had he not committed himself to surgery. He saw everything that was significant. The clotting problem had been dealt with in the liver recipient whom he observed, and the kind of management of clotting during the liver transplant operation which he described became standardized over the years. However, the strategy had a delayed backfire in this case and in the next three liver transplant recipients who followed. During the time when the livers were sewed in, plastic external bypasses were used to reroute venous blood around the area of the liver in the same way as had been worked out in dogs (chapter 6). In the humans who were being given drugs and blood products to promote clots, these clots formed in the bypass tubing and passed on to the lungs. There, they caused abscesses and other lung damage which contributed to or was the cause of delayed death of not only the patient seen by Goodwin (who died twenty-two days later) but in three more recipients who had otherwise successful liver transplants in June, July, and October 1963.

A pall settled over the liver program, and no more patients were entered for more than three years. It was the beginning of a self-imposed moratorium. By this time, other trials had failed at the Brigham (Franny Moore) and in France (Demirleau).

10

Time

The *Time* magazine cover story of May 3, 1963, was about surgery. It recounted the advances already made in this field since World War II and those projected for the immediate future. Franny Moore was featured as the prototype surgeon of the new era, on a stage provided by the Peter Bent Brigham Hospital, and with a supporting cast of the talented physicians and surgeons who worked there. In the main body of the story, a surgeon identified as one of the most articulate men working at the Brigham was quoted as saying that "this little place with only 284 beds has made more contributions to progress, per brick and per patient, than any other hospital in the world."

Above Moore's handsome aquiline face on the cover, with hair covered by an operating room cap, was the caption, "If they can operate, you're lucky." Those with an envious streak hooted, but derision was hard to sustain. The Brigham was nearing the fiftieth anniversary of its founding, and for nearly a third of this time Moore had provided its surgical stewardship. He was not yet fifty years old.

The new development that was most emphasized was transplantation. The identical-twin kidney transplantation of 1954 was highlighted and the operation erroneously attributed to Dave Hume instead of Joe Murray. A description was given of the extension of this successful beginning with identical twins to kidney transplantation using non-twin donors. Moore also pointed out the potential application of the same general technology to other kinds of organ grafts. The three centers in the United States upon which these optimistic hopes were based were identified as the Brigham (under Murray), the Medical College of Virginia (Hume), and ours at the University of Colorado.

The optimistic projections were eventually fulfilled, but they were ahead of their time. Will Goodwin, the urologist from UCLA (whose contributions were not mentioned in the *Time* story), had taken a leave of absence from his academic post in the late 1950s to study kidney transplantation in Boston with Murray and in Edinburgh with Michael Woodruff. He understood how hard it was going to be to safely cross the immune barrier and to control rejection. In his lectures he always warned, "Don't promise more than you can deliver," and illustrated the point with the photograph of an ancient statue of a sparsely clad Greek god. Wrapped around the god's leg was a voluptuous maiden, expressing some unfulfilled desire, the nature of which was left to the amused audience's imagination.

When Goodwin visited Denver in early May 1963, he realized the regularity with which the promise actually was being fulfilled in kidney recipients using the Imuran-prednisone treatment. These were results largely unknown elsewhere. Goodwin advised us to confirm what we already had observed in kidney transplant recipients rather than rush ahead with secondary application to another organ system such as the liver. He also advised me to continue research and clinical work in nontransplant areas of surgery, because he thought that I might be discredited professionally otherwise. In his opinion, the future of transplantation was highly uncertain. This was friendly guidance and reflected his own career development. I did what he advised for the time being.

Throughout the spring and summer of 1963 we curbed our liver transplant activities, but increased our pace of kidney transplantation. By September the kidney series had reached more than thirty. In the meanwhile, I wrote a manuscript describing our systematic use of the Imuran-prednisone drug therapy in our first kidney recipients emphasizing two points: the reversibility of kidney rejection with high doses of steroids (prednisone), and the "adaptation" that seemed to occur in the weeks and months after successful kidney transplantation. It was apparent that something changed in the reaction of the recipient to the graft once the first hurdle had been passed, so that in time, some of the alien kidneys eventually became viewed by the recipient immune system as less foreign and were therefore half forgotten by the body.

In late May 1963 I submitted the manuscript to the *Journal of the American Medical Association* (*JAMA*). As a courtesy, I sent a copy to Loyal Davis, my previous chair at Northwestern who still was the editor of *Surgery, Gynecology, and Obstetrics*. Davis recognized the potential importance of the observations and wrote back some opinions that reflected his maturity and wisdom. A few days later, he flew to Denver where he told me the same things over lunch at the Brown Palace Hotel.

Davis correctly predicted that the paper would be judged to be so radical and contrary to prevailing opinions that, if it were published at all, it would be only after major and time-consuming editorial reviews and revisions. This proved to be the case. The manuscript which I sent to the *JAMA* became a bone of editorial contention and was not published until the spring of 1964. However, Dr. Davis also suggested that the material should be refined, made more highly focused, and brought up to date. If these conditions were met, he offered to consider a streamlined version for the journal he edited.

I followed his advice. Davis published the article in the October 1963 issue of *Surgery, Gynecology, and Obstetrics*. Its title was "The Reversal of Rejection in Human Renal Homografts with the Subsequent Development of Homograft Tolerance." The other authors were Thomas L. Marchioro and William R. Waddell. The introduction read:

Because of the high failure rate after renal homotransplantation, there has been an air of pessimism concerning the possibility of long term function of the grafted kidney. The immunologic processes subserving rejection are generally thought to be so powerful and persevering that consistent success cannot be expected with the use of any of the currently available methods of antirejection therapy.

Recent personal experience in caring for patients with renal homografts [transplants] has resulted in alterations in many of our preconceived notions concerning the management of such patients. It has led to the beliefs that the rejection process can almost never be entirely prevented, but that its effects can be reversed with a high degree of

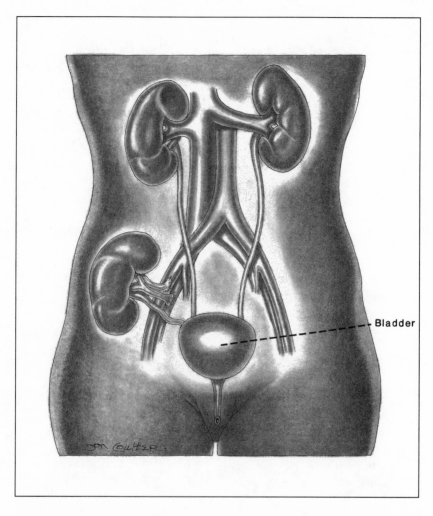

Figure 7. The location of normal paired kidneys (upper) and the pelvic position where the transplanted kidney can be inserted most conveniently (lower).

regularity and completeness. Furthermore, the subsequent behavior of patients who have been brought through a successfully treated rejection crisis suggests the early development of some degree of host-graft adaptation, since the phenomenon of vigorous secondary rejection has been encountered only once.[1]

The article marked the unapologetic beginning at a practical level of a new clinical field. The timing of its publication coincided with the historic Washington meeting on September 26 to which Will Goodwin had arranged belated invitations for Waddell and me. This meeting was held at the National Research Council building, with only about twenty-five contributors. However, the list included almost all the key workers who had brought the field of kidney transplantation this far. The only ones whom I knew personally were Dave Hume and Will Goodwin.

There was naked incredulity about our results. Will Goodwin had warned me that our claims would not be believed. For this reason, we brought the wall charts for all our patients and used these to illustrate what we had learned. Bound like giant scrolls inside a chamois leather cover, these were carried to the center table of the room and examined. There were thirty cases. After the first day, Dave Hume, Kendrick A. Porter (a London pathologist), Roy Calne (who had returned from Boston to England) and two or three others stayed up most of the night reviewing the charts.

At the formal meetings, I found it difficult to speak. It may have been my insecurity in the presence of such important dignitaries which caused me to be uneasy. In addition, I felt like someone who had parachuted unannounced from another planet onto turf that was already occupied. I was the only American transplant surgeon who had no exposure to the Harvard system and experience. However, although I had never been to any other transplant center including the Brigham, I was keenly aware of what had been done by the others who had gathered for the conference.

By this time, I was far along in writing a book, *Experience in Renal Transplantation*, which was to be published the following summer.[2] In the introduction I summarized the encouraging but rare examples of prolonged kidney graft function reported by these men, and concluded:

Despite these encouraging findings, it was not yet possible to obtain consistent success with homotransplantation procedures, either in experimental animals or man. Like the elusive jigsaw puzzle, in which many of the pieces had been fitted into their appropriate slots, the picture was not yet complete. The pioneer efforts of Murray, Küss, Hamburger, and Hume had all demonstrated that a renal homotransplant was capable of protracted function in the occasional case. If this could be achieved sporadically, it seemed reasonable to expect that the proper manipulation of a number of small details might provide a consistently successful solution. Despite this expectation, almost all renal homotransplants had failed when, in the spring of 1963, Goodwin and Martin compiled the known renal transplants from various centers throughout the world. Less than 10 per cent of those patients treated to that time had survived for as long as three months. The courageous and often tragically unsuccessful attempts of the early pioneers provided a vast, although frequently uncatalogued, background of valuable information upon which future progress might be built.

I considered the men mentioned to be the kidney transplant pioneers. What we had done was to complete their story. At the same time, Waddell and I realized that we had more surviving kidney transplant recipients by far than everyone else in the world combined. Determining the eventual outcome of these patients would be important. This was made possible by the creation at the conference of a worldwide kidney transplant registry, which would be based in Boston. The impetus for this extraordinary compilation came from Joe Murray of the Brigham.

The meticulousness of the second registry report[3] made it possible over twenty-five years later in the summer of 1989 to trace the fate of all 342 non-twin kidney recipients who had undergone transplantation throughout the world from the beginning up to the end of March 1964. Twenty-four were still alive, fifteen from our original Colorado series and nine from six other centers. These included three of Dave Hume's original patients at the Medical College of Virginia, two from the University of Minnesota (Kelly and Lillehei), and one each from Boston (Murray), Cleveland (Kolff), Edinburgh (Woodruff), and Paris (Hamburger).[4]

The painful and suspicious questions that were asked at the Washington conference about the credibility of our claims had been resolved. The portrait sketched in black and white in 1963 was enriched with color and detail by 1989, but it was fundamentally the same when the day of reckoning arrived. It was noteworthy that none of the world's twenty-four quarter-century survivors had been given an unrelated donor kidney. Nor was there a single example in the world of a twenty-five-year survival of a cadaver donor kidney allograft at the time of this follow-up report. A cadaver recipient in Paris who had maintained perfect kidney graft function finally passed this barrier on October 12, 1989. The French recipient was thirty-one years old at the time of her transplantation in 1964 under the care of Jean Hamburger, one of the Washington participants.

The early or late loss of the nonrelated kidneys usually was from rejection or from infections following the high doses of immunosuppression that were needed to prevent rejection. By the time of the Washington meeting, we already knew from our own experience that results would be inferior with unrelated donors. The subject caused a spirited exchange between Waddell and Roy Calne, who was opposed for ethical reasons to the use of living related donors. Some years later, I concluded that Calne had been fundamentally correct in his position.

Because liver and heart grafts could be obtained only from cadaver (unrelated) donors, this conclusion meant that what had been learned so far was not an open invitation to go forward with the liver trials or even indiscriminate kidney transplant trials. Better antirejection treatment than the Imuran-prednisone combination must be developed, or else a means had to be found to better match up the donors to the immune system of the recipients (tissue matching).

Our primary mission of liver transplantation had failed. Instead of introducing a new treatment for liver disease, we had succeeded only in making kidney transplantation practical if a living related donor was available. Not long after, Waddell remarked that we had climbed onto the wrong tiger and would find it hard to get off. After a while, I understood how right he was.

» «

Following the Washington meeting, seven or eight of the conference participants came to Denver for a firsthand look. One visitor was Kendrick A. Porter, the pathologist from St. Mary's Hospital and Medical School, London. Porter agreed to write the section on kidney transplant pathology for my book on renal transplantation. His chapter proved to be a classic which was years ahead of the field.

Within a few weeks, the clinical gold rush was on. More than twenty-five new kidney transplant programs sprang up in the United States alone in the next year. Within a few weeks, after publication in October 1963 of our article in *Surgery, Gynecology, and Obstetrics*, Colorado General Hospital was flooded with visitors from all over the world. More importantly, we were inundated with fellowship applications, providing a talent pool that produced many of the leading figures in transplantation of the next generation.

The revolution that had occurred was as unpredicted by most experts as was the fall of the Berlin wall twenty-six years later. Kidney transplantation seemed to have become a clinical service overnight. When mountains are climbed, the triumph can be spoiled by asking who took the first step to the summit, or who took the longest stride. From my point of view, it was hardly worth discussing. What we had contributed was peripheral to our main objective of liver replacement—which had failed.

Besides, victory with kidney transplantation was only an illusion. This was not the summit but only a ledge halfway up. It would not be possible for many more years to safely transplant cadaveric organs of any kind, including the kidney. Well into the 1970s, compilations of thousands of cadaveric kidney cases from multiple programs showed that the one-year graft survival was less than 50 percent in North America. Individual centers tended not to report their own poor results, erroneously believing that everyone else must be doing better.

During the peak of the exaggerations and professional euphoria, public expectations also reached new heights. Many major hospitals had acquired artificial kidney capability, with the result that patients who would have died only one or two years earlier could be kept in good condition while they waited for a kidney transplant. But they were almost entirely dependent on live donors, who were not available for everyone. Legislation allowing the removal of organs from donors whose brains had been destroyed but whose hearts were still beating had not yet been passed—this reform was five years in the future. Desperate potential recipients were piling up faster than places could be found for them for artificial kidney support, a service for which most health insurance agencies refused to pay because it was "experimental."

At the height of the crisis, the option of using animal kidneys was explored. In France and Germany nearly sixty years earlier, unsuccessful attempts had been made to transplant pig, monkey, and ape kidneys to human patients. On February 16, 1963, Claude Hitchcock of Hennepin County Hospital, Minneapolis, secretly transplanted the kidney of a baboon to a sixty-five-year-old woman. The organ functioned for four days before its artery clotted. The case was not made public until long after it was learned that later in the same year, Keith Reemtsma of Tulane University had a far more encouraging experience using the closer-to-human chimpanzee donor. One of Reemtsma's chimpanzee kidney grafts functioned for nine months. Reemtsma also transplanted a Rhesus monkey kidney which was fiercely rejected.

Convinced that his own first failure was due to a defective surgical operation and that the baboon would be an acceptable kidney donor for humans, Hitchcock called me about exploring this possibility for our patients with urgent need. He already had a strong collaboration with workers at the Southwestern Primate Center in San Antonio, Texas, who bred baboons and kept lifetime medical records for each animal. Infecting patients with baboon diseases transmitted through their transplanted kidneys seemed unlikely.

Six patients were given baboon kidneys by our Colorado team, joined by Hitchcock's group. All the organs functioned promptly and maintained function for six to sixty days. However, the doses of Imuran and prednisone necessary to prevent rejection were very high, and eventually nothing could halt this process. The severity of rejection was midway between that of the chimpanzee and Rhesus kidneys in events that were recapitulated two decades later in the Baby Fae baboon-to-human heart transplantation, in spite of much improved immunosuppression.

All these attempts to use the monkey, baboon, and chimpanzee kidneys (heterografts) eventually failed. It was clear that the use of animal organs would have to wait for better and possibly fundamentally different antirejection treatment. It also became obvious that the most compatible animal donor, the chimpanzee, would be excluded from future consideration because of the threat to its extinction, and because its anthropomorphic qualities were increasingly recognized. The killing of such nearly human creatures came to be (and still is) regarded as an outrage. Twenty-eight years later, we are no closer to the practical use of animal organs, in spite of the fact that the gap between grafts needed and those available has increased manyfold.

After the dust settled, a new era began, this one of consolidation, confirmation, and sober reflection about what had been done. Will Goodwin, whose memorandum of May 1963 was quoted in chapter 9, now wrote another one to his UCLA team, reflecting the amazing events in the intervening eleven months. Like the first document, this one was found in Nice, in the memorabilia that Jacques Poisson had saved. After a lengthy description of the papers (many on transplantation) given at the 1964 American Surgical Association (April 1–3, Hot Springs, Virginia), Goodwin concluded:

> It seems to me that we are now in a kind of "second phase." Many have more confidence than before and are beginning to look for longer range successes. At the same time, we should go slowly to study and observe some of these strange things that are being seen, such as peripheral neuropathies and vascular lesions, etc. I would not be surprised if one of the most interesting things that could come out of all of this will be observations of what may turn out to be "new diseases" in some of these long range survivors.

» «

Goodwin's memorandum was prophetic. There would be new diseases in the transplant recipient population. The most obvious were those caused by the steroids that were essential for consistent success. The steroids caused redistribution of body fat and other changes that were so cosmetically deforming that they could be interpreted as nature's revenge for defeating its purpose of rejection. Most noticeable was a ballooning of the face (moon face) and the appearance of a "buffalo hump" between and just above the shoulder blades. The most poignant victims were children whose growth was arrested.

On the thinned and easily damaged skin of the abdomen and elsewhere of patients receiving high-dose steroid therapy could be found stretch marks like those which develop during pregnancy. Cataracts began to develop, and soon the eye clinics were flooded with moon-faced children and young adults who were going blind. The steroids also contributed to the weakening of bones, which could be seen on X-rays to gradually lose their calcium content. Now, the orthopedic clinics were filled with moon-faced kidney recipients whose height was shrinking as their backbones slowly dissolved, whose hips or other joints needed replacement with plastic or metal devices, and whose ribs or other bones might break with a movement as slight as a cough. Muscles wasted away as the nerves supplying them degenerated (peripheral neuropathy). A quarter or more of the recipient population developed sugar diabetes caused by the steroids.

The quality of the recipients' lives was inversely related to the amount of steroid therapy needed to retain function of the transplanted kidneys. It was soon learned that low-dose requirements could be expected only if the donor was a family member. Even under these circumstances, it was tempting to bring to conferences or symposia only those patients who had been recently operated upon, before the ravages of steroid treatment became visible.

The steroid doses were not fixed. As described in our 1963 article, it often was possible as the weeks and months went by to reduce the amounts, and in some cases to stop steroids altogether and rely on Imuran treatment alone to prevent rejection. A few patients stopped both drugs with no adverse consequences, but the majority who tried this, even years later, lost their grafts to rejection. How many concealed suicides were committed by deliberate drug discontinuance is not known. These deaths almost always were classed as being caused by "noncompliance." Doctors, like all other people, do not like to admit imperfections or failure. It was better to blame the patients for their own demise.

This was only the beginning. Lurking within the bodies of these patients were armies of the "germs" which normally are kept at bay by the same immune defenses that now were weakened by the drug treatment used to prevent rejection. The common infections caused by bacteria usually could be controlled in these recipients with conventional antibiotics. Such specific treatment was less effective or was not available for infections caused by bacteria that normally were not dangerous. Funguses, which are natural inhabitants of the body and are commonly found in the soil, were a serious threat.

Worst of all were the viruses, the lowest and most incomplete forms of life. They could invade the recipient cells and live there, either attacking them or waiting patiently for the optimum moment to strike. Infections of the lungs, liver, brain, and other organs became the main causes of late death as we watched the bellwether group of Colorado recipients who made up most of the world's transplant beachhead. As with the cosmetic and physical disability, the risk of infection was proportional to the steroid doses, usually lower in related recipients.

A further specter emerged when one of our earliest recipients developed a malignant white blood cell tumor (then called a reticulum cell sarcoma, now B-lymphocyte lymphoma) in his liver. It was soon apparent that these and other cancers would be seen in increased numbers in these patients. A viral cause was suspected at the outset, but not proved for another fifteen years. At first, I hoped that the tumor was a coincidental stroke of bad luck. In 1968, the connection between antirejection therapy and cancer development was too strong to be denied, and I issued a warning to this effect at that year's meetings of the Swiss Society of Immunology and the American Surgical Association. One of our surgeons, Israel Penn, began a registry of these cancers in transplant recipients; by the end of 1990, more than five thousand had been entered.

Until the summer of 1964, the armies of germs infecting our patients had seemed strangely distant. Now we learned that the doctors and nurses on the wards and in the clinics and laboratories were in the war zone. Like silent snipers concealed in trees, the viruses struck. One Sunday morning after playing for the transplant softball team, I was brought home with a high fever and prostration. Thinking it was a heat stroke, I went to bed. After Barbara had trouble arousing me, she called a physician who drew blood from my arm and started intravenous fluids. When the blood from the needle stick did not clot, she called him back and learned that the blood chemistries showed serious clotting and liver function abnormalities.

I had hepatitis, a diagnosis soon made in several other transplant team members. One of them was my chief research technician, an efficient middle-aged women who had worked for Ben Eiseman before he left for Kentucky. She recovered enough to return to work, but died of liver failure several years later. When Bill Waddell became ill, he recovered quickly but then relapsed. The activity in the research laboratory tripled as we realized that he might need a liver transplant, which we were not yet prepared to try again. Just when he reached his deepest yellow color, he began to improve.

The hepatitis epidemics in artificial kidney and transplant centers were worldwide in the mid-1960s and caused many deaths among the health care personnel. Those who were left mourned and moved on, like infantry men who did not know where the shots came from, or where to hide. Seven years later, when Baruch Blumberg (Nobel prize, 1976) found a way to detect the B hepatitis virus in the blood, we found the answer by analyzing blood samples which had been stored from the beginning of the program. Many of our patients had been virus carriers from the time we first saw them. They were a deadly reservoir from which other patients were infected later.

I recovered and fled from the hospital as soon as I was able to walk out. The noise there kept me awake when I did not want to be, and when I slept it was so deeply that both arms were temporarily paralyzed when I woke up. Feverishly, in the hospital room, I went over the galley proofs of the last chapters of my kidney transplantation book as the summer of 1964 faded, believing that I might not live to see it published. Before long, the first bound copy came to my house. Still yellow and weak from the liver disease, I bought a plane ticket to LeMars and took the prize to my father at 205 Central Avenue S.W. By now, it was Indian summer in Iowa, and I wondered if I would be able to work again. I was thirty-eight years old.

11

Tissue Matching

Even before my bout with hepatitis and recovery from it, I had concluded that the imperfections of kidney transplantation had been so well defined that merely accruing a larger patient series would be a futile exercise. Better immunosuppressive drugs could be developed in the research laboratory. In the clinics, there was the possibility that tissue matching could improve the results, or at least permit the use of lower doses of the drugs. Such attempts for the selection of the best family donors were known to have been made in Paris by the kidney disease specialist Jean Hamburger and the immunologist, Jean Dausset.[1]

In the spring of 1964, while dozens of other centers were scrambling to develop kidney transplant programs, we closed ours for half a year in order to set up the first extensive trial of tissue matching ever attempted. The trial resulted in a controversy about the benefits of tissue matching that has not been completely resolved twenty-seven years later. When the trial did not conform to expectations, the wrath of the government bureaucracy fell on Paul I. Terasaki. His sin was to unveil the truth, and his punishment was expulsion from the tissue typing establishment.

It was predicted by many participants in the Washington conference of 1963 that tissue matching would have to be nearly perfect if kidney and other organ grafting procedures were to succeed permanently with any degree of reliability and predictability. This seemed logical, but what to measure, and how, were still unanswered questions. Presumably, the vigor of the recipient's immune response was dictated by the structure of molecules (antigens) in the cells of the donor tissues which were different from those in the recipient and therefore seen by the immune system as alien.

Paul Terasaki's name was frequently mentioned in discussions of antigen detection. Although I had not met him, he already had perfected a method for this purpose, employing "cytotoxic" antibodies that bound to the antigens in question. His discovery eventually made him one of the world's foremost authorities on tissue typing and matching for transplantation. With such techniques, Terasaki and a French scientist named Jean Dausset (Nobel prize, 1980) were convinced that they could separate out the tissue antigens that provoked the immune response known as rejection. This was the beginning of human histocompatibility research, a new field of indescribable importance and complexity which made intelligible many previous mysteries of the human immunologic system generally, and certain aspects of immune rejection of transplants in particular.

By the end of 1963, the list of seemingly measurable human tissue antigens was long enough to convince Terasaki that matching efforts in future cases might be worthwhile. However, he wanted to begin by comparing the antigens in patients bearing successfully transplanted kidney grafts with those in their donors to see if there was any relation between the quality of the antigen match and the clinical outcome. A positive correlation of good matching and good outcome would suggest that the antigens being studied were the crucial ones involved in rejection. This was Terasaki's hypothesis and that of Dausset. The cells whose antigens were measured were the lymphocytes in the circulating blood. These antigens were thought to be the same in all cells, including those making up the solid organs such as the kidney.

Terasaki realized from the Washington conference report that the majority of the kidney transplant survivors in the world were in Denver, and this prompted his visit to Colorado after the meeting concluded. We rounded up the surviving recipients and their donors (most were blood relatives), took blood samples, and made estimates of the antigen match using the still impure and incompletely classified detection panel. To everyone's delight, many of the most trouble-free recipients were those whose white cell antigens closely matched those on the donor white cells. The clue was tenuous because there were so many exceptions, and also because most of the successfully transplanted kidneys came from sibling donors (brothers or sisters) or from parents who had donated to their children.

Nevertheless, Terasaki and I decided to attempt matching before transplantation as a means of identifying the best donor for the next cases. We made our preparations during the six-month closure of the kidney program and began the matching trial when the program reopened in October 1964. At the time, we were accepting kidneys voluntarily donated by convicts at the Canon State Prison. The number of volunteers for patients who had no family donors was large enough in many cases to have a choice among as many as fifty or sixty. It was difficult to find a perfect or even a good match in spite of the size of the unrelated donor pool, but the best-matched volunteer was selected. In contrast, if there were potential donors within a family, we frequently encountered very complete matches.

The results when the kidney transplantations were actually performed in unrelated cases were disappointing. No difference could be seen in the recovery of patients who received kidneys from relatively well matched versus completely mismatched donors. Only when kidneys were transplanted from perfectly matched blood relatives did rejection-free recovery occur consistently without the need for large doses of prednisone or other extra therapy.[2]

The results were reported as "preliminary" in 1966. In the meanwhile, a cottage industry of clinical tissue typing based on the assumption that matching would have a profound influence on transplantation had sprung up worldwide, mostly funded by contracts or grants from the NIH or other government agencies. In late 1969, I was invited to give a state-of-the-art lecture on kidney transplantation to the American Society of Nephrology in Washington, D.C., on December 2.

One specific charge was to discuss the role of tissue typing for donor selection. By this time, I was alarmed by the continued lack of correlation between clinical outcome and quality of matching in unrelated cases (by now largely cadaver donors), and concerned about my role in starting these epidemic efforts in 1964 and spurring them on subsequently. Well-meaning but unwarranted legislation was pending in Italy and elsewhere that would make it illegal to perform transplantation without certain matching conditions.

My report created a furor. What I did in preparing for it was to collect information on all our patients for whom we also had tissue typing information from the beginning of our Colorado program in 1962 until the present. In looking back, the closeness of tissue match had not been an important determinant of outcome using unrelated donors. It had predicted ideal donors within families, but short of perfect matches, it was only equivocally influential even in families. The evidence was that the antigens being matched were transplant antigens which were inherited by classical genetic (Mendelian) laws, but that the system was so complex (more than we were measuring) that matching would not be the boon we had predicted in 1964. We were heartbroken, but published the results in 1970.[3]

Although he was an author on this paper, Terasaki was not convinced. He thought there was either a "center effect" in which our experience and skill with immunosuppression had covered up a typing influence, or that the sample size was too small to be a significant test of his original hypothesis. He was scheduled to give a paper on typing at the Transplantation Society in The Hague on September 8, 1970, and set out to collect data on twelve hundred cases of cadaver kidney transplantation from other centers. As the day of his lecture approached, the finality set in that our original conclusions were valid.

I was in the back of the auditorium on the fateful day. Anxious and looking smaller than I remembered him, Terasaki walked resolutely to the podium and read his message to a huge and it seemed to me hostile audience. What he said was not only clear and honest—it was wise. He pointed out that what was more interesting than the poor correlation of matching and outcome after cadaver transplantation was the large and unexpected number of patients with very poor matches who had done well. When he finished, there was little applause. As he walked off the stage with serene dignity, I realized that I loved Paul as his friends must have loved Socrates. He was the symbol of integrity.

That night I came back late to my hotel on the waterfront. It was cold and raining when I arrived, and the entrance door was locked. I slept on a lawn chair in the rain, was sick the next day, and returned home through London two days later. At Heathrow Airport there was a large bookstore with stacks of books separating the aisles so that browsers on one side could not see those on the other. What I heard fixed that moment in my brain to the smallest detail, including the book I had pulled out to examine.

I knew the men talking. One was an official of the NIH agency administering the contract that was the main support of Terasaki's laboratory. The other was a military officer stationed in Washington who later left the service and became a department chair in a medical school. What caught my ear was Terasaki's name. The two were planning an emergency site visit to UCLA with the intention of discontinuing Terasaki's laboratory support. Paul's heretical report was not what they wanted to hear, and now the messenger must be killed.

I phoned Paul a few days later and warned him what was coming. The site visit to California occurred within a few weeks. On Christmas Eve, 1970, Paul called me and said that his funding of nearly $400,000 per year had been cut off. He asked if we could help him by buying piecemeal typing services for our patients and of course I agreed. The conversation was as chilling as any I can remember. People were laughing and drinking champagne at a Christmas Eve party down the hall. I walked home slowly through the snow.

Two emergency typing conferences were held early in 1971, the first in Dallas and the second in Europe. Already on the first occasion, there was evidence that Terasaki's analysis was correct, but it was too late to save his laboratory. In April I went to Washington to an NIH policy commission concerned with transplantation. I could not refrain from repeating publicly the utter outrage about the treatment of Terasaki that I already had expressed at the meeting in Dallas. A few weeks later, I was called from the NIH with the news that we ourselves were having an emergency site visit a few days hence. I had little doubt of the purpose. Our largest support grant also was summarily defunded, a negative investment in grantsmanship which was worth every penny of the money we never received. Believing he knew what had provoked the thunderbolt, an associate dean at Colorado contacted me suggesting that we appeal. I told him not to bother.

Terasaki had been right not only about what typing could do, which was considerable for transplantation within families, but about what it could not do unless there was a perfectly matched cadaveric donor. Twenty years later the only controversy is whether matching under all other circumstances means enough to be given any consideration in the distribution of cadaver kidneys. By exposing the truth, Terasaki had made it clear that the field of clinical transplantation could advance significantly only by the development of better drugs and other treatment strategies, not by vainly hoping that the solution would be through tissue matching.

Although it was not appreciated at the time, Terasaki's conclusion breathed life into the still struggling fields of liver and heart transplantation. There were no artificial organs to support these patients while they waited for a well-matched donor. It was a relief to know that the selection of donors with random tissue matching would not result in an intolerable penalty.

Ironically, the supreme practical contribution of tissue typing proved to be the antibody test developed by Terasaki to measure the tissue antigens. The antibodies he used, which kill white blood cells, are not normally present in the blood. At the first Histocompatibility Tissue Matching Conference (June 7–8, 1964, in Washington, D.C.), Terasaki described how these antibodies, if present in the recipient and directed against the cells of the donor, can cause destruction of a transplanted kidney within minutes (hyperacute rejection). He pointed out that the antibodies could be detected by mixing the serum of the prospective recipient with the white blood cells in the blood of the planned donor (cytotoxic crossmatch). His recommendation that this be done is carried out today before every kidney transplantation anywhere in the world.[4] By common misconception, the credit for this major contribution often is given to someone who was in the 1964 audience and reported the same thing almost two years later. Subsequently, this same scientist had the misfortune of serving on the site visit team that closed Terasaki's laboratory in 1970.

Although he was born in California, Terasaki spent his youth in one of the internment camps to which Americans of Japanese descent were consigned during World War II. I know him very well. If he ever complained about his treatment then or later, I believe I would have heard it. During the Watergate days, several years after Terasaki's lab was closed, a young Colorado University physician who was meeting his military obligation in government service stole a copy of the unexpurgated minutes of the fateful site visit to UCLA of November 1970 and sent it to me. In the meanwhile, I had talked to almost every member on that site visit team. To a man, they expressed shock at the outcome and described to me how they personally had fought for Terasaki and preservation of his lab. Now I knew this was not true. Believing it would be petty to add to their shame, I kept the pilfered document in my desk for several years and then shredded it.

Those anywhere in the world who have anything to do with medicine or surgery are aware that Terasaki not only survived but thrived. That he could have triumphed in America in spite of what its bureaucracy did to him may explain why you can find a flag in front of his house on every Fourth of July.

12

Why Not Two Livers?

By 1964 the University of Colorado had become a mecca for clinical kidney transplantation while the liver program had all but disappeared from view. However, our decision in 1963 to temporarily abandon liver transplantation following the initial failures was not the same as capitulation. The liver is an unpaired organ. Instead of removing and replacing it, why not transplant a second (auxiliary) liver in some convenient location in the abdomen? Theoretically, such an operation would be of lesser magnitude because it omitted the very difficult step of removing the recipient liver. Moreover, whatever function the diseased recipient liver still possessed might tide the recipient over until the transplanted auxiliary liver began to function. Even if the new liver failed, there might be a chance to take it out and find another one.

Those with a biblical orientation might have suggested that if God wanted us to have two livers or two hearts, he would have given them to us. No one was thinking this way. The implantation of an auxiliary liver had a special appeal for our team because of our now extensive experience with kidney transplantation. Kidney grafts are essentially never placed in a normal anatomic location, and frequently they are implanted without removing the two natural kidneys. We had developed a technique by which the over-sized kidney of an adult could be transplanted into the right side of the abdomen of a very small infant even though it was ten or more times larger than the normal kidneys of the tiny recipient. It was easy to see how an extra liver could go into the same location.

Transplanting an extra liver in dogs had been described in 1955 by C. Stuart Welch, the senior surgeon at Albany Medical College, New York, who was the mentor of John J. Farrell (see chapter 5). Welch's article was published three years before Franny Moore and I made our first attempts at liver replacement in 1958.[1] When the livers were destroyed a week or so after Welch had put them in, there was no reason to believe that anything other than rejection was responsible. The only lingering question was whether his method of restoring the extra liver's blood supply in its abnormal location was as good as that which nature normally provided. In Welch's operation, a normal volume of blood flow to the extra liver was provided by a double blood supply (hepatic artery and portal venous). The artery supply came from the body's main blood vessel (aorta) and was not fundamentally different in the transplanted liver and the dog's own liver. But the kind of blood sent to the grafted liver through its portal vein was different than normal. This blood was that returning from the legs, pelvis, and kidneys and was not the insulin-rich blood coming back from the pancreas or the blood coming back from the intestine with its high content of digested food. These special kinds of blood continued to be directed only to the dog's own liver, which remained in place.

What Welch had done without knowing it was to create an experimental model of enormous power. The principle of the model was the coexistence of two livers in the same animal with identical conditions except for whatever was different in the venous blood inflow. Welch assumed that the kind of blood coming into the portal vein was not a critical factor in the health of a liver, and because of this, he thought that the extensive damage found in his transplanted auxiliary livers was due solely to rejection. This assumption cost him a truly major discovery. It was an understandable lapse. He had no means to prevent rejection in 1955 when he performed his experiments, and thus no way to verify his assumption.

By the time of our research in 1963 and 1964, we could protect the transplanted extra liver from rejection by using Imuran. The results under these new circumstances in dog experiments were astonishing. Some of the extra livers were not rejected, but nevertheless they shrank to a fraction of their normal size within a few days. We suspected immediately that the liver with first access to the pancreatic and intestinal blood removed something from the portal blood (presumed but not proved to be insulin) leaving little for the other liver—which consequently shriveled up. This was a stunning development because it pointed to further experiments which eventually showed how insulin and other hormones and substances in normal portal blood can modify the liver's structure, function, and capacity for self-renewal (regeneration). Collectively, these liver-hormone relationships became known as the "hepato-trophic concept" and opened up the new field of hepatotrophic physiology.

I presented the experimental findings to the American Surgical Association (ASA) at Homestead, Virginia, on April 1, 1964, along with a complete report of the failed clinical liver replacement trials.[2] Ordinarily, the ASA is not an optimal place to present a series of abject failures, and as a diversionary ploy I may have placed uneven emphasis on the interesting auxiliary liver experiments. If so, the strategy did not work and I had a sense of faint but politely stated disapprobation in the remarks of those who discussed my paper. C. Stuart Welch was one of these. I perceived him at the meeting as overtly angry, but perhaps I was imagining this because I could find little such evidence in his published comments.

The next day I received a call from Denver that my daughter, Becky, had been admitted to Colorado General Hospital with suspected appendicitis. Barbara and I chartered a plane and arrived that evening to find that it was a false alarm. Much later, at home, the phone rang and it was Dr. Welch. He wanted to let me know of further reservations about my work which he had neglected to mention during the discussion. Besides being sleepy, I was offended at first when I realized that he had been drinking. Finally, we said good night.

A few days later he called back and asked me what he had said, which was hard to summarize because I had gone to sleep during the tirade. After that he called frequently, always at two or three in the morning. For him in New York, this was four or five o'clock. Sometimes I could understand him perfectly and sometimes not. After a while, I realized that each call was a *cri de coeur*, especially

when I learned more of his life. Welch had been chair of the
Department of Surgery at Tufts University in Boston before
moving to Albany. While there in 1944, his wife had died a few days
after giving birth to twins. Throughout the pregnancy, she had
been inexplicably ill with recurrent abdominal pain.

When she was operated on, a twisting of her intestine was found
which could have been corrected earlier with a relatively routine
surgical procedure. The young Franny Moore had assisted Leland
McKittrick, a famed Boston surgeon of that era, in performing the
operation. Forty-seven years later (July 1991), Moore wrote me with
the details of the tragedy:

> Stu Welch's wife was a beautiful and very charming person. Towards
> the end of her pregnancy, she began to have very bad abdominal pain. I
> think they thought it was due to some complication of pregnancy. . . .
> The abdominal symptoms and signs progressed, and within just a day
> or two [after delivery], Dr. McKittrick operated on her, with me as
> assistant. We found her entire small bowel and much of her large bowel
> to be black and stinking with advanced gangrene.
>
> It is the sort of thing where, nowadays, I think we would go ahead
> with a truly massive resection and then try to hope that she could get
> along with total intravenous feeding, or that you and other people who
> are heavily involved in all sorts of new ventures in transplantation,
> would be able to give her some new small bowel. . . . As it was [in
> 1944], we simply closed her up, and told her and her husband what we
> had found. She faced up to death with great courage, and went ahead
> and died in about a day. That is really all I can tell you.

Like Moore, Welch was a precocious star in surgery. At the age of
thirty-five he was the youngest surgical chair in the United States and
one of the most respected. His young wife had died from a missed
diagnosis of a surgical condition, something for which he took the
blame. Whether it was really this simple I have no way of knowing.
What I do know is that he remembered it this way. He quit his job and
left Boston. After a while, he settled in Albany where he practiced
surgery and taught at Albany Medical College. He died of a heart
attack in 1980, on the morning of his seventy-first birthday.

It seemed to me, as the late night phone calls became more
friendly and open, that Dr. Welch thought that he had lost every-

thing dear to him. For the most part, this was true. Except for one thing. He was the first person to think of transplanting the liver, or at least the first to try it as he did in his dogs ten years after his wife had died. Was this "irrational thought" born of sorrow? It did not really matter any more. The idea would not be erased from the record or lost in obscurity.

» «

The claim made at the ASA that portal blood has special liver-supporting qualities not found in other kinds of venous blood is accepted now. In 1964 the concept was heretical and provoked the most serious expressions of disbelief by almost all students of the liver. It would require a dozen more years of work to convince the last of the skeptics that the claim was true and even longer to establish that insulin was the most important of the hepatotrophic factors. These were issues of basic science. At a practical level, we were gearing up to attempt auxiliary transplantation and needed to determine quantitatively how much portal blood was needed to ensure the metabolic health of the extra liver, as well as other details of the auxiliary graft operation. The studies, also carried out in dogs, were spearheaded by a young surgeon named Thomas L. Marchioro.

Marchioro grew up in Butte, Montana, where his father before him, and then he, descended into the copper mines by day, knowing nothing of sunlight except on weekends. He worked his way through high school, then college, and finally medical school at St. Louis University. When the time came for surgical training, Tom bounced from the St. Louis University program to the Henry Ford Hospital program in Detroit, and then to Colorado. He was hard to please and was not particularly preoccupied with pleasing others.

When I arrived at the University of Colorado in December 1961, Marchioro was chief resident at the Colorado General Hospital, an appointment analogous to that of Bob Brittain, my chief resident at the VA. I was looking for talent, and both men had it to spare. They were exceptionally skilled clinical surgeons and natural scientists who considered themselves products of the Swan era (Henry Swan was the previous chair of the Department of Surgery) rather than having much new to learn from Waddell (the new chair) and me.

Each played a critical role in the development of the Colorado Transplant Program, Brittain briefly and Marchioro until he left in 1967 to become chief of the Division of Transplantation at the University of Washington, Seattle.

A transplant surgeon was the last thing Marchioro wanted to be until 1962. Strongly influenced by Swan, his ambition was to be a heart surgeon, and he had trained for this. His misfortune was that he was assigned for a year to Lyon (France) during 1960–61 when Swan was removed from the Colorado chairmanship. By the time he returned, a slightly older and very competent Scottish surgeon named Bruce Paton, also a product of the Swan heart surgery program, had been assigned the difficult task of picking up the pieces of the cardiac service. The service had shrunk, and there was no room for another person.

For Marchioro, I was a booby prize, but for me he was the grand prize. I named him assistant chief of surgery at the VA Hospital when he finished his chief residency in June 1962. He became everyone's favorite teacher—residents and students alike. Once he made the commitment to the embryonic transplantation service, no effort was too great to make it work. His indispensable role in the Colorado donor efforts was mentioned in Will Goodwin's report of his visit to Colorado (see chapter 9).

In his studies of portal blood in dogs, Marchioro did two further kinds of experiment, each of which resulted in a classic of the surgical literature. In one, he repeated the experiments reported at the ASA, except that the auxiliary liver grafts were given the recipient's portal venous blood instead of allowing this special kind of blood to go to the dog's own liver. Now the graft retained its size and its normal appearance under the microscope whereas the dog's own liver shrank. When the dog's own liver was removed one hundred or so days later, the auxiliary liver graft was able to maintain life.[3]

The second classic study did not involve transplantation. In these experiments, the animal's own liver was divided into two parts. Half was given the normal portal inflow from the intestines, stomach, and pancreas. The other half was given all of the venous blood returning to the heart from the legs, pelvis, body trunk, and

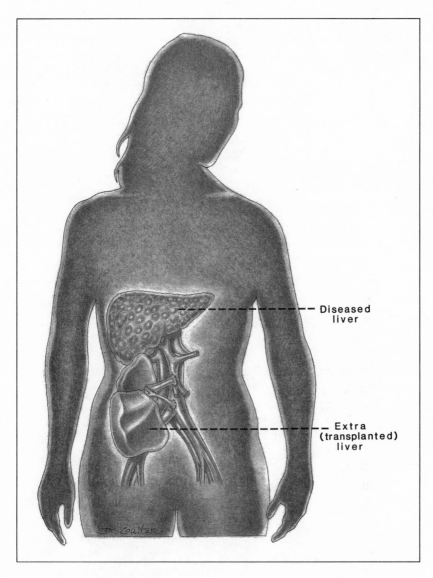

Figure 8. Transplantation of an extra liver within the abdomen but below the patient's own diseased liver.

kidneys. The results from this crucial experiment were unequivocal. The liver fragment given the blood returning from the pancreas, intestines, and stomach grew in size and was healthy. The fragment given the substitute blood shrank to a nubbin. The relative sizes of the two liver fragments adjusted themselves with the mysterious wisdom of nature. One fragment became large and the other small so that the weight of the combination added up to that of a single normal liver.[4]

Efforts to understand how liver size and growth are controlled in these and other experiments would continue in our laboratory for many more years. For the moment, the implications were less sweeping. They gave us the incentive to begin clinical trials with the seemingly less radical operation of auxiliary liver transplantation. We thought that we knew the necessary conditions to transplant an extra liver successfully.

Instead, we failed again in three attempts at auxiliary transplantation during 1965. So did five other teams between 1965 and 1967 in Minnesota, California, Australia, England, and Scotland. One of our three patients lived for thirty-five days. Halfway through 1967, this was the longest survival in the world after either auxiliary liver transplantation or liver replacement. Worldwide, the auxiliary trials had failed because of the inability to obtain good organs, transplant them without surgical complications, control rejection, or prevent lethal infections. Most commonly, it was a combination of these factors.

Providing an extra organ would not be the easy solution to liver transplantation. There were too many weak or missing links for the successful transplantation of the liver or, for that matter, of any organ beyond the kidney. The most pivotal deficiency was inadequate antirejection therapy. If this could be corrected, liver transplantation might succeed, and when it did, the best operation would be liver replacement, not the engraftment of an extra liver.

13

A Counterattack on Rejection

My assumption in the strategy to develop liver transplantation was that advances in controlling kidney rejection would be applicable to the transplantation of all organs, essentially without change. This belief was the reason for developing a kidney transplant program as a pathfinder for the technically more difficult liver replacement. However, at the time K. A. Porter, the London pathologist, visited Colorado in October 1963, no one had been able to demonstrate truly long survival of dogs submitted to liver transplantation.

This disquieting fact, plus the failure of the clinical trials in Denver, Boston, and Paris, caused a growing suspicion that there might be some fundamental difference that made it more difficult to protect the liver from rejection. We began a full-scale evaluation of this question in the autumn of 1963. The dog transplantations were performed at the VA research laboratories in Denver with weekly or twice weekly shipments of the resulting tissues to Porter in London.

Approximately four experiments per week were carried out over the next fourteen months. Considering the complexity of the operations and aftercare, it is hard in looking back to imagine the magnitude of the effort. On the morning of November 22, 1963, we were in the middle of one of these operations when someone rushed in to tell us that President Kennedy had been shot. After a moment of silence, we decided to complete the operation, hoping that we could take a small step forward and honor him. We failed. The dog with the sign "J.F.K." on the cage died several weeks later.

It was not until March 23, 1964, that we produced the first life-time survivor in the world after liver transplantation. This dog lived for almost twelve years before dying of old age. After this, successes came steadily. These were not attributable to any single factor, but were due to accretion of small details in surgical skills and post-operative management. Half of the animals treated with Imuran lived for twenty-five to fifty days, and about one in five had very long survival.[1] The results were similar to those which we obtained after dog kidney transplantation in 1962—with one difference.

In many of the liver recipients it was possible to stop treatment after three or four months without evidence of subsequent rejection. This drug-free state, in which the animal's immune system appeared to have lost its antagonism to the graft, also had been seen in dog kidney recipients but far less commonly. It seemed likely that rejection of the liver might be easier to control than that of other organs. A few years later, much stronger evidence that this was true was provided from pig experiments by a Frenchman named Henri Garnier and in England by workers at Bristol (Peacock and Terblanche) and Cambridge (Calne).

Porter's pathologic studies filled in other missing information. He redefined the features of acute liver rejection and delineated those of chronic rejection. His expertise with two different transplanted organs (kidney and liver) allowed him to develop generalizations about the rejection of all organs which made it unnecessary to start over when hearts, lungs, and pancreases came along later.

Important as these experiments were in establishing the commonality of all solid organs, we did not see in the results a cause for celebration. They settled once and for all the issue of feasibility of liver transplantation but not of practicality. For human cases, all livers would have to come from cadaveric donors. It was clearer than ever that these livers would be more difficult to protect from rejection than the "easy" human kidneys from family donors that had fanned our enthusiasm in 1962 and 1963. We would need some therapy beyond the Imuran-prednisone combination that had made kidney transplantation possible.

» «

It was amazing how fast progress was made when there was no clinical field of transplantation and how difficult it became when transplantation was accorded specialty status and began to develop a collective wisdom. The transition from ground zero to a finite level of expectation had occurred by revolution and was complete by 1964. Hot on its heels came an international organization of which I was the second vice-president. The group was modestly called *the* Transplantation Society. The first American transplant organization, the now powerful American Society of Transplant Surgeons (ASTS) did not come into being until 1975, one year before the British Transplantation Society. As the founding president of the ASTS, my main functions were to give the first presidential address and then self-destruct.

In my inaugural, I reflected on the nature and difficulty of progress, using the work of the medical historian T. S. Kuhn as reference. I described "how progress consists of a series of great and small revolutions against authority. A great advance necessitates the overthrow of an established dogma, and when that occurs the advance itself becomes the new dogma to which advocates flock. It is natural for those disciples to become protectors instead of improvers of the *status quo*, guardians of the past instead of seekers of the future. To make matters formal, they might even consider creating a society which, if unaware of the dangers, could be the means by which the next stages of development were blocked."[2]

This was not idle chatter. I was speaking of the doctrines that I had introduced in 1963 and 1964, whose limitation we had defined almost before they had become dogma. I knew perfectly well by the end of 1965 or even earlier that improved (and of necessity, different) antirejection treatment would hold the key to further real movement in the field. Tissue matching would have a marginal impact, or perhaps none at all, on transplantation from nonrelated donors. Yet the dogmas that were fiercely defended for the next dozen years were, first, that the standard treatment to prevent rejection was the double drug combination of Imuran and prednisone, and second, that tissue matching would be the means by which the greatest future gains could be achieved. The fervor with which these obsolete positions were held and would continue to be by the following generation of kidney transplant physicians and surgeons, and by tissue typers, was an extreme manifestation of the Kuhn Syndrome.

» «

Professional societies can themselves be impediments to progress and the instruments by which old idolatries can inhibit creative movement. Before the formation of these new transplantation societies, their most important potential function—the free exchange of information and ideas—was carried out by the New York Academy of Sciences. Every year, starting in 1954, meetings on transplantation were held in New York City and attended by those who had an interest in this field. The few who came published their reports a few months later in the *Proceedings of the New York Academy of Sciences*, which served as the specialty journal for the field until the founding of *Transplantation* in 1964 and *Transplantation Proceedings* in 1968. Before 1964, the only other outlet for publication was the Transplantation Bulletin, an appendix in the mid-1950s of the *Journal of Plastic and Reconstructive Surgery*. Joe Murray, the pioneer kidney transplant surgeon from Boston, was a practicing plastic surgeon, and so was another key figure, John Converse of New York City.

Those who were there during these antediluvian days credit the arrangements with the New York Academy to two men, John Converse and Felix Rapaport, who were destined to be the first elected president and secretary respectively of the Transplantation Society. Converse was a master surgeon and an acknowledged founder of modern plastic surgery, being chief of this specialty program at New York University. In addition to his powers as a clinician, he also possessed unusual insight into the biologic problems of skin transplantation. He was married to the widow of the movie star Gary Cooper, and he himself could have passed for a screen idol. Even when he was old and ill, his appearance and presence put him above normal men.

One of his star pupils was Felix Rapaport, a person of shorter stature and less photogenic qualities, who joined Converse in research in 1954 at the age of twenty-five. That Rapaport was there at all was a quirk of fate. He escaped Hitler's furnaces and came to the United States when he was fifteen. Many members of his family who stayed behind, including his aunts and uncles, died in concentration camps. While still a medical student at New York University, Rapaport became Converse's partner in the management of the New York Academy transplantation symposiums and conferences. Later, he was one of the earliest clinical transplant scientists and made crucial contributions to the establishment of the human histocompatibility (tissue typing) system. These administrative, work-bench, and clinical experiences equipped him for his long later tenure as editor of *Transplantation Proceedings*, which became the organ of the Transplantation Society after its founding. In 1978, he was elected the ninth president of the Transplantation Society.

» «

The swan song of the New York Academy sponsorship of transplantation occurred in 1966. Fueled now by enthusiasm from the successful clinical trials of kidney transplantation, the annual meetings at the Waldorf Astoria Hotel had swollen to unmanageable size and complexity. The time had come for formation of the Transplantation Society. In his address on February 22, 1966, the founding president of the new society, Sir Peter Medawar, combined his last talk to the old organization with his first remarks to the new one. He predicted that the next advance in antirejection therapy would be with a substance called antilymphocyte serum (ALS). The history of ALS was a long one and could be traced back to the turn of the century.

Ilya Ilyitch Metchnikov, a Russian pathologist who was working then at the Pasteur Institute in Paris, envisioned using ALS preparations to deliberately destroy the cells which he suggested might be responsible for certain human diseases. In 1899, Metchnikov wrote:

The time is not remote when medical art will actively intervene to maintain the integrity of the whole organism, the harmony of which is broken by the preponderance of certain cells, mononuclear cells in the atrophies, several other elements in the malignant diseases. Therefore, I undertook the study of the effect produced by the resorption of macrophages. To attain this end I initially injected guinea pigs subcutaneously with an emulsion of rat spleen or lymph nodes ground up in saline solution. Forty-seven days after this injection, guinea pig serum agglutinated and dissolved rat leukocytes. Mononuclear cells were the most sensitive and were converted into transparent vesicles. Later the granulocytes underwent the same changes and finally the mast cells.[3]

In his experimental studies Metchnikov had immunized guinea pigs by injecting into them cells obtained from rat organs (the spleen and lymph nodes) which contain large numbers of lymphocytes. More than a half century later these same lymphocytes were identified as the cells that reject transplants. After immunization of the guinea pigs, he demonstrated that their serum came to possess something that would destroy the lymphocytes of rats. He concluded that he had found a way to target and kill specific cell lines by raising a substance (antibodies) against these cells in another animal species.

Neither Metchnikov nor anyone else of that time knew anything about transplantation, or that these targeted cells were the same ones responsible for graft rejection. However, with a flash of clairvoyance Metchnikov had identified the fundamental reason for human disorders called *autoimmune diseases*: psoriasis, multiple sclerosis, sugar diabetes, ulcerative colitis, and many others. Long after Metchnikov's death, his idea of eliminating the cell lines guilty of causing these diseases was shown to be sound. The pursuit of this fantasy was through transplantation (see chapter 25).

ALS preparations for experimental skin grafting were first used about three decades ago at Yale University (Byron Waksman), Edinburgh University (Michael Woodruff), and at Harvard (Anthony Monaco and Paul Russell). A tidal wave of publications followed, including those from Medawar's English laboratory. In these experiments, rabbits were immunized against the lymphocytes of mice, guinea pigs, or rats. The rabbit serum was injected inside the abdomen of the treated animals. Skin grafts placed between mice, between guinea pigs, or between rats survived for prolonged periods instead of being promptly rejected.

One reason for the importance of Medawar's lecture on ALS was his enthusiasm. Having discovered the antirejection effects of the steroid drugs many years earlier (see chapter 8), Medawar realized immediately that the ALS preparations were far more potent than anything he had worked with. He thought that ALS therapy should be tried in patients. However, there were some practical barriers, one of which was the resistance to change by clinicians who were reluctant to alter the double drug therapy with Imuran and steroids which they recently had been taught and of which they now were fervent disciples.

Their concern had credibility. The infusion or injection of raw animal serum into humans was not a particularly palatable idea, especially when the dosage into the abdomen would be several gallons if the available experimental information was applied to clinical practice. In addition, an animal larger than the rabbit would be a preferable host to raise the antibodies against human lymphocytes. The horse was a candidate. Finally, there was no reason to give the whole animal serum to patients when the antibody activity was presumably limited to some small fraction of which the location was suspected but not proved.

I was thrilled by Medawar's lecture because we were far along in research on ALS that was designed to achieve what he was passionately advocating. We were gearing up for clinical trials. The suggestion for this project had come from K. A. Porter, who was aware of rat experiments on ALS being done in Britain.

Beginning in the summer of 1964, we had selected the horse as a serum donor, identified the gamma globulin (one of the protein fractions) in the horse serum where the desired antilymphocyte antibodies were located, learned how to remove and purify this fraction (which we called *antilymphoid globulin*, ALG), and devised test-tube analyses which would allow us to estimate its potency.

The leader of this research team was Yoji Iwasaki, a Japanese surgeon who today is chair of the Department of Surgery at Tsukuba University near Tokyo. When Iwasaki returned home, he sent another surgeon, Noboru Kashiwagi, to take his place in Denver. Kashiwagi now is professor of experimental surgery at Kitasato University. Every step in the process of manufacturing ALG was tested in the dog with both kidney and liver transplantation. The lymphocytes for injection into the horse were removed from these tissues in the same way that Metchnikov must have used two-thirds of a century earlier.

Finally, everything was ready to treat patients. In June and July 1966, the first patients in the world to be treated with ALG could be picked out of a crowd of their transplant peers at the Colorado General or Denver VA hospitals. The ALG was given into the muscles of the buttock and caused such severe pain and swelling that the patients constantly walked the floors trying to rid themselves of what felt like a charley horse. They sat crookedly on chairs and formed their own support group to exchange tall tales, and especially complaints. The injections were given every day for one or two weeks, and every other day for another two weeks. Chalk marks appeared on the patients' walls noting surreptitiously how many shots had been given and how many remained before the gauntlet would be finished.

The trial was a success. Rejection was practically eliminated during the period of ALG therapy if treatment was started at the time of transplantation. If ALG treatment was delayed, it could be used effectively to reverse established rejection. The amounts of Imuran and prednisone (especially the latter) were reduced.[4] This was the beginning of the triple drug antirejection therapy (Imuran-prednisone-ALG) that marked the new plateau from which transplantation of all whole organs would develop for the next dozen years. The introduction of triple drug therapy meant that liver transplantation could start again, and not far behind would come the heart, lung, pancreas, and intestine.

As always happens, improvements were made in ALG therapy. Purer preparations of human lymphocytes could be obtained by collecting them from the large lymph channel called the thoracic duct that returns lymphocytes from the lower body to one of the neck veins (J. Traeger of Lyon, France, and Rudi Pichlmayr of Hannover, Germany) or by culturing lymphocytes in test tubes. The technique of lymphocyte culture was developed by George Moore of Roswell Park Hospital in Buffalo and applied by John Najarian, Richard Condie, and Richard Simmons at the University of Minnesota. Also, the ALG could be given intravenously instead of into the muscle, eliminating the injection pain which for some patients was almost unendurable.

Although the ALG was useful in preventing or treating rejec-

tion, its limitations also were defined. Unlike Imuran or prednisone, it could not be used for chronic treatment because the
patient's immune system soon began to react against the injected
horse protein. What we had accomplished was a significant but not
a quantum improvement in patient care. The main penalty for use
of ALG was a higher incidence of virus infections, including those
associated with new cancer formation.

The ALG story is not finished yet. Ben Cosimi, one of our
Colorado medical students, assisted with the development of ALG
for human use before leaving for the Massachusetts General Hospital in July 1964 to begin his surgical training. His dream was to
produce a more practical and safer ALG, an objective which came
within reach when G. Kohler and C. Milstein of Cambridge
University (Nobel laureates, 1984) developed their so-called hy-
bridoma technology. This method is too complex and peripheral to
our story to discuss in detail beyond saying that clones of single
immortalized cells could be created, all of which produced exactly
the same antibody (a monoclonal antibody) that bound to and
inactivated the target lymphocytes only, without damaging innocent bystander cells. The first patients to receive this kind of ALG,
called OKT3, were treated by Cosimi at the Massachusetts General
Hospital in 1980.

The possibility still is being actively pursued of narrowing the sub-
population of lymphocyte targets or other cell types involved in
immune reactions in order to create safer and more specific versions of
these so-called monoclonal antibodies, each for a well-defined therapeutic purpose. This means that Metchnikov's once absurd vision is
more real now than on the day he had it almost a century ago.

» «

When a new treatment is tried, something changes in the atmosphere of the hospital wards. Doctors, nurses, and patients alike
become scientists with senses alert, looking for signs of danger and
signs of benefit—looking for anything new. It is a good time for
learning but sometimes what is learned has no relation to what is
being sought.

The summer of 1966 was like that. In June, Burl Osborne, a
young journalist from the state of Washington, came to Colorado

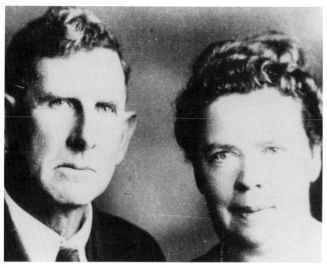

Thomas Patrick Fitzgerald and Catherine Ann Mangan, my Irish grandparents.

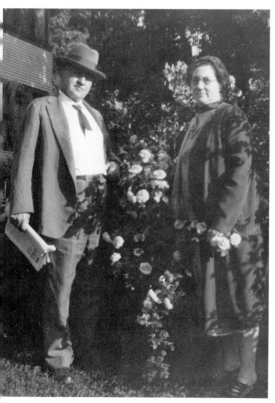

John V. Starzl, publisher of the LeMars *Globe Post*, and Margaret Theisen, my paternal grandparents.

My mother, Anna Laura Fitzgerald (R), with her sister Caroline.

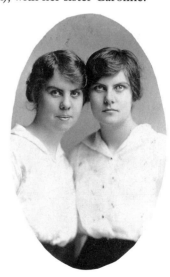

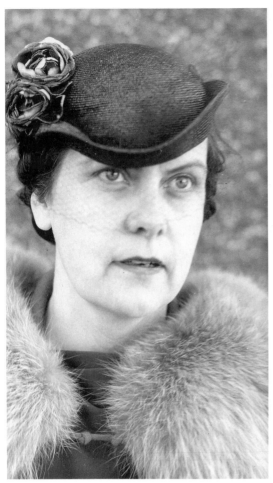

Mother, about 1939.

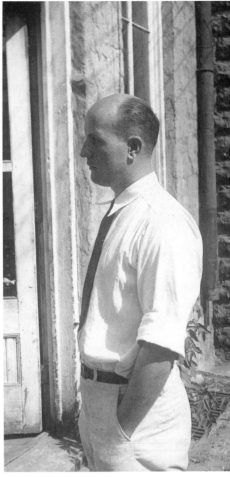

My father, R. F. Starzl, about 1935.

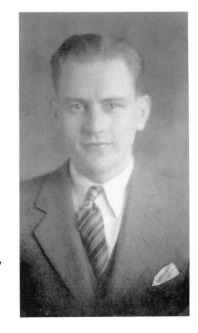

Uncle Frank Starzel in his early twenties, about 1925.

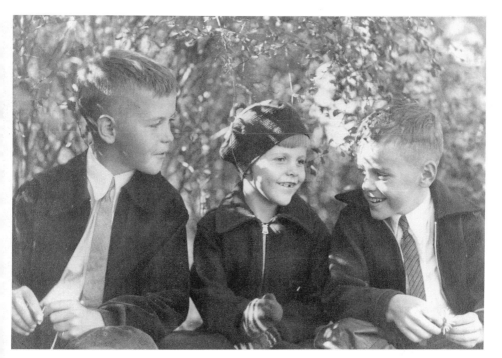

With my brother John (L) and my sister Nancy.

Christmas 1975. Becky and Tim are on my right; Barbara and Tom on my left.

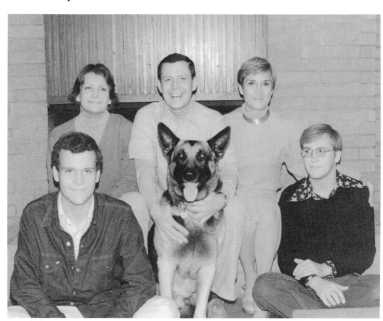

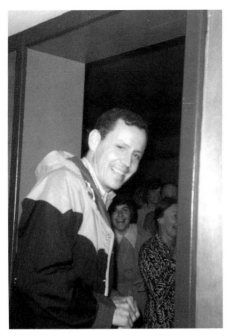

The surprise party to celebrate my fiftieth birthday, March 1976.

The Arctic expedition, June 1972. *Photo by Charles Putnam*

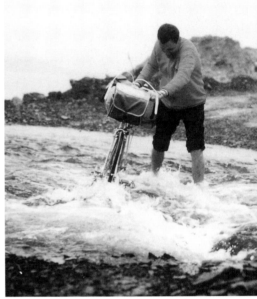

On the way to Long's Peak in the Rockies, 1977. *Photo by Joy Starzl*

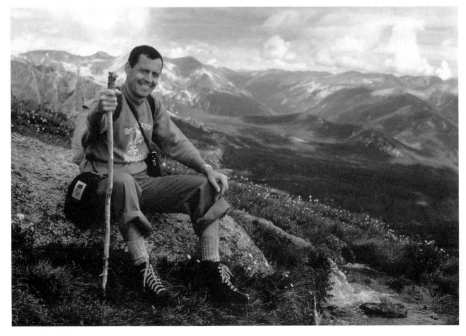

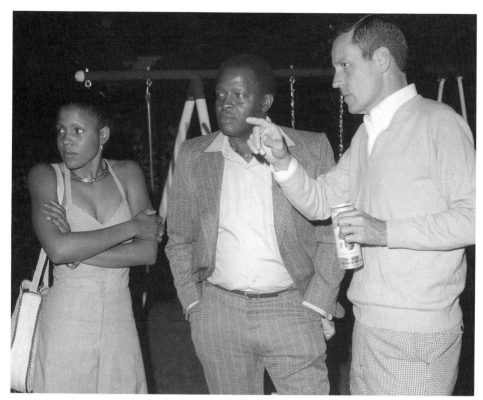

With Joy and her father, James Conger, 1977. *Photo by Paul Taylor*

With Joy (and someone else's car) in Rome, November 1980.

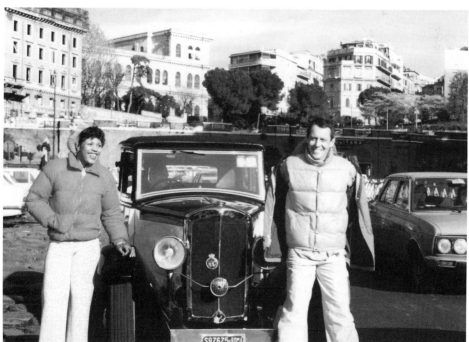

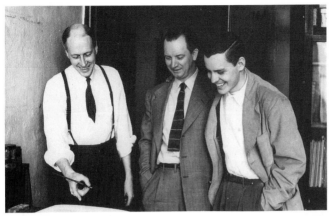

With Horace W. Magoun (L) and Donald Lindsey, Chicago 1950. *Neuroscience History Program, Brain Research Institute, UCLA*

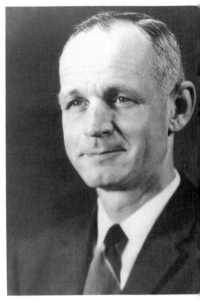

William R. Waddell, about 1960.

Paul Taylor, with a dog that lived over thirteen years after liver transplantation. *Medical Illustration Laboratory, VA Hospital, Denver*

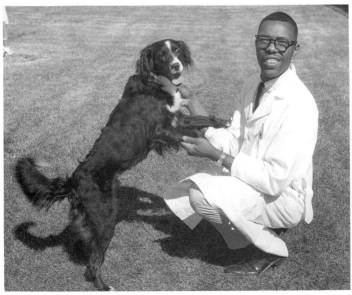

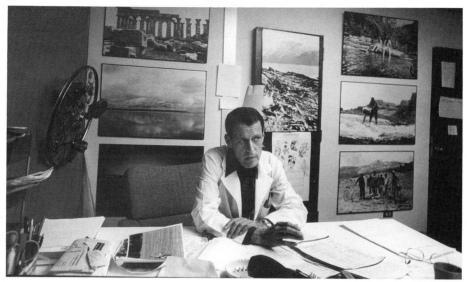

The chairman's office, Denver 1976.
Photo by Carl Iwasaki

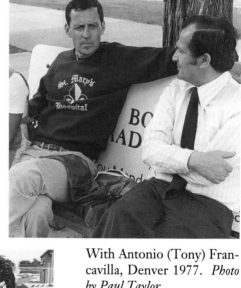

The Denver organ retrieval team in
Sioux City, Iowa, September 1980.
From L to R: Shun Iwatsuki, myself,
Richard Rubenstein (a Sioux City
surgeon who cooperated with the
visiting group) and Gerald Jurkovich.

With Antonio (Tony) Fran-
cavilla, Denver 1977. *Photo
by Paul Taylor*

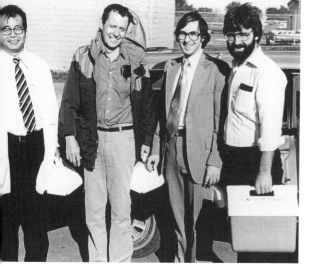

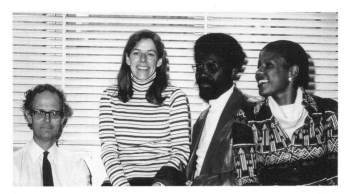

Kendrick A. Porter (L) in his London laboratory, November 1977. With him are (L to R) his secretary, Anthea Phelps, Paul Taylor, and Joy.

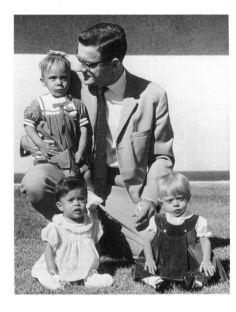

Carl Groth with the first survivors of liver transplantation, Denver 1967. Julie Rodriquez sits on his knee; the others are Kerri Brown (L) and Paula Hanson (R). *Medical Illustration Laboratory, VA Hospital, Denver*

With Shun Iwatsuki on the beach at Malibu, 1980, after deciding not to move the transplantation program to UCLA. *Photo by Paul Taylor*

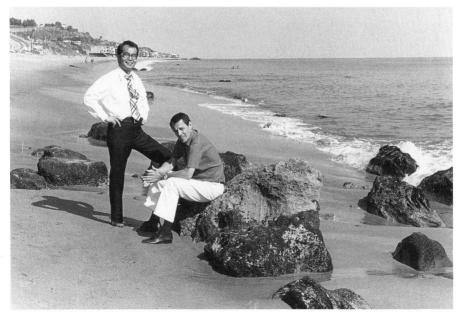

General Hospital for a kidney transplantation from his mother. He arrived just in time to be the third person in the world to be treated with triple drug antirejection therapy that included ALG. Shortly before he came, something terrible had happened to Mary Cunningham, a twenty-three-year-old woman from Fort Collins, Colorado, whose transplantation was a few days too early for the new treatment. Both of them, or the two together, taught me something which took more than fifteen years to fully learn. By the time it sank in, Mary was long since dead.

Until that summer, I must have subconsciously viewed the transplant recipient as a delicate piece of fragile glass, existing in a separate and low-function world. Mary, the thirty-first patient in our kidney series, had received a kidney from an unrelated donor on September 3, 1963. The graft worked well, but at each clinic visit the steroid effects deepened. Her face rounded, acne marred her once smooth skin, a small mustache appeared on her upper lip, and her body slowly transformed into an amorphous lump. The price of survival was too high.

Mary's boyfriend saw her as she had been, not as she was. He wanted to marry her, and one day in clinic they timidly asked my permission. I tried to point out the unknown future and asked whether they would want to have a baby, not knowing what the chances were of her living to raise the child. They said yes.

After this, Mary started to change back, slowly regaining her original form and face. Was she reducing her steroid dose? I believe she did, although she denied it. She began an exercise program and seemed happy for the first time since the transplantation. She told me that she might have a baby with or without being married.

Then the graft failed, sending her back briefly to the artificial kidney which she hated. On May 18, 1966, she received a second kidney graft, this one from a cadaver donor, giving her a matching scar on the other side of her lower abdomen. The new organ did not work, and on June 7 a third cadaver kidney was placed, this one in the bed of the first graft, which was removed. It functioned, but now Mary's lungs collapsed and became clouded with pneumonia.

A tube was placed in her wind pipe through an incision in the front of her neck (tracheotomy). Other desperate measures were taken to give her enough air. I stayed with her and tried to reinflate her collapsed lungs with a bag that helped breathing when I squeezed it with my hands. She did not try to move. When I looked up, her eyes were filled with tears and after a short time, she was dead.

Except for children, it was always a protection not to call patients by their first names. It made things easier if something like this happened. I do not know why Mary was Mary instead of Miss Cunningham as she should have been. She had slipped through the net, which was becoming more porous every day. Here was a friend, and the question would always be whether we could have done better.

Burl Osborne came to the hospital a few days later, confident that he would win. Except for having renal failure, he had led a charmed life. When his own kidneys failed, he was lucky to be in the state of Washington where chronic artificial kidney treatment had been started by Belding Scribner. The technology had spread to Burl's city of Spokane, where a young physician named Peter Ivanovich (later professor of medicine at Northwestern) operated a satellite dialysis unit. Ivanovich called me because Burl had had heart stoppages requiring closed cardiac massage, one of these being followed by a convulsion. Ivanovich was concerned that one of these incidents would be fatal or cause brain injury and was anxious to proceed with transplantation as soon as possible.

Because he had been hired for his position with the Associated Press in Spokane by my Uncle Frank (see chapter 2), my anxiety was higher than usual on the day of Burl's operation, July 27, 1966. His new kidney worked well and, except for complaints of sore buttocks from the hated ALG injections, his recovery was uncomplicated. Being an able journalist, he knew a good story and wanted to write one about ALG, as well as a second story on the total Colorado program. He may have been angry about my resistance to this and my conviction that our confidential relationship with him superseded his ambition to disclose what he had learned personally. He honored our request, but was never comfortable with what he claimed was an abridgement of freedom of the press. He went back to work quickly.

The next time I saw him, he was on his way to Aspen for a ski vacation. Although moon-faced from steroids, he was bursting with energy and confidence. "Please don't go," was my advice. I could imagine that his bones, thinned and weakened by the steroids, would crack with the first hard fall. He went anyway, and did so every year until I left Colorado at the end of 1980.

By the time I saw him in 1980, he had advanced through the ranks of the Associated Press and was managing editor, with an office in New York City. He was being interviewed for a new job as executive editor of the Dallas *Morning News*. The health division of the newspaper and Burl himself were concerned about his staying power and the extent to which his ancient kidney transplantation would affect his performance both immediately and in the future. They sent me X-rays of his chest, which showed some old scars and irregularities that had been there on earlier examinations and were unchanged.

My advice was different than that which I gave Mary Cunningham and had tried to give Burl fifteen years earlier when he struggled to escape from my restrictions. Now I told him that he should fly as far and fast as he was able, and assured him that if his wings came off I would try to catch him. My advice to the *Morning News* was to judge his candidacy in the same way as for any other healthy and talented executive being considered for recruitment. There were no guarantees for anyone.

Not long after this, Burl came back to Denver as a journalist. His mission was to find out why I was leaving the University of Colorado to go to Pittsburgh. Many people were looking for a conventional explanation such as fiscal irregularity in my department, a power struggle within the school, or estrangement with the university governance authorities—dean, chancellor or regents. The reasons were much more complex and personal. Burl sat with me for a morning while I talked with a reporter for the university newspaper, the *Silver and Gold* (published in Boulder), who had written an article full of speculation about such questions and more. I wanted to have the opinion of a responsible journalist on whether to take legal action and that was why I asked Osborne to join us. After the reporter left, Burl told me that the question was not whether to bring a libel suit, but only for how much. This would be a suit against an instrument of my own university. I told him that I could not do it. The reporter printed a retraction and later joined the staff of the *Rocky Mountain News*, a member of the Scripps-Howard newspaper chain.

Privately, I told Burl that I was leaving Colorado for two reasons. First, I did not believe liver transplantation could go forward in a center that did not see a future for this kind of treatment and would not take the steps necessary to make it feasible. Beyond this, I confided that there were personal reasons to leave Denver, and what these were. When I asked him if he regarded my plan to go to another university as foolish or unrealistic, he laughed and reminded me of my earlier advice to him: "Do what you want, and go as far and fast as you can."

In June 1991, Burl Osborne, publisher and editor of the Dallas *Morning News*, passed the magic quarter-century mark after his kidney transplantation. Many have made it by now, but it is still a significant event medically. His life has been a great success, and I have watched it from a respectful distance. He has reciprocated with mine. Perhaps he has done more than if he had run the race of life without the handicap.

I can not remember calling Mr. Osborne anything but Burl. Like Mary Cunningham, he had slipped through the net and become a friend, but unlike Mary I had not treated him like a frail vessel to be shielded from life's insults by a solicitous physician. I was his doctor, but in the long run, who helped whom?

14

The Donors and the Organs

As 1966 dawned, our moratorium on liver replacement had entered its third year. It seemed certain that improved antirejection treatment soon would be available with ALG. Whether this alone would allow resumption of the suspended liver trials was anything but clear. Two additional issues needed resolution, and both were on the agenda of the first symposium on the medical ethics of transplantation which was held in London at the Ciba Foundation house March 8–11, 1966.[1] One of these topics was human experimentation. The other was organ donation.

For all practical purposes, organ transplantation still was synonymous with kidney grafting. Kidney transplantation burst onto the scene so unexpectedly in the early 1960s that little forethought had been given to its impact on society. Nor had its relation to existing legal, philosophic, or religious systems been considered. Procedures and policies were largely left to the conscience and common sense of the transplant physicians and surgeons involved, who had acquitted themselves well. However, it was clear that these new procedures, which had been a curiosity only two or three years earlier, probably were going to be used widely and would be extended to other organs. Twenty-five participants were invited, including seven from the United States: Willard E. Goodwin (surgeon), David W. Louisell (lawyer), Joseph E. Murray (surgeon), Keith Reemtsma (surgeon), George E. Schreiner (physician), C. E. Wasmuth (anesthesiologist), and me (surgeon). The American universities represented were California (Berkeley and UCLA), Case

Western Reserve (Cleveland), Colorado, Georgetown, Harvard, and Tulane.

The appropriate conditions for human experimentation was the foremost concern because the medical atrocities of World War II were still fresh in the collective mind. Three of the European participants (David Daube, Regius Professor of Law, Oxford; Hugh Edward de Wardener, nephrologist at Charing Cross Hospital; and Michael Woodruff, professor of surgery, Edinburgh) had experienced violations of their own human rights almost beyond description during years spent in concentration or prisoner-of-war camps. Woodruff was a star prosecution witness in the Asian war crimes trials.

Two policy statements that were part of the postwar reaction to the European and Asian atrocities were index documents for the Ciba proceedings. One was the Nuremberg Code and the other was its successor, the Helsinki Declaration. The Helsinki Declaration was shorter and easier to read. It divided human experimentation into two categories. The first was advanced or innovative but unproven therapy that was being tried because it could be of direct and immediate benefit to the person who received it. This was primarily an attempt to treat, not to study. The second category was investigation that might benefit humankind but would not directly benefit the person undergoing study. In this case, the purpose was the acquisition of knowledge about humans, using humans as research subjects. The intention was not therapeutic.

The nature of surgery almost always limits its activities to the therapeutic category, or at least this had been the position of transplant surgeons in relation to their recipients. However, there was a potential conflict of purpose with the transplant donor, and this became a critical issue at the conference. In the early 1960s, the most convenient and usually the only donors for many patients needing kidneys were family members. An organ that could save the life of another person was removed from a healthy and well-motivated human being, a process well within the framework of conventional Judeo-Christian ethics. The act was compared to leaping into a lake to save someone who is drowning. But concerns about the conditions under which these donations take place already were troubling in 1966 and haunt us to this day.

The legal (and probably moral) basis for living donations dates back to a 1954 Massachusetts court ruling that permitted the identical-twin kidney transplantation by Joe Murray. The legal opinion reflected the probability that identical twins were so close, emotionally as well as in every other way, that the loss of a kidney by the donor would be less devastating in the holistic sense than the loss of an identical twin sibling. Similar reasoning in subsequent court cases was upheld and extended to other kidney donors, including parent-to-offspring and other intrafamilial combinations. This was the rationalization for the frequent use of family donors in the bellwether Colorado kidney transplant series in 1962–63.

This lofty justification notwithstanding, examples of donor abuse within families were being found. If a prospective donor was deficient in some way, usually intellectually, the family power structure tended to focus on his or her presumed expendability. In addition, I and others had seen refusal of donation lead to ostracism within a family, or donation made as a reluctant sacrifice to someone for whom there was little or no affection. The use of captive donors such as minor identical twins (in Boston) or volunteer convicts (in Colorado) was seriously questioned. The possibilities arose of donor coercion, commercialization, and injury or death of the donor. A donor death already had occurred at one of the premier centers represented at the Ciba meeting.

Although I was one of the first to use the expedient of living kidney donation and have never had a donor die, I was shaken by these discussions. The concept of living donation seemed less and less acceptable to me as the years went by. After the Ciba conference, I tried to avoid the practice without oppressing my colleagues who believed in its probity, and in 1972 I stopped using kidneys from any living donors.

Obtaining organs from people who are dead was the alternative. At the London meeting in 1966, the concept of *brain death* was broached for the first time by Guy Alexandre of Louvain, who described the removal of kidneys from "heart-beating" cadavers. Isolated examples of this practice in other European countries were reported. At first, this idea appalled me because I envisioned that the care of a trauma victim could be jeopardized by virtue of his or her candidacy to become an organ donor.

These fears were unfounded. The chances of a seriously injured patient being properly cared for were actually greatly increased when death was defined by the disappearance of brain function rather than by the criteria of cessation of heartbeat and respiration that had been used since ancient times. Under the circumstances that existed before, when someone with a serious brain injury was brought into the emergency room, the physicians often were obliged to make an on-the-spot decision about the patient's capability of survival. A negative decision precluded resuscitation since it was almost impossible to discontinue artificial lung support (ventilator) without being accused of a crime.

Dave Hume (Richmond) and Norm Shumway (the heart surgeon at Stanford) later would be charged with murdering such brain-dead donors whose organs were removed. The cases were dismissed. With the wide acceptance of brain death in the Western world, all injured patients who come to the hospital in a helpless condition could have a fair trial at resuscitation. Then, in an orderly way, it can be determined whether these people already were dead but with functioning hearts and lungs, or if they had a chance of restoration of brain function. The quality of care and the discriminate application of such care to terribly damaged people was one of the great fringe benefits of transplantation.

These legal and social reforms were not in effect during the first trials of liver transplantation in 1963 and would not be until 1968. Rather than trying to maintain a strong heartbeat and good circulation in the cadaver donors, the legal requirement before the end of 1968 was the opposite. Because all such donors were incapable of breathing if the brain actually had been destroyed, they were supported by ventilators. The steps to donation began with disconnection of the ventilator, which the public called "pulling the plug." During the five to ten minutes before the heart stopped and death was pronounced, the organs to be transplanted were variably damaged by oxygen starvation and the gradually failing and ultimately absent circulation.

The strategies that could be used to minimize the organ injury under these circumstances were limited, and those who were forced to use them correctly regarded them as cynical. As soon as the heart stopped and the donor was pronounced dead, the external heart message which I had watched being developed a dozen years earlier at the Johns Hopkins Hospital (chapter 4) was started along with restoration of the breathing machine.

The objective now was to restore the heartbeat and circulation, hoping that the damage to the organs just inflicted could be stopped or even undone. Usually, the heart could not be restarted, and then the technique of perfusing the whole corpse observed by Will Goodwin in 1963 in Denver could be used (chapter 9). No one was comfortable with these maneuvers. We feared that by following the letter of the law, we were violating its spirit and jeopardizing the lives of the organ recipients in the process. Was this elaborate sham necessary or moral?

A much earlier opinion, written by Pope Pius XII and introduced into the record of the 1966 London meeting by Raffaelo Cortesini of Rome, suggested that it was not. In this document Pope Pius had defined death as the departure of the spirit from the body (cessation of brain function) rather than loss of the pump action of the heart. Although this opinion concerned the discontinuance of mechanical support in patients who were brain dead apart from their consideration as organ donors, its applicability in transplantation was evident. The Catholic church would be an ally in the reforms that were crystallized in the so-called Harvard Ad Hoc Committee report two years later.[2] Public support for this report, which advocated acceptance of brain death, was overwhelming.

The United States and other countries quickly passed laws that gave legal sanction to what society had already decided. Death would be defined in terms of brain function from this time onward. Transplantation had changed the face of the law. Warren Burger, later to become chief justice of the U.S. Supreme Court, remarked at a medical ethics conference in 1967: "It is not the role and function of the law to keep pace with science . . . the law does not make discoveries as you do; the law evolves and evolves slowly. It responds rather than anticipates."[3] By the late 1960s the law had responded.

» «

Acceptance of brain death in 1968 was a boon to transplantation. The problem was that our new liver trials were being planned in 1966, not 1968. Paul Taylor, a black man who had been hired in the research laboratories for some pedestrian metabolic studies in 1962, also had been swept away by the transplant passion. He became a key player in all the laboratory studies. Now he would become an organ procurement officer whose task it was to visit hospitals throughout the region and identify victims of accidents or disease whose organs might still be useable.

The elaborate and self-defeating steps that still were required by law in order to be pronounced dead made it necessary for the donors to be at the Colorado General or VA Hospital, in an operating room adjacent to the kidney or liver recipient. Some of the bereaved families were willing to fly the bodies of their loved ones from as far away as California, breathing machines and all, in order to allow donation. After removal of the liver, time was still a critical factor. We believed that even if we were able to remove a relatively undamaged liver, we would not be able to preserve it for much longer than two or three hours unless some kind of blood flow could be supplied after it was removed.

The person who agreed to try to improve preservation in this way was Lawrence Brettschneider, a thirty-year-old surgeon and lieutenant commander in the U.S. Navy who was detached to Colorado for two years, beginning in the summer of 1966. Before long, Brettschneider began to assemble a complex machine that soon would be used to preserve human livers. A similar device had been used previously to preserve dog kidneys by John Ackermann and the South African heart surgeon, Christiaan Barnard.[4] How I met Barnard is worth explaining because apparently he was secretly planning a heart transplantation long before he performed this historic operation in Cape Town in December 1967. I was one of the necessary steps in his preparation although I did not know it.

During 1965, a young faculty member named J. A. (Bertie) Myburgh from Witwatersrand University, Johannesburg, came to the United States on a fellowship which he split between the universities of Utah and Colorado. After he returned home, his university offered me a visiting professorship endowed by a couple who owned a chain of stores as well as a national soccer team. The tenure of the Janey and Michael Miller Professorship was to be one month, during which Myburgh wanted me to help him set up the first kidney transplant program in Africa.

After spending the last two weeks of August 1966 training the Johannesburg nursing and surgical teams in the morgue, we carried out two kidney transplantations, using family donors. Myburgh went on from this start to make many contributions to transplantation surgery. A very talented man, he soon was appointed chair of his surgery department.

During the last few days of the visit, I was scheduled to fly from Johannesburg to Cape Town as the guest of the thoracic surgeon, Christiaan Barnard. The trip was canceled at the last minute because it was said that Barnard suddenly had picked up and gone to America for an extended stay. A short time after my return to Colorado, he showed up in Denver.

This was no casual visitor. He spent the better part of a year in the United States at three centers, first in Richmond with Richard Lower, who had developed heart transplantation in dogs with Norm Shumway at Minnesota and Stanford. Lower and Dave Hume (the surgery chair at Richmond) told me later that Barnard had seemed interested mainly in learning how to treat rejection. They assumed that he was going to start a kidney program in Cape Town and so did I.

During his visit to Colorado, Barnard was especially focused on the ALG that we were using for the first time in patients. I told him candidly that we were planning to go ahead with heart transplantation in Denver, but not until we were successful with the liver. Charles Halgrimson, a senior resident in surgery, had spent one year working in the VA research laboratory perfecting this operation, which is a far more difficult one in dogs than in humans. A chest surgeon named George Pappas had been recruited to the VA with the promise that heart transplantation would be the next item on our agenda. If Barnard had any such plans of his own, he did not mention them. Brettschneider and Barnard had a special affinity for each other. Both had an engaging manner with men and women alike. After he left us, Barnard went to Stanford to visit Shumway, whom he had known since their earlier days at the University of Minnesota.

The liver preservation apparatus, a modification of the Acker-mann-Barnard machine, was simple in concept. It was primed with chilled blood that was pumped through two plastic tubes, one to the liver artery and the other to the portal vein so that the preserved liver had a double blood supply after its removal from the body. After passing through the liver, the blood drained passively down a terraced cascade over which the liver was suspended and then back to a reservoir and pump to start around the circuit again.

The special feature of the system was its oxygen delivery. The liver as well as the blood draining from it were kept inside a high pressure chamber similar to those used to prevent (or treat) the bends in deep sea divers. The so-called hyperbaric chamber was built by the Bethlehem Steel Corporation in Pennsylvania. During its use, the oxygen was kept at three atmospheres (sea level is one atmosphere). In this high oxygen environment, the cold blood in the system always was red, meaning that it was full of oxygen.

It was possible with this device to preserve dog livers for as long as a day, an enormous improvement. Brettschneider presented his results at the surgical forum of the American College of Surgeons in October 1967 and in a more detailed report the following year.[5] He achieved celebrity status overnight and found himself on the Euro-pean lecture tour, visiting exotic places which for him had been only pictures in books. He was elected to membership in the prestigious Society of University Surgeons at a precocious age. Those in academic life feared that his remarkable potential could not be reached when he returned to the active military duty to which he was committed.

Brettschneider accepted the acclaim he deserved. His initiative had been responsible for the project, and his passion for it had seen it through. However, there was a darker side to his meteoric rise that was known only to a few of his colleagues in Denver. Because he was left-handed he complained that most special instruments of that period were constructed for right-handed surgeons. In addition, he had an acquired handicap known as "baseball finger" which is caused by an abnormal attachment of one of the finger tendons following an injury. He believed that these limitations precluded his personally doing the actual surgical experiments. The donor operations were performed by Pierre Daloze, an exceptionally gifted French Canadian fellow who subsequently became chair of the surgery department of the University of Montreal (Hôpital Notre Dame). I did the recipient operations, which were progressively more difficult with each additional hour of preservation time.

When Brettschneider returned to the navy, it was assumed that he had surgical skills of which he was not capable. He became prone to violent outbursts of anger. Ben Eiseman, the Denver surgeon who was himself a naval officer and a friend of Brettschneider, recommended to Admiral David P. Osbourne, the commandant of the U.S. Naval Hospital in Bethesda, that Brettschneider's request for discharge from the service be honored. After this was done in 1970, Larry had short-lived academic appointments at George Washington University, Tulane, Loyola, and the University of Oregon.

While Brettschneider was at Tulane, Ted Drapanas, chair of the department of surgery, sent him to an orthopedic surgeon in New York who treated baseball players with the kind of injury that affected the index finger of his left hand. After each of several operations, the reattached tendon was torn off again. Brettschneider left Tulane and took positions in Chicago, Portland, and finally Vancouver (Washington). At the end came oblivion at his own hand in the spring of 1978, only ten years after his star had burned so brightly. He put a gun in his mouth, and with the defective finger, pulled the trigger.

When someone dies in this way, those left behind ask how did they fail. Brettschneider had been gone from Denver for more than a decade, but the haunting possibility remained that the seeds of his ruin were sown at the height of his achievements, and even were caused by them. Perhaps it was the realization that he could not rise this high again.

Or was it possible that the seeds were sown even earlier? After Larry was dead, the chair of the Department of Anatomy at Colorado (and chair before that at Syracuse where Brettschneider went to medical school), told me of a faculty panel that had considered defaulting Brettschneider's graduation for some behavioral aberration. An extenuating circumstance carried the day in Brettschneider's favor: he had participated as a volunteer in the LSD experiments that were being carried out by the armed forces on many American campuses in the 1950s. Those who knew him well said he was never the same person again.

The Brettschneider method of liver preservation was the best one ever used up to his time, and it may have been superior to anything that has come along since then. However, the hyperbaric chamber was cumbersome and extremely heavy. The pilots who flew us in small planes to donor cities on the other side of the Rocky Mountains were terrified that it would roll through the side of the aircraft like a lead ball, or explode from its high internal pressure. Consequently, its use was abandoned after brain death was accepted in the late 1960s. Yet it played a role. This was the technique that we used to preserve all of the first successfully transplanted human livers.

15

A Liver Summit Team

In planning a perilous journey, it pays to know your companions and not to have too many of them. "Perilous" might be verbal overkill for the liver transplantation we had in mind, but in 1967 it came close to the truth for all concerned. For the surgeons, it seemed apparent that liver transplantation was not going to be a ticket to an academic career. The worldwide impact of the Colorado program had been in kidney transplantation, but this was fading now as other competent renal programs opened, many of them headed by our former fellows and faculty in the United States and abroad. The institutions to which they went were not anxious to recapitulate the agony of liver transplantation which was slowly staining the Colorado kidney transplant triumph of the early 1960s.

I could see this myself when I was invited to consider more than a half dozen surgical chairs between 1964 and 1968. More than once, members of the search committees asked openly or tacitly for a pledge to start a kidney transplantation program, but with the proviso that I not push forward with liver transplantation. The concept of transplanting any organ beyond the kidney was contrary to institutional interests and purposes in most places. This would be a pervasive attitude until the 1980s.

Tom Marchioro, the Colorado surgeon who beyond all others had earned a place on the human liver transplantation team, would become a casualty of this climate. He was destined to leave Denver less than one month before success was finally achieved. He had promised to become director of the Division of Transplantation at the University of Washington on July 1, 1967. In Seattle, he was expected to marry kidney transplantation technology to the artificial kidney program already in place. There were no plans for a liver program. At the time of the negotiations for this important job, the prospects of clinical liver transplantation in Denver had seemed far in the distance. Now they were imminent. Marchioro's promise to Washington was as good as his word. He packed up and left, leaving behind the dream that he helped to create.

I flew to Seattle a year later (June 1968) and stopped at the new Marchioro house. Tom's life was fuller than it could have been in Denver. He created the kidney transplant center and became a fixture and pillar of the University of Washington School of Medicine. In 1977, he was elected the third president of the American Society of Transplant Surgeons. Perhaps it was more my disappointment than his that he was no longer in the liver transplant chase and never would be again. When it was over, and the story was put together, it was easy to see how much he had done and how profoundly his five years in the struggle (1962–67) had shaped the course of events.

Tom Marchioro's face looked like a piece of metal so tough that the divine sculptor could not find a chisel strong enough to work out all the creases. This was an illusion. I knew before he left Denver of his unease at the fame which his work had brought his way already. Late one afternoon in the parking lot of the VA Hospital, he told me of his wish to go to an Indian reservation for the U.S. Public Health Service and serve those people whose rights he thought had been violated. He was not comfortable with the pressures and politics of academic life. He disliked writing scientific papers, in spite of the fact that thoughts and phrases came naturally and logically in either English or French. He was the opposite of vain, which was one reason that he was so respected.

Marchioro had one more bullet to shoot in liver transplantation. In a classic study in hemophiliac dogs carried out in Seattle, he showed that this bleeding disorder—called in humans the "disease of royalty" because it affected the male lineage from Alexandra, one of the daughters of Queen Victoria of England—could be cured by liver replacement.[1] This was of therapeutic interest eventually and meant that the deficient clotting factor was produced predominantly by the liver. However, the clock ran into the 1980s before a human hemophiliac was cured by liver transplantation.[2]

» «

Marchioro's shoes were filled by a Swede named Carl Gustav Groth whom he helped train. The world talent pool had opened up following the September 1963 conference on kidney transplantation (see chapter 10). Not long after, Curt Franksson, the professor and chair of surgery at the Serafimer Hospital, Stockholm, visited Denver. The Serafimer Hospital (since closed) was the oldest of the hospitals making up the teaching network of the Karolinska Institute, one of the world's foremost medical centers. It also was where Franksson had started his country's first, and at the time of his Denver visit its only, kidney transplant center.

While in Denver, Franksson proposed sending Groth, one of his young protégés, to Colorado for a fellowship in kidney transplantation. Groth had not yet completed his formal surgical training, and in addition he was preparing a Ph.D. thesis which he would defend publicly in Stockholm during early 1966. The dilatory pace of these plans, stretched out over nearly two years, did not reveal any sense of urgency. As a first step, Franksson invited me to give a series of conferences on kidney transplantation in Sweden in the spring of 1965 which would be held in Stockholm, Uppsala, Lund, Malmö, and Gothenburg.

When my wife, Barbara, and I arrived in Stockholm on May 22, 1965, our host was Carl Groth, in whose parents' flat we stayed. This was the first time either of us had been to Europe. Stockholm was much colder than we had expected, and at first we looked forward to the next stops in London, Paris, Strasbourg, and Rome. In contrast, Groth (and his wife Birgit) were warm. They were enthusiastic about their trip to America even though it would not be until the end of the year.

Groth was born in Helsinki in 1933. Some of his vivid childhood memories were of the winter siege of Helsinki by the Russian army in 1939 when the resolute Finnish Resistance held the vast Soviet forces at bay. The sounds of a bombardment leave fine lines on a child's brain like India ink on paper long after its texture decays. In

1944, Carl's father, a businessman, immigrated to Stockholm with his family. Carl's brother later became a diplomat and in 1991 was Swedish ambassador to Denmark. Carl went to medical school at the Karolinska Institute. Whether these facts are relevant may be debatable, but when describing steel, it pays to know what fires have tempered it. Groth had emerged friendly, open, and durable.

By the time Groth finally arrived in Denver in January 1966, I had given him phantom status, imagining that he had been engaged in some kind of academic or administrative minuet in preference to rushing over. It was not clear what were his special skills. Like me, he was entering transplantation without a formal background in immunology and thus without the pessimism which is fashionable among some of the learned.

Instead, Groth understood blood flow. His Ph.D. had been in rheology.[3] As young men do who learn a discipline, he selected research in his new field of transplantation that would tie in with the research in the field he had just abandoned. Not long after arriving in Colorado, he contributed a key piece of information about a fundamental event that occurs during liver rejection. When this process started in dogs, he showed that the liver blood flow fell drastically to a fraction of that at the outset. Part, if not most, of the tissue death caused by rejection was due to the choking off of the transplanted organ's blood supply. A strategy of the immune system army was to cut the graft's supply lines.

Groth correlated his flow measurements in dogs with the microscopic and electron microscopic studies carried out by K. A. Porter in London on liver samples taken at various times after liver grafting. What emerged was a dynamic view of rejection that could be used to explain complications after liver transplantation in animals and in patients. This led to further studies with X-ray imaging techniques that allowed the amount of flow of blood to the transplanted livers to be seen without opening the body. Groth's instincts and prior background had led him to an insight about the management of problems of blood flow—including both bleeding and clotting of blood vessels—that had contributed to, or caused the death of, some of our first patients.

At first, these inquiries into liver grafting were secondary to

Groth's primary responsibility to master kidney transplantation, something which was simple for a person of his ability. Except for fine tuning, management of the kidney recipient was as standardized by now as it would be until better drugs became available a dozen years hence. The tissue matching and ALG trials were well underway by the time he arrived and needed tending more than innovation. Groth realized that the time had come to reopen the liver trials. He was not only prepared for the challenge, he was determined to see it happen. If anyone could replace Marchioro, it was he.

May in Denver is a pleasant time. Long before this, the golf courses and tennis courts (which we did not use) were active, and the bicycle pathways (which we did) were humming. The swimming pools began to open, which is where Groth and I began our 1967 spring training for what we knew was coming. Day after day we exercised, growing stronger, darker in color, and more confident. The Crestmoor Swim Club was the place for strategy sessions and for debate with other team members about whether to start the liver program again. The political damage that could be done by more failures had become an open issue. Groth was like a fresh mountain climber who reached a base camp occupied for the most part by disconsolate and exhausted people who had been there too long. They did not believe, as Groth and I did, that success was possible. Groth rescued us.

Large by any ethnic standards, Carl Groth could not pass easily for a Scandinavian. His features were too strong and primitive, like those of a caricature drawn in charcoal on cream paper. Instead of being blond, his hair was almost black. He towered over most adults, and his size (six feet, one inch tall, 220 pounds) seemed gargantuan alongside the tiny liver recipients whom he was destined to protect a few months later.

The adversary was death. Once the battle was joined, I wondered more than once whether anyone else saw the symbolism of his constant vigil. Sometimes, the vision was of the sentinel always alert to the circling wolves just beyond the flickering camp fire. Or he was a soldier in white, interposed between the invader and his native Finland. No man's land was the intensive care unit (ICU) on the third floor of the Colorado General Hospital. Groth's fuel came from inside, except for lemonade, gallons of it, which was brought to the ICU station at each change in the nursing shift. By this time he had sent his family back to Stockholm and was prepared for the supreme commitment of his life.

» «

Others fell in line. The power of the team came from its diversity. It was a world team, devoid of nationalism, and would always be that way. More than two decades later, I performed what had become a routine liver transplantation on a famous old man who for many years had helped make the guiding policies of his government. Not privileged by high birth, or even living parents, he had spent his orphaned childhood in tents and around camp fires in desolate and primitive places. When he was a youth, and for years after, he bore arms with distinction.

He later became for his grateful nation an architect of peace and social reform. He was treated with deference by kings, prime ministers, and presidents, but not by a virus which had damaged his liver years before and left marks that changed into a cancer. After crossing the Atlantic on the Concorde, I met him in a London hospital the night before an operation which I had been asked to attend. He spoke with dignity and no regret about his past life and what lay ahead. Those who were with him loved him.

The next day at operation, the cancer could not be removed from the liver that itself was shrunken and cirrhotic from the old virus infection. A few weeks later, he came to Pittsburgh for a liver transplantation from which his recovery was rapid. Many prominent people visited his room, but the most important to him was an American general with whom he had an initially stormy but later warm relationship during a troubled period long ago in his country's history. These two old comrades reminisced quietly and drank tea while the entourage waited at a respectful distance.

He was ready to leave the hospital, and one by one those who helped care for him came to say good-bye. Referring to the general and to the medical team, he asked me, "Where do you find people like this?" Caught off guard, I told him, "They grow wild like weeds in America." This was incorrect. I should have said "in the world," because the resolve, intelligence, and skills to bring liver transplantation to a reality and to maintain it there were international in 1967, before that time, and still. If the world could function like this on simpler matters, there would be no wars.

16

A Pyrrhic Victory

The struts were in place for another attempt at liver transplantation: better antirejection therapy, improved means of organ procurement and preservation, and insight about what role tissue typing would play—or more correctly, would not. In the animal laboratory, dog recipients were living in their fourth year after receiving the livers of nonrelated mongrel donors. These accomplishments did not silence the opposition to further trials. Those who were opposed believed that what they said was inherently correct and virtuous, but in all fairness so did I. I publicly defended the impending liver trials and also what had been done in kidney transplantation, which was not yet generally accepted therapy.

The most important debate forum was the forty-eighth annual session of the American College of Physicians, held in San Francisco on April 12, 1967. It was called "A Colloquium on Ethical Dilemmas from Medical Advances."[1] In addition to me, the speakers were Warren E. Burger (soon to be chief justice of the U.S. Supreme Court), René Dubos (microbiologist), David Krech (psychologist), Chauncey Leake (pharmacologist), Peter Medawar (Nobel laureate, 1960), Joshua Lederberg (Nobel laureate, 1958), and Samuel E. Stumpf (college president).

I was the youngest and least experienced of the group. Most of the others spoke about how modern technology could control both the numbers and the genetic constitution of great masses of people in a deliberate effort to improve the quality, performance, and comfort of the human race. They were concerned with birth control,

abortion, genetic manipulation, and the use of performance enhancing and/or mind altering drugs. My presentation was last. It
seemed to me that transplantation was being handed down like a
hot potato from speaker to speaker until it reached Medawar, who
was next to last.

In connection with this division of labor, he announced that, "not
to be outdone in magnanimity, I have made over all my rights in the
field of transplantation to Dr. Thomas Starzl." It was an uneasy
moment. I began by making

a distinction between the noble aims of these society-oriented programs
[described by the others] and the humbler but by no means ignoble
objectives of the vast majority of practicing physicians and surgeons. . . . It is doubtful if many doctors who actually care for the sick
and the infirm plan their actions on the basis of the predicted effect
upon society. Instead, the dominant tradition is for the physician to
provide the best care of which he is capable for those who either seek his
services or are assigned to his responsibility; by and large this is done
without regard for the conceivably broader issue of whether treatment
is justifiable on social grounds.

His reasons may include pride, altruism, compassion, curiosity, a
spirit of competition, even avarice, or a combination of all these things.
Whatever the motives, the reflexes that follow are sure and respond
similarly to the needs of the productive members of the community, the
insane and feebleminded, children with incurable birth defects, condemned criminals, or even soldiers who moments before were members
of a hostile army.

The foregoing viewpoint is a narrow one, but there is no reason to
believe that it should be abandoned in the face of advancing technoc-
racy. It has shielded the ill from the caprices and the moral judgments of
other men through centuries of evolving philosophical, religious, and
legal doctrines. It has placed the concept of the sanctity of human life on
a practical foundation, since the responsibility of one person for another
could not be more clearly defined than through the doctor-patient
relationship, irrespective of the reasons for the contract entered into
between the two involved parties.

Has this ancient creed of medicine been ravaged by the scientific
explosion in which we are now involved? Examination of this question
as it applies to organ transplantation is inevitable, first, because of the
widespread lay publicity that has accompanied such efforts and, second, because the harsh term "purely experimental" has consistently

been applied to these procedures by virtually all workers in the field as well as by interested observers.

The designation of "experimental" is perfectly correct. Few endeavors have ever yielded such a rich and diversified harvest of both fundamental and practical information, have so united basic and clinical scientists in the pursuit of a common goal, and have defined and stimulated such large areas of potentially fruitful new research. Nevertheless, the primary purpose in these human cases was therapeutic, and it is important to realize that this objective has been met to a degree that may not be generally appreciated.[2]

Here I provided a three- to five-year follow-up for our Colorado kidney transplant recipients of 1962–63, whose high rate of survival was still unknown by many in the profession, or else not believed. I described the deficiencies that still existed in immunosuppression and the need for the ALG trials which already had started (see chapter 13). I summarized the failed liver replacement and auxiliary liver cases, including the fact that all the recipients had died in less than five weeks.

I went on to say:

The clinical trial of new therapeutic methods is based more firmly than ever on prior animal experimentation. Virtually all practices in cardiac as well as in transplantation surgery have been transferred, almost without change, from the laboratory to the clinical ward or operating room.

Not infrequently the transition has been made with haste and with an air of urgency that, the generous may concede, was fed by the needs and wishes of desperate patients who had the misfortune of not becoming ill at a later and more convenient time. Historically, the decisions to proceed have often been wrong. Nevertheless, they have almost invariably been based on the hope, however fleeting or erroneously conceived, of potential benefit to the individual patient.

Right or wrong, the actions are eventually subjected to implacable scrutiny, principally by other members of the scientific community but also by intelligent and informed outsiders. Inaccuracies in reporting, claims that cannot be reproduced, and procedures that neither relieve suffering nor prolong life are rapidly identified. Harmful practices are snuffed out quickly; homeopathic ones may suffer a lingering death, but they also ultimately disappear from the scene.

The system is ruthless and without pity and demands a policy of nonconcealment from those who would innovate in medicine. It is not sufficient to report only successes. Failures must also be fully documented, no matter how painful and humiliating these may be, in order to prevent repetition by others of the same mistakes. In general, such openness has characterized efforts in the field of transplantation.[3]

This was a statement of intention three months before the liver trials were to begin again. How well it was received I cannot remember, or perhaps I could not judge accurately even at the time. Back in Colorado, the lines were drawn. Henry Kempe, the chair of pediatrics, would support the trials. The Department of Medicine would not. Consequently, all of the next seven patients were infants and children. Eventually, adults would be treated, but never by referral within the Colorado system. The referral of adults would have to be direct from outside physicians to the transplant team.

The mortality from the failed early trials and that which occurred later did not mean that liver transplantation was causing deaths. These patients were under a death sentence already because of the diseases that had brought them to us. Even now, I continue to receive letters from parents or family members. These always start by saying that they know I won't remember Jimmie or whatever was the patient's name. Then they express thanks for the fact that we had made an effort instead of letting their children die, off in a back room without hope. Those opposed to trying always claimed that these little creatures had been denied the dignity of dying. Their parents believed that they had been given the glory of striving.

They were wrong about one thing. That I would not remember.

» «

Almost exactly one year later, on April 17, 1968, I reported the results of the new liver transplant trials to the American Surgical Association, which met that year in Boston. All seven of the newly treated children had passed through the previously lethal period during and just after liver transplantation. Four had died after 2, 3-1/2, 4-1/3, and 6 months, but the other three were still alive and would remain so for long enough to demonstrate convincingly the potential value of this kind of treatment.[4] In discussing the paper, Franny Moore remarked that "liver surgery as of this day has an entirely new look." His remarks were prophetic, but there were warning signs of the limitations to liver transplantation which would inhibit its widespread use for another dozen years.

All other complications were trivial compared to one that already had caused the death of the four patients. This was the development of gangrene in a portion of the transplanted livers, the other part of which continued to function properly. The dead portion of the liver was infected with the bacteria that normally live in the intestine but are kept there in quarantine by the barrier of the intestinal lining, by the resistance of the normal liver to their attack, and by the body's total immune defenses. Once these germs had escaped from the intestine and populated the susceptible dead portions of the transplanted liver, they were free to migrate onward to other parts of the body including the lungs, brain, and kidneys.

These sinister invaders, who struck without warning, were met head on by Carl Groth in the ICU, which he dared not leave. Heart stoppages requiring massage, sudden breathing failure needing ventilator support, blood pressure collapse, convulsions, visits to the operating room to remove dead fragments of liver tissue—these defined Groth's days and nights for eight months.

In the end, the four children died anyway. They were all girls. Numb with grief, their mothers took their frail bodies home, leaving behind the haggard Swedish surgeon, who had found in himself the lasting sorrow which inevitably is there no matter how great the self-discipline. That vulnerability always is the touchstone for the next step up in the improvement of patient care.

There were three patients left to be cared for. The reason for the transplantation for the first and seventh liver recipients in the series was cancer of the liver. Those children were nineteen months, and sixteen years old. The nineteen-month-old girl, whose name was Julie Rodriquez, underwent transplantation on July 23, 1967, and became a metaphor for courage and human progress. At the time, it was thought that an ideal use of liver replacement would be for patients with cancer that originated in the liver and could not be removed with any lesser procedure.

It was not yet realized that the majority of such patients already had tiny and undetectable deposits of tumor spread elsewhere which would continue to grow. These recurrent cancers could be seen on Julie Rodriquez's chest X-ray after three months; soon afterward, recurrent cancer was found throughout the abdomen, including her transplanted liver. The abdominal cancers were partly removed at re-operations 3-1/2 and 7 months following transplantation. Anticancer chemotherapy had no effect.

Yet this beautiful child seemed healthy most of the time. Doomed now, she became a familiar sight in the small parks near Colorado General Hospital where she went with her parents and doctors to play with the dogs who had undergone liver transplantation long before. The animals were brought out by Paul Taylor from the laboratory. The big people talked quietly and frankly to the other big people. Julie talked to the dogs, who watched her as if they understood.

After 400 days, she died. Dietrich Grunewald, a Swedish artist living in New Mexico, created a symbolic portrait called *In Memoriam Julie Rodriquez, January 2, 1966, to August 26, 1968*. It shows a child bathed in sunlight, picking long-stemmed flowers. This hung on the wall of the transplantation ward at Colorado General Hospital for five or six years until it was defaced during the careless moving of equipment. After having it restored, I brought it home. It has a position of honor in my bedroom, placed by a window where it catches the first rays at dawn. When I die, I will leave it to the person who is closest to me. Still pock-marked by the earlier damage, it is the dearest possession I have.

Terry Kent, the seventh patient, who was sixteen, recovered quickly from her transplantation. A powerful girl, she transferred her academic records to Denver after her transplantation on March 17, 1968, and enrolled at the George Washington High School where she was an outstanding student. Nearly a year later, recurrent tumor appeared in her new liver. On March 31, 1969, a second transplantation was performed. She never left the hospital again and died on May 23, 1969, of widespread cancer.

This left only Randy Bennett, the sixth patient in the series and the only boy. His original diagnosis was biliary atresia, the disease which ultimately became the main indication for liver transplantation in children. He was two years old at the time of his transplantation on

February 9, 1968, and was four and a half when he died on July 29, 1970, of chronic rejection and an attempt at retransplantation.

He had stood on the crumpled shoulders of Bennie Solis and the earlier children in the 1967 series. By the time he died, another child, Kimberly Hudson, was a half year into a new life that has now continued into the twenty-second post-transplant year. Kim Hudson also had biliary atresia, but in her removed liver was found a small cancer which had not been suspected in advance. It never came back.

Exhausted by his effort, Groth returned to Stockholm and to his family in March 1968. On the way out, he helped complete a study in dogs by Larry Brettschneider. This was based on Groth's observations in the children who developed partial gangrene of the liver graft. The Brettschneider study showed that an important factor predisposing to liver infection was undertreatment with immunosuppression. The consequence was the development of rejection. Because of the reduction in liver blood flow caused by rejection, which already had been demonstrated by Groth in animals, the stage was set for oxygen starvation of the transplanted liver and a consequent lowered resistance to bacteria. Paradoxically, the best way to prevent this was more vigorous antirejection treatment in spite of the fact that this weakened the immune system and the overall body resistance to infection.

Before leaving, Groth had his own stay in the adult ICU. He developed a heart condition called auricular fibrillation. With this disorder, the conduction of impulses from the upper to the lower heart chambers is disturbed. The orderly initiation of beats by the upper chambers was replaced by an irregular pattern that caused the lower chambers to beat unevenly and too rapidly. This was the same conduction system that I had studied at the John Hopkins Hospital fifteen years earlier (see chapter 4). Groth's rhythm was restored to normal by electrically shocking the heart. He has had this problem from time to time since. For many people it would be a handicap. For him, it is something to be endured if necessary and ignored when possible.

Groth had not yet made his last contribution to liver transplantation (see chapter 22). He still is in the field and in 1983, he became the chair at the Karolinska Institute of the first Department of

Transplantation in the world. He is famous now and full of honors, but if any moments in his life were more precious than those of the summer and autumn of 1967, I would be surprised.

» «

The survival of Julie Rodriquez and the next children in the series became known worldwide by September 1967. The ripple effect went far beyond the liver. Until then, a seemingly impenetrable barrier had precluded extension of transplantation operations beyond the relatively simple kidney. Suddenly, a second organ was on the horizon, a vastly more complex one in its function and in the technical requirements for its engraftment. In fact, the liver was the most defiant of all organs. If it could be transplanted, anything was possible. The smoldering embers in other speciality centers burst into flames.

In December 1967, Christiaan Barnard of Capetown performed his famous first heart transplantation, followed shortly by the beginning of Norman Shumway's clinical heart program at Stanford. After frantic phone call requests and emergency shipping arrangements, we became the suppliers of homemade ALG for these and other heart programs that followed like a swarm of locusts. One of the first of these was at the University of Pittsburgh under the direction of my old Hopkins friend, Hank Bahnson. The first successful lung transplant was performed on November 14, 1968, by F. Derom of Louvain. Pancreas and intestinal transplantation was begun at the University of Minnesota under the direction of Richard Lillehei and William Kelly.

Most of these attempts failed. When the rush of enthusiasm was replaced by reality, only a few diehards were left. Further clinical development of hearts would be at Stanford. The pancreas would depend upon Carl Groth in Stockholm, Jean M. Dubernard of Lyon, and David Sutherland of Minneapolis. Clinical lung transplantation lay dormant for almost fifteen years until Joel Cooper of Toronto finally established its practicality. Intestinal transplantation was abandoned for almost two decades.

For liver transplantation, the moment of professional responsibility was now. By early February 1969 we had treated twenty-six patients with liver replacement of whom the last nineteen cases started with Julie Rodriquez. For one, a chimpanzee was the donor. In addition, there were four more recipients of auxiliary livers. Of the thirty patients, six had either lived for one year or were expected to, which they did. As it turned out, all six were dead within two and one-half years of their transplantation, three from cancer recurrence and the other three from chronic rejection.

A grim conclusion was unavoidable. Liver transplantation was a feasible but impractical way to treat end-stage liver disease. It was important to make this complete picture available so that the next stage of development could be planned. This would require a book, a companion piece to *Experience in Renal Transplantation* which I had written five years earlier. Every clinical attempt made at liver transplantation in the world and every experimental paper written on the subject up to early 1969 would be included.

The task was too large to do alone. As had happened before, and would again, a collaborator was waiting. This one was Charles W. Putnam. What had brought Charley to this crossroads was a strange tale. One summer afternoon in 1964, Charley came to the Denver VA laboratory and explained that he was a twenty-one-year-old premedical student at Hamilton College, New York, scheduled to begin his senior year. He had earned money doing forestry work during earlier summer vacations but now he wanted to be a volunteer in our research program. According to him, no job would be too menial and he meant it. He had walked in at a moment of incredible activity when all the critical inquiries were being made that led to resumption of the clinical liver transplant trials and were applicable to other kinds of organ transplantation.

Far from being a volunteer flunky, he became a leader. Not long after he entered medical school he published his first scientific article. Every summer after that, Charley came back, first from Hamilton and after 1966 fresh from each succeeding year at Northwestern University where he had become a star medical student. When the liver transplant trials were restarted in 1967, Putnam was Groth's main assistant in caring for the children, although he was not yet a junior medical student. After Groth left, Charley was the person who knew the most about every detail of the clinical as well as experimental liver programs.

Charley spent much of his junior and senior years at Northwestern in transit. Every Friday night he flew to Denver, and at the end of the weekend he took back material for follow-up research in the Chicago library. He was a natural bibliophile with the integrity, obsession for accuracy, and curiosity found in these people. By the time he graduated from Northwestern Medical School and came to Colorado General Hospital to begin his internship on July 1, 1969, the book *Experience in Hepatic Transplantation* was finished. It had taken eighteen months. Putnam, a beginning intern, was co-author of a book that defined a new field.[5]

Charley Putnam was voted the best intern, the best resident, the best teacher, and after his surgical training was completed, the most promising young faculty member in the Department of Surgery. In 1975, he became the University of Colorado nominee for the Passano Foundation Young Scientist Award. Perhaps I was so blinded by Charley's scientific talents that I did not realize that he had other objectives. Above all, he wanted to be a teacher. To him, the highest achievement would not be what he could do, but what he could transmit to others. He preferred to lead young surgeons through difficult decisions and operations rather than do the work independently.

Also, there was a love story. Charley wanted to marry a young woman who had been one of my first kidney transplant recipients in 1963 when she was eight years old. He needed to make a real home for her. The ceremony was in the mountains late in the day as the sun set. By now she was a beautiful woman and a nurse practitioner. Later, she went to medical school and became a physician in her own right. Career stresses finally broke the union, but at the time it was like an allegory of transplantation with the surgeon marrying his most loved patient. In 1977, Charley moved to the University of Arizona where he is professor of surgery and director of the residency training program. In 1990, he received the Excellence in Teaching Award.

The book that Charley and I had labored over portrayed liver transplantation more pessimistically than was warranted by the events of the next ten years. Yet, more recipients died than lived throughout this time. Altogether, 170 patients were treated between 1963 and the end of 1979. Only 29 still survive. What they have done with their new lives would fill a separate book.

Was it worth this much trouble to save so few people? This is what I was asked more and more. In England, the same question was being asked of Roy Calne, who started a liver transplant program in May 1967, the only other one in the world. Like ours, it was controversial. Of his first five patients, only one left the hospital alive.

The number of people who had made the prodigious effort to bring liver transplantation this far was still small. Those at Colorado who worked on either the kidney or liver teams absorbed the extra work into their regular duties. Specialty support also was limited. Few anesthesiologists had the skills or possessed the determination to handle these difficult cases. Anesthesia techniques were developed by a young Mexican-American named J. Antonio (Tony) Aldrete, who was grooming a talented twenty-five-year-old Chilean named Andres (Andy) Zahler Mayanz to be his assistant. Zahler, who was completing his residency at the University of Colorado, and Aldrete were a strangely compatible pair. Like brothers with different temperaments, their sum added up to more than the parts. Aldrete, the headstrong and outspoken leader, blended perfectly with the shy and taciturn Zahler.

Chronically fatigued already, they began a drive on October 16, 1968, from Denver to Leadville to carry out some studies on high-altitude lung function. Whether they fell asleep at the wheel could not be reconstructed later because both were so severely injured when their car fell into a mountain pass. Aldrete recovered. Zahler suffered a lethal brain injury and died on October 24, 1968. His parents, Mr. and Mrs. Jorge Zahler, who both are lawyers, had been told by their son that he wished to be an organ donor in this unlikely eventuality. Accordingly, his liver and kidneys were removed after death and transplanted.

I often wondered later if this was part of the silent mortality of transplantation. Charley Putnam and I put Andy's picture at the front of our new book, which had a green cover. It was all that we could do. We guessed that this might be what he would want the most.

17

Icebergs and Hammer Blows

It might have been best in 1970 to declare victory and quit. In the United States, the 1970s became an era of national humiliation and introspection. There was the unfavorable end of a hated war, the forced resignation of a president, and the slow decline of American technologic and economic superiority. In my small world, as in the real one, disintegration lay ahead before fresh pathways or half-forgotten old ones could be found. This would be a bleak decade. Or was it all a mirage, and only a prelude to the next great surge?

The decade of the sixties had been pure magic. At its beginning, I had been known to no one, probably including myself. By the end, the awards, prizes, honorary degrees, and memberships in elite organizations were almost too numerous to list. The demand for lectures on kidney and liver transplantation, often in exotic and distant places, was never ending.

A small voice reminded me I should not take this new status seriously. The patients who came to the kidney and liver transplant clinics were too few and too unhappy to justify complacency. The medical literature was filling up with what I now called "see what a big boy am I" reports. Many of these reports, which confirmed and extended what had been accomplished in the 1960s, came from new teams entering transplantation and trying to establish credibility. Others came from groups which were trying to avoid the appearance of premature obsolescence. Exaggeration became rampant. Few things were more disquieting than the recurrent debates between those touting the virtues of kidney transplantation versus artificial kidney support when both were highly flawed forms of therapy.

The possibility of finding new antirejection drugs seemed remote during this period, but there were older agents which had not been adequately tested. Cytoxan (cyclophosphamide), the anticancer agent used by Will Goodwin at UCLA in 1960, was an example. Although his patient died after five months, she was the first patient in the world to have such extended survival after kidney transplantation using drugs alone (without X-ray therapy).

An exhaustive reevaluation of cytoxan was carried out at Colorado from 1969 to 1971, using it as a substitute for Imuran in seventy-five kidney, sixteen liver, and one or two heart recipients. The effectiveness of the drug cocktail based on cytoxan was equivalent to that with Imuran, which was of theoretical interest but not a practical advance. I presented the results and conclusions in Chicago at the senior forum session which is a featured attraction of the yearly American College of Surgeons congress. The talk was scheduled for the morning of October 13, 1970.[1]

Will Goodwin was scheduled to discuss the work. The night before, he learned that his son, Peter, had been killed with another young man in a mountain climbing accident. Those coming up behind them heard a shout and looked out to see the two bodies pass by in flight, linked together in their last moments as they had been in a deep friendship for a long time before.

I knew Peter well. During every Christmas season from 1963 to 1967, I and my family joined a small group of ski companions at the Mountain Chalet Lodge in Aspen, Colorado. The members included Robert McNamara (the secretary of defense), Kennedy family members, other prominent members of the Kennedy administration, Barbara Tuchman (the author), and an assortment of successful businessmen and executives. Will Goodwin, a friend of McNamara's since their college days at the University of California at Berkeley, had arranged for my introduction.

McNamara had been appointed to the cabinet by John F. Kennedy in 1960, and he was retained by Lyndon Johnson until the autumn of 1967. Each New Year's Eve for five years we joined Bob and Margy McNamara and the Goodwins for dinner with our children. Peter was often there. Eighteen or twenty years old at the time, he had inherited his parents' good looks and disposition, and in addition, he was endowed with a shock of golden blond hair that arrested the attention of anyone who saw it. He and McNamara's son, Craig, were active opponents of the Vietnam War, but this subject and other matters concerning government never were discussed.

Between Christmas seasons, we had other adventures. On March 13, 1966, Goodwin and I joined McNamara and Joe Murray (the Boston transplant surgeon) for a week of skiing in Zermatt, Switzerland. As usual, news reporters and photographers were everywhere, tracking McNamara's every move. After several days, we hired a snow caterpillar which carried us about twenty miles through fresh snow to the top of a ridge separating Switzerland from Italy. By the time we arrived and the caterpillar had turned back, a blizzard started. The rest of the group decided to ski into Italy, but I had obligations in Denver and started to ski back to Zermatt through the snowstorm. Later I learned that McNamara, Goodwin, and Murray had been trapped in a rescue lodge halfway down the mountain on the Italian side. Although they were convinced that I would not be able to make the solitary twenty-mile journey back to Zermatt, I arrived there at two in the afternoon and caught the train for Geneva. From there, it was on to Paris, and home. In the meanwhile, one of Goodwin's children had come down with a serious infection of the lining of the brain and spinal column (meningitis) and was in a hospital in Boston. By the time the group on the Italian side was rescued, the child was recovering.

A favorite game in all of these trips was trying to guess who among the figures dotting the periphery were security officers. During the Christmas season of 1967, an incident occurred while we were eating lunch at The Hut on the top of Aspen mountain. A woman hurled a ketchup-encrusted hamburger at McNamara screaming that she hoped he would choke on the blood of the young men who had died in "his" war. It is impossible to describe how distraught he was.

The assailant did not realize that McNamara already had resigned as secretary of defense and was scheduled to become president of the World Bank. Much earlier, McNamara had come to the conclusion that the Vietnam War was futile. He had informed

President Johnson of his views in a long letter in November, a month
or so earlier. As recounted in the memoirs of Clark Clifford,
Johnson refused to accept this opinion and replaced McNamara.[2] I
stopped going to the ski rendezvous after this, although I saw Bob
McNamara from time to time in Aspen. From what I observed,
McNamara was one of most deeply moral men whom I have ever
met. Yet, who knows with what twisted yardstick history will
measure him?

In February 1970 while on a ski trip, I saw Peter Goodwin for the
last time at the public library in Aspen. It is an attractive place with
a number of unusual books and artifacts. While browsing around, I
noticed Peter studying the architectural design of some old bridges.
He was absorbed in the task, but was glad to see me. We talked for
an hour, and I learned that he was living in a snow cave outside the
city. He seemed happy and healthy, but being alarmed by his
primitive life style, I called Will after returning to Denver. Apparently, the camping out was for Peter a challenge which he had met
before. He was at peace.

Because Peter had been killed the afternoon before my report on
cytoxan eight months later, I was surprised to see his father waiting
for me when I entered the auditorium. Goodwin was pale and his
hands shook, but he explained that Peter loved the mountains and
died with a friend at his side. What more could someone ask? He sat
in the front row while I gave my talk. I could see that he was not
listening.

There were two thousand people in the audience. When I had
finished, Goodwin walked hesitantly to the podium and began to
speak, his voice cracking slightly. If he mentioned the word cytoxan, I do not remember it. He talked instead about mountain
climbing. "There are people in the world," he said, "who make it a
better place . . . sometimes you cannot see them, but if you listen
carefully, you know that they are there. You can hear their hammers
placing the pitons with which the rest of us can scramble to the
highest peaks. If they win, we all do. If they fall, it is a sad and
glorious thing."

Afterward, someone mentioned the complimentary discussion. I
told him that Goodwin was not talking about me. "Who then?" he

asked. I never revealed that Goodwin had stayed to pay tribute to his son. By this time, Will was on a plane going west. I am not sure that he ever was the same again.

As for transplantation, Imuran (or cytoxan in its place) and prednisone therapy, even with the addition of ALG, was not good enough if nonrelated (cadaver) organs were to be safely used. A deadly inertia set in which would last for a decade in transplantation, as if the reservoir of creative ideas had been exhausted during the frenetic 1960s. What could be done next? All that seemed to remain were loose ends.

» «

It may have been the inability to make progress with antirejection treatment that turned my attention back to the gnawing question of what was so important in the blood draining from the pancreas and intestines and secondarily passing through the liver on its way to the heart. My instinctive belief that nature would not create a system this complicated in normal animals or people without a purpose had been responsible for my involvement in transplantation in the first place (see chapter 5). The instinct had gained substance when it was shown that an engrafted auxiliary liver would wither without this special kind of portal blood, but we still did not know why. As it turned out, the auxiliary transplant experiments (chapter 12) enabled us to expose secrets which had resisted all previous efforts at understanding. However, even with the key in the lock, pushing the door open to see what was inside would require most of the 1970s.

The Swedish surgeon, Carl Groth, played a catalytic role in starting this process of discovery. Like me, Groth was left with a sense of incompleteness after the bittersweet clinical liver transplantation trials of 1967 and 1968. When he returned to Stockholm in March 1968, he realized that the imminent reforms in the United States that would define brain death would take years for acceptance and legal enactment in Sweden.

Because liver transplantation could not be effectively pursued at home without these conditions, he came back to the University of Colorado as an associate professor from May 1971 to September 1972. Activity in the once busy VA laboratory had slowed to a snail's pace, first because the time of the surgeons was consumed in the booming clinical program of kidney transplantation, and second because there were no promising research leads with which to make a major change in the transplant field.

Groth reorganized the laboratory, and in so doing, he became an intermediary between me and an Italian medical doctor, Antonio Francavilla, who was a specialist in diseases of the gut and liver. Francavilla had come to Denver on a one-year scholarship to study liver disease and to do research related to liver transplantation. His English was worse than imperfect. I could not understand a word he said.

Aside from this breech in communication, or perhaps because of it, Francavilla became increasingly angry with each passing day of his wasted visit. Alarmed by his agitation, which had the dimensions of a volcano preparing to erupt, I asked Groth to interview Francavilla and go over with him the chapters about auxiliary liver transplantation from the green book on liver transplantation that Charley Putnam and I had published the year before. In these chapters we summarized everything known about the "goodies" in the portal venous blood which seemed so important to the health of auxiliary liver grafts. A few days later, Groth returned with the opinion that Francavilla was a gifted chemist who might shed new light on this question.

Assured by this opinion, I designed a series of difficult surgical experiments which were carried out in 1971 and early 1972. In essence, these consisted of operations that divided the dog's own liver into two fractions, each differing only by the kind of venous blood which was delivered to its portal vein. In some animals, all the portal blood to one liver fraction was returning from the pancreas, intestines, and other abdominal organs while the blood to the other fraction was returning from the legs, kidneys, and trunk. This was an extension of earlier work done with Tom Marchioro (chapter 12). In other experiments, one piece of liver was given only the blood from the pancreas and the other piece was given intestinal blood. At the end of two months, these liver fragments were compared using two yardsticks. One, to be applied by Ken Porter, the London pathologist, would be the comparative structure of the liver. The other would be a comparison of the chemical composition of the fragments.

Originally, the surgeon Israel (Sol) Penn was asked to take the assignment of performing the experimental surgical operations. Penn also had difficulty communicating with Francavilla. In addition, he may have concluded that this was going to be a boondoggle in which I was trying to involve him in order to appease Francavilla without wasting time myself. Most importantly, Penn was not particularly interested in the project. By this time he had started his now famous international registry for the identification and study of patients with the new tumors that were developing in transplant recipients under immunosuppression. Penn escaped by passive resistance. He did not show up at the laboratory when the experiments were scheduled.

If I wanted this research done, I would have to do it myself or with someone other than Penn. Groth was unavailable. He had learned from Stockholm that his mother was to be operated on to remove one of the most serious of all cancers, from which the chances of cure were small. The tumor involved the lower part of the esophagus and upper stomach. Whatever the outcome might be, his place was at home. Groth would never live outside of Sweden again. His mother is well twenty years later.

Eventually, I did the experiments with Charles (Charlie) Halgrimson, a gifted surgeon who came to play a key role in management of the affairs of the Department of Surgery throughout the 1970s and beyond. The surgical techniques of routing specific kinds of venous blood to different parts of the liver were sophisticated, but we mastered them quickly and delivered the specimens to Francavilla or shipped them to Porter in London.

The chemical footprints in the liver tissue that Francavilla would track were no less distinctive than the microscopic changes in structure that would be studied by Porter. Francavilla measured the chemical composition in the livers, or portions of the livers, which were given three different kinds of portal blood. A few days later, Francavilla came to the operating room, trembling with excitement.

"It is insulin," he announced, referring to whatever it was that made natural portal blood so important for the liver. The portions of the liver that looked the most healthy were those which had received insulin-rich blood returning from the pancreas. This liver tissue had a high concentration of enzymes (small proteins) and a complex sugar (glycogen) which were known to depend upon the action of insulin. The liver portions that appeared to be shrunken were depleted of these substances. We realized that this was a major development, providing Porter's results revealed anything that would correlate with the chemical patterns.

Before we had the answers from Porter, the research team broke up. Francavilla returned to the University of Bari in Italy. I left for the Arctic.

» «

The idea of seeing the Arctic firsthand, not from the air or from a car, was an item left over from the romantic 1960s. In fact, the expedition was the last event of that earlier era. On returning from the trip to the north, I was scheduled to become the chair of the Department of Surgery at the University of Colorado.

Why? Becoming a chairman is one of those natural events of academic life, more to be questioned if it does not happen than if it does. It is a common professional strategy in surgery and other medical disciplines for someone who has made a contribution, even a modest one, to use it to advance in rank or to acquire the administrative power and privilege that comes with a chairmanship. Such people are valuable because they perpetuate information that is already known. Their knowledge is translated into recipes that can be applied without deep thought to the care of the sick.

Some of the finest men and women I know have made this transition. They become defenders of the contribution for which they were responsible or, more commonly, which they have learned and embroidered slightly. If they are ethical and unselfish, they buttress the medical educational establishment, which depends upon them for continuity and administrative organization. In fact, they *are* the establishment, and they tend to honor each other in ceremonial ways—for which they expect reciprocation. Dave Hume, the Virginia transplant surgeon, defined this as aging, which he did not measure in chronologic years. He dreaded it more than dying.

Chairing the department would be my job for eight years, beginning on July 1, 1972; transplant surgery would be relegated to a hobby. Department chairpersons are voluntary servants of the university. These jobs are not imposed. They are accepted and often they are sought after. The clinical chairmanships at Colorado had the reputation of first frustrating and then taming those who took them. Bill Waddell was an example. After eleven years in office, he resigned his administrative responsibilities in September 1971. There was no public versus private explanation for someone as straightforward as Waddell. He simply said that he was worn out with the administration of a department that had inadequate public and financial support and was precluded by institutional and legal statutes from supporting itself fiscally through the generation of surgical fees.

The fiscal restraints and administrative complexity of our department were far more formidable in 1971 than when Waddell had come ten years earlier. Still, a unique academic oasis had sprung from the desert and this was worth salvaging. After first declaring myself a noncandidate for Waddell's vacated chair, I changed my mind in early 1972 and accepted the position. Whether the vacant horizon in transplantation caused me to take this job as a conventional way out, whether it was personal vanity, or whether, as I rationalized, there was some actual justification is hard to say even in hindsight.

However, I stipulated that my tenure would be limited to eight years. This proviso was important because I knew that I would have to temporarily turn over the kidney transplant program to someone else. The responsibilities of the chair were too wide-ranging to allow continuation of my transplant activities. Management of the kidney transplant service was delegated to three capable surgeons over the next eight years. I would perform liver transplantation no more frequently than once every three or four weeks.

Having set these conditions, I flew in late May 1972 to Alta, Norway, the most northerly commercial airport in the world. There I joined the other expedition members—my sons, Tim and Tom; Charley Putnam, the former Northwestern medical student who by now was a surgical resident at the University of Colorado; and Paul Taylor, the organ procurement coordinator.

We each had a ten-speed bicycle with thorn-proof tires; a maximum of forty pounds of equipment, including down clothes; a light-weight sleeping bag; an equitable share of tent components (adding up to two tents for five people); a small supply of food; $100 in our pockets; and one book (mine was a biography of Fridtjof Nansen, the Norwegian explorer). By the end of June we had traveled south to Helsinki, more than two thousand miles away.

On the flight home, the airline pilots pointed out the giant icebergs far below in the north Atlantic Ocean—oblivious to man and his follies, contemptuous of ships that could avoid but not control them, and melting at their own pace as they wandered toward the sea lanes.

These were like the mounds of knowledge that drifted through my life in the decade of the 1970s, not knowing or caring about the carnage all around. In a sea of chaos, the iceberg is stability, and therefore it is king. My biggest iceberg for almost fifteen years had been transplantation. A smaller one, which would become dominant for the next six years, was waiting in my office in Denver. It was in an envelope postmarked London which had arrived while we were gone. The sender was K. A. Porter.

While I tried to resolve administrative problems, Ken Porter's letter lay neglected in my new office until the middle of July 1972. The days were spent from morning to night in committee meetings devoted mostly to arguments about the division and management of money. When finally opened, the letter contained some of the most exciting information I had ever received. Francavilla's earlier chemical measurements had been of bits of liver tissue containing millions of cells that had been exposed to different kinds of portal venous inflow. Porter's studies were of the individual cells in these tissues.

Charley Putnam (who had joined the project) and I poured over Porter's observations as if they were biblical scripture. They showed that the liver tissue which had not been given blood from the pancreas and which had Francavilla's chemical signs of insulin deprivation contained liver cells (hepatocytes) which were shrunken and looked abnormal. In contrast, liver cells nourished with blood coming from the pancreas were normal. Francavilla's chemistry results and Porter's findings fit perfectly. The conclusion seemed inescapable. It looked as if the principal liver-sustaining (hepatotrophic) substance in normal portal venous blood was insulin.[3] It was like finding the Holy Grail after a search of nearly fifteen years.

Finding the Holy Grail was almost easier than finding time to write a paper to announce it. Nearly three months passed before completing what would have been possible in three uninterrupted days. In addition, there was little time to do the next experiments to expand the original findings and fill in the details.

» «

A year went by. In May 1973, twenty-nine years late, I finally was able to go to my high school graduation ceremony from which the war had kept me in 1944. I received the degree and gave the commencement address. I brought my son Tom with me so he could see my father whom he had met at the age of three but could not remember. Because of the complexity of my father's medical needs, it had become impossible to keep him at home.

He was transferred to the Sacred Heart Hospital, which I knew well from my high school days. A general practitioner named Wendell Downing, who also was an able general surgeon, had allowed me to watch several operations, pointing out anatomic structures as he worked. Dr. Downing remembered my affection for his beautiful daughter, who died in childhood of a disease that would not have been fatal if it had come a few years later.[4]

The hospital had a large domiciliary ward, occupied mainly by old patients who, for the most part, were completely bedridden but alert. Hearing of my visit, some of them asked to see me. I could not fight back the tears when I found Mrs. Mabel Dorr, the mother of one of my friends who had lived a few houses away from ours. She had been a robust young matron when I left LeMars thirty years before. Thin as a rail, her body had been twisted into grotesque shapes by rheumatoid arthritis. When I heard the cheerful "Hello Tommie," I knew it was the same person. At the head of the bed I noticed a hanging sculpture of Christ on the cross and wondered why Mrs. Dorr's redemption had been forgotten.

My dad was down the hall. When his first stroke paralyzed one side in December 1955, he learned to walk again and to speak well enough to resume his weekly radio show. The second stroke in July

1962 removed all voluntary motion except for crude movement of a shoulder. With an overhead device that allowed the limited shoulder motion to control a finger, he could point to the letters on an alphabet board and spell words one by one. Bobby Joynt, my high school classmate and now a famous neurologist, had used the term *pseudobulber palsy* to describe this terrible condition.

I had visited my father frequently since the complete paralysis and usually could guess halfway through a word what it was going to be. This allowed him to double or triple the speed of communication. It was the unspoken language of two old hand-set printers. In 1964 and 1969 I had brought to him from Denver the first copies of my books on kidney and liver transplantation. We had talked through the alphabet board about his pride.

His ruined and rudderless body could do one more thing. When he was propped up in bed, the same searching finger could find the keyboard of the typewriter. Gone was the machine gun staccato that could be heard while he churned out science fiction by night and reams of news copy by day. Every few seconds, there would be a single tap. When a letter came to me, I knew that it had taken him a week to write it. Already fluent in German, he now learned six more languages, including Turkish and Russian, and found pen partners overseas to whom he wrote his tortured letters and from whom he patiently awaited a reply.

When Tom and I walked in, he was studying. Tom learned the alphabet game as the afternoon wore on and found out that Dad had never left the hospital since his admission. We arranged to transport him on a stretcher to the high school auditorium. Accompanied by Tom, he was taken to the stage and concealed by the curtain just behind the lectern where I was to speak. When moved by emotion, he cried easily and made unintelligible moaning sounds.

A few minutes after I began my remarks, I heard the sounds, louder than I thought him capable, muffled by Tom's pleas that he be quiet. The audience buzzed and I hurried on with my platitudes, cutting passages wholesale. Dad explained afterward on the alphabet board that his joy at the moment was uncontrollable. My oration was extremely well received, largely, I suspect, because of its unexpected brevity.

Our task now was to take him back to the hospital. While we moved from the ambulance to the hospital, it began to rain lightly on his face, and his eyes filled with water, not from rain but from tears. How easily we forget the beauty of small things. He wrote later that he had not felt the rain in ten years.

The sentence was life imprisonment. Although his brain remained in its dungeon for almost fourteen years, the messages that were smuggled out through the typewriter never contained a hint of sorrow or bitterness.

» «

My father's life was creeping toward suspended animation, but so was mine. Then, on September 30, 1974, an old friend rescued me. I went to see Robert J. (Bob) Glaser, who had been dean at the University of Colorado when I was recruited there in 1961. He was the architect of the utopian full-time Colorado system, which soon would enter its death throes because of internal strife. What better person to see than the man who had created the perfect medium for my own transplant fantasies more than a decade earlier? Glaser himself was war weary, having been through the task of educational reorganization of the Harvard hospitals and a stint as dean at Stanford. Now he was director of the Kaiser Foundation, a charitable trust that promoted medical education and research.

Glaser's office was in Palo Alto, California. Grayer now, he still radiated energy. This always was incongruous because he had been so crippled by a childhood disease that a less indomitable person would have been immobilized. The force of his personality must have alienated some who should have been his natural allies but turned away in anger. However, he had been unfailingly kind to me and uncritical in the past, and was again. We talked quietly and earnestly for an hour. His advice was unequivocal. "Do not escape from one chair by fleeing to another. Fulfill your eight-year promise, maintain your skills, and at the end of the time return to what you were doing before."

He also offered to try to arrange a temporary life raft to make this possible. He was an advisor for the Senior Faculty Scholarship program of the Josiah Macy, Jr., Foundation. This New York based group dispensed its highly prized scholarships to established senior academicians who wanted to learn new technologies or recharge their ebbing energies. Although the deadline for applications already had passed for the next academic year, Glaser gave me a form and urged me to send it to him, saying he would process it personally.

He was successful. By the following May (1975), my wife, Barbara, our three children (Tim, Becky, and Tom), and I were on our way to London for a sabbatical at St. Mary's Hospital and Medical School. My research plan would be carried out with the pathologist K. A. Porter, the portal hepatotrophic project being our first priority. During the eighteen months before leaving Denver, numerous additional experiments lasting from four to sixty days were carried out in dogs, using the same general techniques as in the original study. However, we introduced variations that allowed us to measure the role of the pancreas (and insulin) in permitting the liver to grow back after its partial removal, or in permitting it to carry out special functions such as the production of certain kinds of fats that circulate in the blood (including cholesterol). The tissues from the last of these experiments were shipped to England in advance and were in various stages of processing in Porter's laboratory by the time we arrived.

As it turned out, the year in London became foreshortened to a piecemeal four and a half months because of administrative crises which erupted in Colorado each time our family (or I only) settled into our living quarters in Paddington, the district of London where St. Mary's Hospital is located. The first crisis occurred in August when the selection committee charged with finding a new chair for the Department of Medicine was unable to locate a candidate from another school who was willing to come and who could be afforded. A well-known specialist in kidney disease who already was at Colorado had solicited the job. The dean, Harry Ward, wanted to appoint this man but could not obtain the concurrence of the selection committee. Ward asked me to come back to serve on this committee and to engineer the appointment, which I did successfully. The English interlude before our family returned to Denver had been less than three months.

In November I returned to London, this time staying in the student quarters, only to be called back after a few weeks because of the resignation of the entire Colorado anesthesia department. The operating rooms had closed down, and Dean Ward asked me to co-head a selection committee to find a new chair for that department. Tony Aldrete, the pioneer transplant anesthesiologist, was recruited back from the University of Louisville, and within a few months full services were reestablished.

» «

In spite of the interruptions, we had confirmed unequivocally by the autumn of 1975 that the most important of the portal blood factors, which we had termed "hepatotrophic," was insulin coming from the animal's own pancreas. When the operation invented by Nicholas Eck caused the liver to shrink or the brain to be damaged as had been described by Pavlov (see chapter 5), it was in part because the operation damaged the liver by routing the insulin around it. As a final step, we showed that these effects could be prevented by instilling insulin directly into the liver after performing Eck's operation.[5]

There was an explanation also for the results of the auxiliary liver transplant experiments of a dozen years before. When an extra liver was transplanted, its fate and the fate of the recipient's own liver hinged on which organ had first access to the body's insulin supply. The liver with the best access thrived and used up most of the insulin the first time through the organ, leaving the disadvantaged and insulin-deprived liver to shrivel up.

The whole story was astonishing simple. Only a few years earlier the renowned physiologist and surgeon, J. L. Bollman of the Mayo Clinic, had written: "In the eighty-three years since it was first reported the Eck fistula has been reasonably successful in hiding its secrets as well as giving rise to many additional questions fundamental to an understanding of the functions of the intestine, liver and brain."[6] Now these secrets were stripped bare. The rapidity and accuracy with which this had been accomplished depended, first, upon the design of the experiments, and second, upon Porter's studies of the liver cells and the effect on these cells of different conditions of blood supply.

Because the smallest unit of life is the cell, a textbook of biology is by definition an ode to the cell. The pity is that a scientist must write the ode, using a special language that is incomprehensible to most readers. The glorious panorama of cell life then becomes a maze of unfamiliar words like hieroglyphics on an ancient scroll to be read only by scholars. Except when they are explained by someone like Lewis Thomas, who sprinkled magic on tongue twisters such as "rough endoplasmic reticulum" and "mitochondria".[7] These were the factories, electric light companies, fire brigades, police forces, and other components of the tiny world of the cell. It was the world that Porter watched quizzically through his microscope, painstakingly compiling notes or photographs and making drawings on a standard thickness paper of the silhouettes of the cells or cell parts.

These silhouettes could be cut out later as children do with paper dolls. But unlike a child, Porter weighed these paper dolls on a precision scale, derived the size of the whole or partial cell, and painstakingly recorded the values. Like his father before him, Porter was an artist. Only the subject was different. Instead of landscapes and human faces, his object of affection was the cell, which he did not consider lowly. The tapestry that we now could see had been woven by him.

» «

The English summer of 1975 left another mark. The second priority for the sabbatical was to review with Porter the reasons for success or failure in each of the first ninety-three cases of liver transplantation in Colorado. All the available tissues from the cases were sent to London in advance, as well as the clinical records. For every patient, we would assign a grade for the quality of the liver which had been used, the proficiency with which the recipient operation had been performed, the severity and original cause of the preexisting liver disease, the presence or absence of infection before and after transplantation, the control of rejection, and the amount and timing of antirejection treatment. Case by case, we poured over the details, trying to decide why some patients had thrived and why others in seemingly identical circumstances had died.

The conclusion was that the antirejection treatment we were using had too slender a margin of safety. There could be no quantum advances in liver transplantation under the present circumstances. When we gave enough Imuran and prednisone (plus a short course of ALG) to control rejection, the patients were dying of infection. Too little drug therapy was equally lethal because of rejection. There might be some improvement in certain details of the operation, particularly the reconstruction of the ducts that drain bile from the liver. The futility of trying to save patients who were near death by performing liver transplantation was obvious. Less ill candidates would be preferable. However, operating at an earlier stage of liver disease was not ethically justifiable in view of the fundamental imperfections of the available immunosuppression.[8]

It was important to compare these findings and conclusions with those from the English experience. By 1975 only two liver transplant programs remained in the world from the rampage of the late 1960s which had followed our first successes—our center and the combined Cambridge–King's College unit. The Cambridge University component of the English team was at Addenbrooke Hospital, seventy miles from King's College Medical School and Hospital in London. Roy Calne was the surgeon. He lived in a small house on Barrow Street in Cambridge from which he could walk or cycle to his laboratories and office, or commute to London if necessary on the M-1 highway. The trip took about seventy minutes by car. The medical liver unit at King's College Hospital was run by Roger Williams, one of the world's foremost hepatologists. In 1967, these two men created an inter-university collaboration which had functioned as unity for eight years by the time of my visit.

My son Tom and I left London on our bicycles, heading for Cambridge. We were joined there by Barbara, Tim, and Becky, who took the train. When we arrived, I learned that all the medical problems we were seeing in Denver were the same in Cambridge, if not worse, because ALG was not being used in the English trials. In addition, there was growing resistance to these procedures, particularly from the English anesthesiologists, some of whom regarded the efforts as macabre and refused to participate. Yet Calne also had long-term survivors who had returned from the brink of the grave to a normal life. These spectacular successes fueled his enthusiasm.

Roy Calne was not a wilderness explorer but no doubt he could have been. Some years later, David Winter, the director of the American trials with a better antirejection drug called cyclosporine, made the point. People like Calne, he said, had been the ones to walk on the moon. Determination and courage were the first principles. These had to be combined with intelligence and skill. Nature created the magical alloy in Calne, and then disguised it in a small and stocky frame as if the material had run out. As an afterthought, a mop of curly black hair was plastered on top of a powerful face which featured a prominent nose. Then the template was destroyed so that there could be no clones. This might be an item too hot to handle if it came in multiples.

Calne had been working in transplantation since 1959. His first published work was a historically important description of the prolongation of kidney graft survival in dogs with 6-mercaptopurine (see chapter 7). Like me, his first transplantation experience in humans was with the kidney. In 1966, his interest had turned from the kidney to the liver, and from this time on he made a series of creative and important contributions. He and his associates developed new experimental models, including those in the pig and rat, which greatly facilitated research in the liver field and raised questions about the immunologic behavior of the liver. Some of this early work still is the foundation for important basic research.

Calne had no intention of turning back. He was only forty-six, and there was plenty of time to make things better. On the late summer day in 1975 when we completed our visit, packed up our bicycles, and returned to London, there was no way to predict how this might be done or when. Until that time came, the fate of liver transplantation would depend upon an unspoken trans-Atlantic alliance between Cambridge and Denver without which further efforts could not have continued, much less succeeded, on either side of the ocean. These mutually supportive moral and scientific bonds pulled liver transplantation into the mainstream of medical practice but not until the decade was finished. By then, Calne had been knighted.

Not long after the Cambridge visit, I was scheduled to give a lecture at an international conference on childhood liver disease in

Paris, hosted by the Josiah Macy, Jr., Foundation. Even in Europe, our method of family travel was viewed as eccentric. My three children and I headed southeast from London on our ten-speed bikes and took a channel ferry from Folkestone to Boulogne. Halfway to Paris, in Normandy, we crossed the path of World War I armies. A statue stood in the center of every village with a list of those who had fallen. Throughout the countryside we saw artifacts of what must have seemed like the end of the world to those who were there in 1916. Traveling at the rate of nearly one hundred miles a day, we soon entered Paris.

My assignment was to predict what role liver transplantation would have in the treatment of biliary atresia, the disease leading to the original unsuccessful transplantation in Bennie Solis (see chapter 9). This same disease had been cured in Kim Hudson, who was in perfect health in the summer of 1975, five and a half years after liver transplantation. There were other examples of success, although these were still small in number. In Paris, I would describe the conceptual potential of liver transplantation for these children but emphasize its present unattainability at a practical level. It was always the same — a description of the perfect world of liver transplantation as it could be, but at the same time the world as it really was.

We made a final bicycle tour through Ireland. After taking a boat from Bristol to Dublin, and a train from Dublin to Westport on the west coast of Ireland, my sons and I cycled up the Donegal coast and came back through Letterkenny into Northern Ireland. Londonderry was under siege. When we reached Belfast, the bicycle shop where we planned to make repairs had been destroyed by a bomb. During the middle of our trip, four rock musicians traveling in a van were murdered south of Belfast, near the border. Every place we went, soldiers and police searched our gear. It was time to leave Ireland, and as it turned out, time to leave England. The summons from the Colorado dean of medicine was waiting in Paddington.

» «

On March 12, 1976, I left Denver for London to make a final attempt to complete my sabbatical. It was the day after my fiftieth birthday party. On March 11, I rode home from the Colorado

General Hospital on a bicycle as I had done almost every day for years. The garage door flew open and disgorged more people than I imagined our small house could hold. My Uncle Frank, his wife and his children, two of my children and all of my closest friends were there. I cannot remember being more genuinely touched.

I had planned only a short trip to London. The endless list of urgent administrative problems had doomed my hopes for a year off to pursue my research. The morning after the birthday party, it was snowing heavily. Barbara drove me through the blizzard to the airport. When we left the house, I had no idea that I would never be back. After the plane arrived in London, I received the first of the urgent but ambiguous phone calls with news that our oldest son, Tim, had been admitted to the hospital from Western State College in Gunnison, Colorado, where he had been a student.

I knew what had happened without being told. The marriage had lasted for almost twenty-two years before Barbara's forbearance ran out. Her rival, Mistress Surgery, had been too strong. If I could have explained to her what I have already described in this book and what was apt to come, it might have helped. More likely, it would have made things worse. After she had graduated from Cornell University, she had been selected by a major American corporation for an executive development program in New York. She gave this up and bravely struggled for the next two decades to retain her self-identity. Her decision to move on must have been one of despair.

There was no reason to stay in London. As I left, I delivered to *The Lancet* our last manuscript from the hepatotrophic project showing that insulin alone could prevent the effects of Eck's fistula. The editor of this journal was Ian Douglas-Wilson. I had met him before and knew him only as an older, rather austere gentleman, balding, and with such thick glasses that it was difficult to understand how he was able to see manuscripts, much less read them. He knew a lot about Eck's fistula and liver physiology and already had published a brief report in 1975 on our preliminary experiments showing the insulin connection. Now, in March 1976, the definitive manuscript included more data and extensive controls that answered completely some criticisms which he had received in "letters to the editor" the first time around.

The interior of *The Lancet* office on Adam Street was so unimposing that it was hard to envision it as the nerve center of one of the most prestigious medical journals in the world or in history. Douglas-Wilson's office was threadbare. I sat on a stool while he read. When he finished, he said that he was interested but would send it "across town" for a confirmatory opinion. Then he asked me to join him for lunch at a nearby tea room. Shyly, he asked why I looked so sad. I told him that I was going back to the United States the next morning to see my son in the hospital and to find out what was going on with Barbara, my wife. We shook hands, gravely I thought, and I took a taxi to Heathrow Airport to begin the long trip home. I have not seen Ian Douglas-Wilson since that time.

The thing that surprised me was that he did not forget. First came letters of encouragement, then a note about his retirement, and later accounts of his volunteer activities in computerizing and organizing the record system of a hospice, notes on gardening, and a description of his wife's serious illness. This went on for years until the mid 1980s. Perhaps he knew by then that I was all right and that is why he stopped writing. For my part, I was glad to learn recently that he is still well and will read this book because he will realize how important it was to have his quiet friendship. Whenever anyone tells me that the English are stuffy and cold, I smile and wonder if they know what they have missed.

When I arrived in Denver, I met with Barbara's younger brother, an airline pilot, who told me of her plans to marry a wealthy Middle Eastern businessman, which she did the following August, the day after the uncontested divorce.

» «

I did not know how to break the news to my father. A few days after returning from London, I received a letter from him. It was written with his special typewriter in the way described in his obituary a few days later: "the strokes had reduced him to eyes alive and a single operable finger with which to communicate on an electric typewriter. When we entered [his] room . . . we were at first puzzled by what seemed to be sounds coming from a radio but not music or a play or anything that would constitute a broadcast. The mystery was solved when it was explained to us that Mr. Starzl had lived for so many years with the noises of his newspaper office that they were being transmitted into his room from a mile or so away so that he could still feel part of his former working world."[9] His letter contained instructions about where he wanted to be buried and expressed hope that my work would continue.

The commercial planes traveling to western Iowa from Denver had already left. Knowing that morning would be too late, I rushed to Stapleton Airport and chartered a two-seat propeller plane to LeMars. We flew through a rain storm in Nebraska, and when the plane passed over the hospital on its way to the landing strip, it was heard by his wife, Rita, and her twenty-year-old daughter, Cathy (my half sister), at the bedside. It was 2:30 A.M.

When I came into the room, my dad was frightened and breathless. He had not slept for three days because he knew that if he did, he would never wake up. He wanted to talk one more time. His printer's instinct helped him to find enough letters on the alphabet board to get through. Then, I held his hand and told him to close his eyes and rest, which he did forever.

At 5 A.M., his doctors gave me his chest X-ray, which showed a blood clot in the main artery to both lungs. They asked me if we should support his breathing artificially with a ventilator. I told them no. He died that afternoon. The moving finger would write no more.

» «

A few weeks after the burial, I received an urgent phone call with the news that my sister, Nancy, was dying from liver disease in a northern California hospital. With the transplant coordinator, Paul Taylor, I organized a resuscitation team to try to save her. Carrying with us a liver preservation unit in case transplantation became a possibility, we were paged as we raced through the Stapleton Airport. She too was dead.

After my father and sister died, Tim left the hospital and moved in with me at my new apartment five blocks from Colorado General Hospital. Soon after, we drove to Gunnison to pick up his belongings. His room had been left untouched after his sudden departure two months earlier. The signs of suffering were there—a plain mat on the floor of the bare and dirty room, notebooks full of his writing about Eastern philosophy, and unfinished letters written to me or his mother. It was May, the month which can be the most beautiful one of the year in the Rocky Mountains. While we were driving back, Tim asked me to stop the car. He said that he could not tell if it was moving or if the mountains and road were in motion. The distinction would be hard for him to make for many more months.

Who knows how angels reach their destination? This one was a dark-skinned graduate nursing student from Kashmir (India), who lived down the hall in our apartment building with a female resident in medicine at the university. Encounters at the elevator changed to traffic between the apartments and, as the summer changed to autumn, to a wedding on the terrace of my apartment overlooking the mountain range far to the west. Inch by inch, my roommate-son had been brought up by this beautiful lady from the recesses of his private hell.

The new couple moved to Boulder, where Tim enrolled for the fall term in the Graduate School of Philosophy of the University of Colorado, and later the Business School. The thesis for his first master's degree was on Oriental philosophy. Now, all three of my children were on the same campus because Becky and Tom also had returned to their student lives. In the meanwhile, our house in Denver, which had been home for sixteen years, was sold.

» «

It would be misleading to call the hepatotrophic project the offspring of my sorrow. Instead the discoveries about the liver-supporting qualities of portal venous blood and their tedious confirmation in the years that followed were symbols of value and permanence. The hepatotrophic concept was a delicious little thing—not dramatic like transplantation, not emblazoned on the front pages of the newspapers, and not the subject of emergency policy meetings by a government agency.

In fact, the hepatotrophic concept was not even welcome in many quarters, nor was it accepted for a long time. It was contrary to almost mystical beliefs that all blood was metabolically equivalent. Once established, the dogma became encrusted during nearly a century by layers of irrelevant experiments from which invalid conclusions were reached. The accrual of enough evidence to deflate the fallacies required almost a decade of effort, not sporadically, but day to day.

In its own way, the accomplishment was more magical than the achievements in transplantation, and in some ways more difficult. Fifty years from now, long after all of our names are forgotten, a medical student will read about Eck's fistula, or other similar operations which change the portal vein blood in animals and humans, and they will know without a moment's thought why things happen that do after these procedures. To make this possible, we had placed our own handful of new information onto the giant pile of knowledge which has grown so fast in the years of my lifetime that no one knows or even cares any longer where it came from—except the people who put it there and who learned about themselves in the process.

Everyone concedes that transplantation is an iceberg. If the hepatotrophic concept is not another intellectual iceberg, I do not know what one is. It was smaller and less menacing than transplantation, to which it was related. It came along at exactly the right moment.

18

Smokey

At the surprise party marking my fiftieth birthday on March 11, 1976, the usual comments were made about the good fortune of surviving this long. If I had known in advance what the following six weeks would bring, I might have wanted not to reach the landmark. The world would never be the same again, but I could not withdraw from it. The prospect of returning to the operating room was uninviting. After a month passed, an urgent call for help came to my office from John Lilly, chief of pediatric surgery. He was operating on a five-month-old child with severe liver disease caused by drinking a Jamaican herb tea. The liver scarring had caused blockage of the portal vein, swelling of the thin-walled veins in the wall of the esophagus, and so much leakage of body fluids into the abdomen from the back pressure that management was no longer possible.

The child needed a portal venous bypass around the liver to decompress the dammed-up blood. The procedure, which was the same as Eck's fistula, did not seem possible to Lilly. He shamed me into trying. After many hours of tedious effort, the operation was successful. Fifteen years later, in April 1991, a letter postmarked Denver arrived. In it was a manuscript that Lilly had submitted to a surgical meeting, entitled "Acute Budd-Chiari Syndrome in Infancy: Treatment by Portacaval Diversion." The article described how this infant had become a normal teenager. Lilly's report concluded by saying, "To our knowledge, she is the youngest survivor of portacaval diversion for acute Budd-Chiari syndrome."

One by one, my patients would save me by letting me help them. The rescuers came in waves.

» «

One year later, in March 1977, I assembled a research group to clarify some details of the portal hepatotrophic project which would require approximately six months. One of the recruits was a young black woman named Joy Conger who owned an unusual black poodle named Smokey. We soon learned that the dog and his mistress came as a package.

People who came together in Denver for research applicable to the care of patients tended to form bonds greater than simple friendships that fade with time. With few exceptions, they sought each other out later in life at meetings, helped each other professionally and personally, and kept track of each other in an unusual way. They maintained high standards, as if to do otherwise would be to betray a commitment long since made. There were no restrictive covenants for admission to these groups nor any sense of the high versus the low born. The VA research team that gathered in January 1977 epitomized these flexible criteria.

There were two Italians, Tony Francavilla and a fifty-one-year-old man named Giuseppe Mazzoni who was chief of surgery at a regional hospital in Valmantone (twenty-five miles from Rome) that was affiliated with the University of Rome. A third member was a young surgeon named Joseph Benichou who had spent his earlier life in Algiers and moved to France at the time of Algerian independence. Benichou's passion was liver transplantation. While in Denver, he had completed a study on liver preservation that allowed livers to be safely preserved for six to twelve hours. The work opened up for us the possibility for the first time of shipping livers from city to city after their removal. Benichou now is a professor of surgery in Paris.

The anesthesia and aftercare of the dogs was entrusted to a twenty-eight-year-old man who had spent the preceding fourteen years at Canon State Prison for murdering his parents during a camping trip in the mountains. They had abused him from an early age until the time of the tragedy, when he was fourteen. During his prison confinement, the man had continued his education by correspondence, graduating from his university courses with a 4.0 grade point average. Because he could not obtain a parole without an assured job, John Kane, a Denver attorney and friend of mine (now a federal judge), asked me for help. Kane's request was supported by Brant Steele, a professor of psychiatry at the University of Colorado who had studied the case and also was sympathetic to the prisoner. After distinguishing himself in the laboratory job, the young man gained admission to medical school with my help. When I said good-bye to him before leaving Denver in 1980, he was still a medical student, planning to provide family practice care for the poor after his graduation. This is what he has done.

The technicians responsible for the chemical analyses were Joy Conger and a young Korean woman named Sokie Bae. Sokie Bae, who had a sophisticated background in theoretical and practical chemistry, later went to medical school in Japan and is now a physician. Joy joined us "on loan" from the Clinical Research Center for transplantation at Colorado General Hospital. She lived with Smokey and her younger sister, Julie, in an apartment in Aurora, an eastern suburb of Denver. Beyond this information, we knew little about her except that she was skillful, intelligent, and always smiling.

Those who worked with Joy liked her, and some of them had a faintly protective attitude because of her seeming physical vulnerability and a tendency to bruise which she said was the result of a childhood illness. She had spent most of the first two years of her life in the isolation of a sterile room in an army hospital in Wiesbaden, Germany. She was confined there because of a disease called *aplastic anemia* which is caused by failure of the bone marrow to make red or white blood cells or the tiny particles (platelets) which contribute to normal blood clotting. Her survival and spontaneous recovery were considered miraculous because in the mid-1950s, before the availability of bone marrow transplantation, almost all such children died. Thus, when she came to work at the Clinical Research Center with a black eye or bruised arm, as she did frequently, the aplastic anemia seemed at first to be a reasonable explanation.

Another cause for concern was Joy's work schedule. In addition to the position at Colorado General Hospital, she always had a second job. These included being a waitress at a fast food restaurant, clerk at a convenience store, security guard at the Stapleton Airport, and janitor at the United Airlines training building. She had withdrawn from college after two years and was trying to save enough money to go back. Being five feet four inches tall and weighing 110 pounds, she did not look big and strong enough to have this kind of life and smile too.

It turned out that the smile was a mask. On one of the first Mondays of the new project, the special radioactive chemicals (isotopes) that were needed for the planned experiment had not arrived. With the day free, the lab crew was off to the ski slopes of Winter Park within minutes. There, equipment was rented for Sokie Bae and Joy, who had never skied before. By six that afternoon we had returned. Mazzoni and I dropped Joy off in Aurora and went back to our apartments. During the night, someone smashed the head and tail lights of my car. In the morning, and for the rest of the week, Joy did not come to work. On Friday I told Tony Francavilla to replace her.

Then, late on Friday afternoon, she came to the laboratory to talk to Francavilla, her face obscured with huge dark glasses and her head covered with a bandanna. Francavilla reported that her mysterious absence was because she had been beaten so badly that her eyes were swollen shut and her face was almost unrecognizable. The assailant was the man she had been seeing socially, and the punishment was retaliation for making the ski trip without authorization. Francavilla wanted to go to the police. Later, we drove to her apartment. She was hiding in the bathroom where she was being taken care of by her sister.

Joy was a battered woman. As is typical in such cases, she was too frightened to fight back and too ashamed to seek or accept help. In any event, there was no one to turn to. Society at large was not yet aware of (or had not accepted) the pervasiveness and seriousness of physical and psychological abuse of women. When I asked the professional advice of friends—one a police officer and the other an experienced professor of psychiatry—both said to avoid involvement. These men believed that victims of these deadly assaults somehow were gratified by them. How else, they reasoned, could the repetitive nature of such incidents be explained?

The experts had placed the problem in the hands of the amateurs. The foreign legion in the laboratory sprang into action with a rescue operation that took eighteen months and was not completed until August 1978 when Joy moved to Texas where her parents lived. During the whole time, there was a sense of danger which was deepened by more incidents—each more alarming. What happened to Smokey, Joy's black poodle, seemed like a symbolic warning. This little dog was the only living thing she could love without reservation and without fear of exploitation, jealousy, and abuse. Smokey ate delicacies when Joy lived on mashed potatoes to save money, endured claw manicures while she developed work calluses on her hands, had coiffures at the kennel while she had her hair done by girlfriends, and wore a rhinestone collar and ankle bracelets in contrast to her bare and callused hands. Smokey gave back all that he had—which was utter devotion.

When he came to the laboratory, Smokey's every move mirrored Joy's. He reacted fiercely to the presence of other dogs, an instinct which proved fatal. One evening in the spring of 1977 she took him for a walk near her apartment. Two large animals, hearing Smokey's challenge and unrestrained by a leash, tore open his abdomen and snapped his neck. He died in her arms. Joy buried Smokey in the vacant lot across the street from her apartment, read a prayer, and put up a cross. Many puppies were brought to the laboratory by those who wanted to help. She refused them.

When her father came for Joy and her life's belongings, there was a collective sigh of relief that could be heard from Seoul to Rome. She would be back, she said, but as the months went by, I knew that she could not return to Denver. When the American College of Surgeons met in San Francisco in October 1978, I talked to Jim Maloney, my old roommate at Hopkins and now chairman of surgery at UCLA. I told him about the vacuum that Joy's absence had created in my life. I told him that for the first time since moving to Colorado seventeen years earlier, I would consider leaving in order to be on neutral ground to which she could come.

Maloney and I talked for several hours at Tommy's Joint, a

restaurant up the street from the San Francisco convention center. The professional and administrative discussions were very brief. What I really wanted to know was his reaction to the fact that Joy was black and his prediction of the reception she would receive if she came as my wife. As far as Maloney was concerned, Southern California was color blind. She would be accepted on her own merit. Within a few weeks, I visited Los Angeles with several colleagues to see what could be done for the further development of transplantation in the UCLA environment. This was the first of three such visits over the next fifteen months.

The move that Jim Maloney and I discussed in 1978 came to pass in 1981 but to another city, Pittsburgh. By then, I realized that the scars left on Joy from abuse were deeper by far than anyone realized and had ancient origins during her childhood illness and itinerant life as the daughter of the professional soldier whom I came to know. Retired now from the army, James Conger, her father, raises cattle on a 160-acre farm in East Texas near the small town of Quitman. The land has been in the Conger family for nearly one hundred years. Tony Francavilla and I explored its far recesses in 1986. After passing around a picturesque pond and through the trees just beyond, we came upon two giant metal scarecrows, gracefully bowing to each other in gentle rhythm as they pumped the precious oil from beneath the earth.

Joy's mother, Ollie, is with James now, but in 1978 and for a long time before and after this, she lived separately in Dallas and worked in a teacher's credit union. When she was young, she enrolled in Tuskeegee University in Alabama, but was married soon after and withdrew. Her father, Lucky McMillan, taught school in Arkansas and Texas for nearly forty years, and beyond him one of her forebears was an early faculty member of the Meharry University Medical School in Nashville, Tennessee. Ollie's foremost ambition was to have one of her three children graduate from college. She fought for this and lost, but only temporarily. Joy will make this dream come true if she can. She became a student again in 1989 at Chatham College in Pittsburgh, majoring in human services. Her thesis is on the factors causing the abuse of women. Some day soon, she hopes to open a home for battered women in Pittsburgh.

No one on the VA research team of 1977 claims that they saved Joy. The obverse was true. Tough as steel and flexible as a willow, this slender and graceful lady saved us, one by one. I cannot say how she did it with the others. With me, it was with gentleness and patience. The year after Smokey was killed, she brought me a tiny snake plant which I did not want because it would be too much trouble to care for. I took it anyway to avoid hurting her feelings. She said to call it Smokey. Smokey grew out of its container, and then succeeding ones, until now at the age of fourteen, it dominates all of the many other green things that grow in our house.

When the plant was young, I had lost all trust and perhaps all hope. There was no one to talk to. Then one night, a strange thing happened. I had a vivid dream, not like other dreams which have a broken sequence, cannot be reconstructed, and are quickly forgotten. This one had no gaps and left an imprint as memorable as a moving picture. I was sitting with my Irish mother in our large living room in LeMars. The Philco radio was there, with a green photoelectric eye for focusing the frequency bands. She was young again, but I could see the beginning of worry lines at the corners of her mouth that deepened with each new year of her life as I grew up. I wondered if I had put them there.

She said that she was proud of what I had done and not ashamed of anything she had seen, granting the imperfections that I shared with other humans. The conversation was a long one and very explicit. There was much more ground to cover when she stood up and excused herself, saying that she would come back some day if necessary. Then I woke up with the sunlight in my eyes.

This was not the kind of dream I would tell to another physician or even to a good friend. It was too real. That day I had lunch with Joy and told her that I had had a visit from my mother.

"I thought that she was dead," she responded.

"She is," I said, "but she came in my sleep."

"What did she say?"

And so I told her. This was someone I could talk to.

19

The Kidney Wars

After more than a four-year absence from the field, my resumption of kidney transplant activities began with a ceremonial function. On August 25, 1976, I was invited to give an overview of the present status of kidney transplantation for the Transplantation Society meeting in New York City. I wore a bright red tie. Afterward, an old friend, Erna Moeller of Stockholm, who had a vague idea of the disruptions in Denver, remarked how the tie symbolized coming back to life.

In preparing, I began with the state of the art as it had been in 1972 and tracked what had changed since then. Scientifically, there was almost nothing new. This became the main message of my talk. I expressed concern about the intellectual growth arrest which had overtaken our once scintillating new specialty. It was not a problem of resources. The scientific inertia had developed at the same time as economic plenty arrived and may have been related to it.

When I left the field four and one-half years earlier, kidney transplantation was fiscally impoverished—lacking a sponsor and designated "experimental" by insurance companies that wanted to avoid responsibility for its costs. Consequently, aside from government-funded research centers and a few designated VA hospitals (ours in Denver was the first), renal transplantation could be offered only to the most wealthy recipients.

Across the parking lot, our Clinical Research Center at Colorado General Hospital was the largest one in the country devoted to transplantation. The ability of this and other similar units to meet the needs of indigent citizens or even of the population with money was overwhelmed by the end of the 1960s. Stories were common of desperate acts to finance the dialysis or transplant care of loved ones in private centers. Failing these efforts, crimes sometimes were committed to raise money. A national scandal was in the making.

During this bleak period (early 1971), John Fordtran, a doctor from Dallas, came to see me in Denver with his son, Billy, whose kidneys had failed because of an inherited disease. This was no ordinary physician. Fordtran was one of the foremost specialists in the world in diseases of the digestive tract. He was chief of the Division of Gastroenterology at Southwestern University Medical School. Even with the special advantage of unusual access to health care, he was going to have to consider leaving his cherished but modestly paying academic post for private practice or some other more remunerative position because of the financial liability ahead. Eventually, this is what he did. Two of Billy's siblings had the same disease and also would need transplantation in the future.

Fordtran's wife, Jewel, volunteered to donate one of her kidneys in an operation scheduled in June. As she prepared herself for her ordeal on the evening before, chance intervened. That afternoon, a fatally injured teenage accident victim with the same blood type as Billy arrived in the emergency room of Colorado General Hospital and later was pronounced brain dead by the new criteria which had begun to be accepted less than three years earlier by the legal and medical professions. Knowing that their son could not recover, the teenager's parents had given permission for organ donation.

With a cadaver kidney at hand, I talked to Jewel and John Fordtran about changing our plan for Billy's care. The new strategy would be to cancel the living donor operation and use the cadaver kidney instead. The appeal of sparing Jewel a trip to the operating room was great. The argument against this was that results with cadaver transplantation were far inferior in 1971 to those with kidneys from living related donors. Because only Jewel had the right blood type for donation, there could be only one parental kidney among the three offspring with present or future need. Who should have the kidney and when were questions not answered by the formulas that direct decision making in medicine.

Jewel and John sought guidance in prayer. When they finished, Billy was given the cadaver kidney — which has functioned perfectly for two decades. Few of that era could expect to do this well.

» «

The economic plight of patients and their families was relieved in 1973 by the federally mandated End-Stage Renal Disease (ESRD) program. The new system originated in 1972 with an amendment to the Social Security Act. It was one of the most noble examples of health care legislation in history and a step toward "socialized" medicine. In fact, it *was* socialized medicine for end-stage disease of one organ, the kidney. This legislation created overnight a national network for the care of patients with kidney failure. The government would pay the bill for both dialysis and transplantation.

At the same moment, the federal flow of gold created a potential economic aristocracy of medical kidney specialists who provided artificial kidney services, and a disincentive for transplantation. In Denver, for example, where the only artificial kidney facility had been at the University of Colorado with Joe Holmes, a dozen private facilities sprang up overnight. There were too many centers to be profitable if their patient ranks were thinned by systematic removal of patients for transplantation.

Consequently, potential recipients were "sequestered" on dialysis units. One way of doing this was to tell them horror stories about transplantation, which all too often were true. The shocking cost of the national ESRD program mushroomed to over $2 billion per year over the next ten years. Although 90 percent of these costs were for artificial kidney centers and not for transplantation, the size of the bill was not forgotten by health care planners when the time came later to consider how to finance the transplant care of recipients of livers, hearts, and other organs.

Thus, what had been a crusade when I dropped out of kidney transplantation in 1972 had become a business by 1976 — a very large and often unpleasant one. Competition was naked among physicians and/or surgeons who had "regional concessions" for dialysis and transplantation. Ruthless struggles raged for control of various franchises within the ESRD program, including cadaveric organ procurement agencies. The competition between hospitals for the economic and public relations advantages of transplant programs sometimes had the appearance of corporate warfare.

It looked to me as if the patients whom we had set out to save fifteen years earlier had become pawns, dehumanized now by joining a captive population with limited options set by an entrenched bureaucracy. The supreme degradation for a patient must be to feel that the expression of a demand or a deviation from docile behavior can jeopardize his or her own care. This was not my imagination at work. The concept was confirmed in letters from or conversations with physicians or their assistants openly stating their proprietary relationships with their patients. They had forgotten that doctors are the servants, not the masters, of patients. Or that patients belong to themselves — not to doctors, to systems, or to hospitals.

The new bureaucracy had created a second problem. A large cash flow can contribute to the fixation of therapeutic practices at an unsatisfactory level. Because a major change requires inconvenient or expensive retraining, one refuge may be blind adherence to, and even insistence upon, historically important but dangerous, morbid, and ineffective treatment practices. This is what had happened in kidney transplantation. Despite its inadequacies, antirejection treatment was frozen into an administrative matrix that did not exist five years before. The lack of progress reinforced and perpetuated dependence upon living, related kidney transplantation with its generally less formidable immune barrier.

It was disillusioning to see how the new system was governed by reactionary kidney specialists and newly arrived surgeons who became wealthy from the flow of federal money and whose riches then made them into a powerful lobbying force against policy changes. Many were people who lacked insight into the process of scientific inquiry and who had a minuscule record of discovery and contribution to the field. To justify and continue the national program that was in place, it was necessary to minimize its shortcomings. Only those who were genuinely inexpert could do this convincingly. By not realizing that what they said was untruthful, they were able to boast with a clear conscience.

My talk in New York about these issues was interpreted by some as a symptom of personal woes and depression. This was not true. The purpose was to improve things. To make change, I had to identify publicly whose dogmas were being challenged. They were my own. Two years later, in November 1978, I went to New Orleans to receive the David Hume Memorial Award, the highest distinction of the National Kidney Foundation. It was given for the development of the double and triple drug treatment strategies using combinations of Imuran, prednisone, and ALG which I had introduced during an earlier generation and which I was asking to have reexamined. In accepting the award, which I treasure as much as any I have received, I analyzed once more how the field had reached an impasse that could be broken only by harsh self-assessment and fresh ideas.

In addition, I asked if the integrity of the field had been undermined by persistently optimistic claims in kidney transplantation that were deceptive at best and potentially fraudulent at worst. Very few centers published their own results with cadaver kidney transplantation, and those that did reported unsatisfactory graft survival and high patient mortality. The public received a far more optimistic message. When I finished speaking, I had the impression that the award would have been rescinded if another vote were taken. I was subverting business.

The problem with focusing on the defects of kidney transplantation in 1978 was that there was no obvious way to make things better. The fundamental issue was the poor safety and ineffectiveness of the antirejection treatment. There were two possible avenues for exploration. A team at Stanford had devised a promising modification of the X-ray treatment that had been found to be unsatisfactory when used in a less discriminating way nearly two decades previously. The new procedure, called "total lymphoid irradiation," subsequently received a limited trial at the University of Minnesota.

The second avenue was the mechanical removal of the lymphocytes—the cells responsible for rejection—by tapping into a large channel in the neck through which a heavy concentration of these lymphocytes flow on their way back to the heart. A surgeon named Curt Franksson had introduced this technique, known as "thoracic duct drainage," in Stockholm in 1963, and it had been used sporadically since then. We conducted extensive further trials in Denver in 1978 and 1979.

Both total lymphoid irradiation and thoracic duct drainage improved the results after kidney transplantation. However, their use was superseded and then aborted by the arrival of a new drug called Cyclosporin A (later called cyclosporine in North America or elsewhere ciclosporin).

» «

In May 1978 I met Roy Calne again at the Jerusalem Hilton Hotel where we were on a program together at an international surgical congress. He was just starting clinical trials in kidney transplantation with cyclosporine. It was too early to predict what would happen. We talked for a long time about the second and third waves of transplant surgeons who were resistant to change. Change, it seemed, would depend upon those who had opened the field. The professional risks were too great for younger surgeons whose careers could be ruined by deviation from "standards." This would be a job for risk-takers.

Cyclosporine had been discovered by workers at the Sandoz Corporation, a Swiss pharmaceutical company, and shown by one of their immunologists, Jean Borel, to weaken immunologic responses in a variety of test systems, including skin transplantation in mice.[1] The conditions for new drug development were vastly different in the mid and late 1970s than in the early 1960s. Basic immunology had undergone a revolution apart from transplantation. New technology made it possible for Borel to show at the outset that cyclosporine inhibited only part of the immune apparatus. Like a doting parent, he had carried out a one-man crusade within his company to save his precious drug from abandonment.

The drug affected primarily a subgroup of lymphocytes (T-helper cells) which control the actions of other cells that work together to destroy transplanted organs. The possibility was implicit that the narrower range of immunosuppression with cyclosporine would allow transplantation to be performed without unduly depressing all immune functions. The nonspecificity of previous therapy had frustrated the further development of transplantation for almost fifteen years after the breakout of 1963. Three groups in England had been doing research with cyclosporine, and all had confirmed and extended Borel's claims.

Cyclosporine already had led a charmed life. David White, a young immunologist at Cambridge, heard Borel speak about the drug at an immunology meeting in Britain in 1976 and had obtained a small supply. The ability of the drug to prevent heart rejection in rats was so great that these experiments, which were performed by a Greek surgeon named Alkis Kostakis, were not believed by Calne at first. By the time the Cambridge workers had pressed on with kidney transplantation in dogs, Sandoz Corporation executives had decided to discontinue developing the drug because of its cost and their perception that the limited market would never permit them to recoup these expenses. White and Calne flew to Basel and successfully appealed the decision, allowing an experimental supply to continue. Further experiments led directly to the first human trials in kidney transplantation at Cambridge, beginning in the late spring of 1978.

That the transition from the laboratory to the clinics came in Roy Calne's department in Cambridge was not surprising. Calne was a true pioneer with a steady record of contributions since 1960. However, rumors or reports of new drugs and immunosuppressive techniques had come to be viewed with reflex skepticism by 1978. Every new lead worldwide for a dozen years had fanned enthusiasm at first, followed by disappointment. When Calne and I talked in Jerusalem in May 1978, his comments about cyclosporine were guarded. What had been learned about cyclosporine by the first week of September added an entirely new dimension. Calne presented these results at the biennial congress of the Transplantation Society in Rome. By this time, cyclosporine was seen as the most promising new antirejection agent to emerge in years.

I was among those in Rome trying to obtain cyclosporine for a pilot clinical trial in the United States. However, fulfillment of these Italian autumn dreams was not automatic. Calne's first clinical experience revealed that the most serious side effect of cyclosporine in humans was damage to the kidneys. This meant that the transplanted organ, if it was the kidney, could be the victim of the very drug being given to prevent its rejection. Attempts to use the drug in England and France for bone marrow transplantation also led to frequent damage of previously normal kidneys.

The prospects of obtaining the drug for American trials appeared to be fading until the arrival in Denver of David Winter on a warm spring day in 1979. Winter had authorized pilot trials with cyclosporine at the University of Colorado and at the Peter Bent Brigham Hospital in Boston. He had a green light from the U.S. Food and Drug Administration (FDA).

The name Dave Winter cannot be found in either the early or late publications on cyclosporine, and for that reason it will soon be forgotten unless this book is read. For reasons of his own, he declined authorship on all the work from the U.S. trials with cyclosporine, for which he bore the responsibility. Winter was the director of clinical research for American Sandoz with an office in East Hanover, New Jersey. He was exactly the right man for the times.

In his previous life, Winter had been director of life sciences for the National Aeronautics and Space Administration (NASA) where, among other duties, he was responsible for the medical care of the astronauts. He knew how those remarkable people had been chosen who would walk on the moon and go other places where humans are not supposed to be. He understood that the heart was as important as the head in breaking new ground. He chose carefully where his cyclosporine trials would be, and after this he depended on the judgment of those he selected to stay the course or to change direction if need be. In many ways, Winter was the opposite of previous emissaries from Sandoz with whom we had been talking. His approach was flexible.

When we heard that we could have a supply of cyclosporine, the next question was how to use it. As we made plans, the phone bills between Denver and Cambridge mounted. My prime source of information was David White, the scientist responsible for bringing cyclosporine to Cambridge and for the first animal experiments there. One by one, White read me the pathology reports from the human kidney graft biopsies (tissue samples) obtained during the pilot trials. On the basis of these, I concluded that the transplanted kidneys in the English patients had suffered a double injury, first from the drug and second from incompletely controlled rejection.

If this interpretation was correct, it would not be acceptable for us to treat with cyclosporine alone, which was the strategy being recommended in Cambridge and eventually adopted for the trials at the Brigham. Instead, we would combine the cyclosporine with steroids. This had been the secret with Imuran nearly two decades previously (see chapter 10). The steroids would allow dose maneuverability downward with cyclosporine in case kidney toxicity was suspected. An additional wild card was the preparation of half of our first patients with thoracic duct drainage before transplantation. These deviations from the original Sandoz protocol needed high-level authorization. Dave Winter had to make a decision upon which his own career could ride. After hearing the arguments he granted permission without hesitation. Another name was added to the roll call of quiet heroes who risked everything for a small step forward and asked nothing in return.

If the Colorado cyclosporine trials had been delayed for even a few extra days, it might have been impossible to go forward. Calne's definitive report on his first thirty-two kidney transplantations was published in the November 17, 1979, issue of *The Lancet*.[2] The journal did not arrive in the library until after we had started. There was nothing in it that we did not know, but the article was seen as vindication of their negativism by those who were opposed to the Colorado trials. None of the English patients had normal kidney function, five had died, and three had developed white blood cell cancers.

Opposition to the Colorado trials was not muted. On January 7, 1980, an unusual letter went to all members of the Colorado Society of Nephrologists over the signature of a physician from Colorado Springs. He said he was writing at the suggestion of a senior physician at the University of Colorado. The letter read:

> The exact figures regarding mortality and morbidity have been difficult to obtain, and the protocol for post-operative immunosuppressive therapy does not seem to be consistent and is considered by some to be excessive.
>
> Because of the many rumors and accusations regarding the transplant program at the University of Colorado, [the senior university physician] asked me to write to the nephrologists in the State regarding

their experience with the transplant program. He would also like to invite comments on any potentially immoral and unethical situations.

I would suggest that you forward your recent transplant experience and any other comments to [him] at the University of Colorado. Thank you very much for your cooperation in this matter.

When confronted with the letter by Richard Weil (a transplant surgeon) and me, the university physician who had engineered it explained that he was trying to smoke out the sources of the outcry so that he could defend us from our critics. I was willing to reserve judgment, but when the letter found its way to the desk of Dave Winter, it was interpreted by him as hostile. The consequence, when I departed for Pittsburgh at the end of 1980, was exclusion of the University of Colorado from the new age of transplantation that had been spawned there. Cyclosporine would not become available again in Colorado until December 1983, after the FDA had released it for general use.

The death rattle of the Colorado transplant program was being heard at its moment of greatest triumph. The kidney trial was a stunning success through the rest of the winter and early spring of 1980. The one death among the first twenty-two recipients was from a heart attack that did not seem related to the cyclosporine. Cadaver kidney graft survival was 85 percent. The eleven patients who had been prepared with thoracic duct drainage had an extraordinarily easy recovery and almost no evidence of rejection. The other half without thoracic duct drainage did almost as well.

However, negative reports about cyclosporine were coming in from European centers and from the Boston trials. The drug's charmed life was to be tested again. In March 1980, we were warned by David Winter that the Sandoz Corporation might not go forward with the drug trials. Our reaction was amazement. Cyclosporine, used with steroids, already had revolutionized our kidney transplant program. We were on the eve of beginning its use for liver transplantation.

The urgency of making public our positive kidney transplant experience was obvious. I spoke about the problem to Loyal Davis, who still was the editor of *Surgery, Gynecology, and Obstetrics*. I asked him to consider expediting a report on cyclosporine-steroid therapy before more harm was done. Enfeebled by age and heart disease, the ancient warrior agreed. The article came out during the 1980 meeting of the Transplantation Society that this year was convened in Boston over the Fourth of July holiday.[3] It was in the nick of time. Further English trials in London at the Royal Free Hospital had been stopped because of more white blood cell tumors, severe kidney damage, and several deaths. At the Brigham, the results were no better than with Imuran and prednisone, and only a handful of cases had been entered.

During the middle of 1980, two more American kidney transplant trials with cyclosporine were started. Again, Winter's instincts were true. One choice was the University of Minnesota program headed by John Najarian, Dick Simmons, Dave Sutherland, and Ron Ferguson. Before starting at Minnesota, Sutherland assigned a surgeon named John Rynasiewicz the task of reviewing all the cases in Cambridge and in Colorado. From what he learned, they decided to go with the cyclosporine-steroid cocktail, Denver style.

Rynasiewicz, an unusually pleasant young man with blond hair and a magnificent physique, spent two months in Colorado compiling information and interviewing patients, physicians, and nurses. A year later, he had lost nearly one hundred pounds and was completely bald. Dying now from leukemia, he made one last trip to the American Society of Transplant Surgeons annual meeting in May 1981 to see where his efforts had led. From what he heard, he may have derived some peace of mind. The last time I saw him was at the Drake Hotel in Chicago. He was standing in a coffee room with his back to the wall, using it for support as he patiently explained to shocked friends who had not recognized him what had happened in his life.

Winter's second choice was the University of Texas, Houston, where Barry Kahan also adopted the Colorado therapy. Over the years, Kahan became one of the world's experts on cyclosporine. Both new trials were positive. The cyclosporine era of transplantation was launched.

20

A Tale of Four Cities

Throughout 1979 and 1980, Joy Conger, the missing member of our research team, was a thousand miles from Denver at the Parkland Hospital in Dallas where President Kennedy died. There, she had joined the research team of John Fordtran, the medical doctor whose son had received a cadaver kidney transplant in Denver in 1971. I no longer had any illusion that she could or would return to Colorado.

My discussion with Jim Maloney in October 1978 about moving to UCLA also was receding into the background. A few days after we met in San Francisco, I had visited him in Los Angeles along with several members of the Colorado transplant team. We did not see how the program could be transferred intact and dropped the negotiations. Almost exactly one year later, in October 1979, I made a second visit to UCLA with most of the same Colorado people. By this time I had made arrangements for the cyclosporine trial, which could be conducted at the location of my choice.

During this second visit, it looked as if getting these trials off to a quick start at UCLA would be difficult or impossible. Failure to do so would be a breach of our moral contract with Sandoz. In contrast, all the ingredients were in place in Colorado, including three transplant wards and several research laboratories. The collaboration with the anesthesia department, which was essential for the further development of liver transplantation, had never been stronger. Finally, a physician named John Franks had just obtained funding of $1.8 million per year for five years for our federally financed Clinical Research Center (CRC). This was where the liver recipients would be treated.

Estimates of the time necessary to duplicate elsewhere the resources developed layer by layer over the years in Colorado were as long as two or three years. We had no choice. A few weeks later, in November 1979, we began the cyclosporine kidney trials in Colorado and I notified Maloney that we could not come to California. The matter was finished. What followed would be a lonely Christmas. I did not go to Dallas for the holiday with Joy. It seemed best to let these memories fade.

Although the decision now had been made to pursue the cyclosporine trials in Colorado, no one imagined that this would be easy. The school of medicine and its Colorado General Hospital were chronically short of money. After years of bickering within the faculty about the division and deployment of resources (the polite word for dollars), two new administrative leaders were in office and were committed to straighten out the mess. That they came was a tribute to their fortitude and self-confidence in view of the sad and usually brief tenure of a string of their predecessors, of whom Dean Harry Ward was the most recent. In the end, the new leaders fought each other.

They were John Cowee, chancellor, and M. Roy Schwarz, dean. Cowee, a lawyer, had been chancellor at Marquette University Medical School, Milwaukee (later renamed the Medical College of Wisconsin), during a volatile period in the life of that school. Schwarz was recruited from the University of Washington. A trained anatomist, he possessed an M.D. degree of which he was proud. Although he had not gone on to an internship or further training, he had a lively interest in clinical affairs to the point of frequently providing advice and judgment about patient management. His skyrocket career was based largely on the organization of outreach medical education programs, managed from Seattle and extending as far north as Anchorage, Alaska.

Both men appeared to agree that the full-time system, which used the income from fees generated by physicians and surgeons to subsidize basic science development and weak clinical departments, should be changed. This was not so much an idealistic reform as a practical one; the clinical faculty would be more eager to see private patients because they would generate money for their own income from which a percentage would be remanded to a dean's fund. The strict full-time system with fixed, relatively low salaries for clinicians was being abandoned.

Nothing could have been less interesting to me personally than this convulsive transition, although I knew how important it would be for my successor as chair of the Department of Surgery. I gave the job of negotiating the new conditions to Charlie Halgrimson, the vice-chair of our department. It turned into a nightmare of arguments about percentages of fee rebates to the dean's fund, reallocation of state salary lines, criteria for judging industriousness and faculty effectiveness, and all the other matters that break down teamwork. I knew that my stipulated tenure as chair would be finished in six months and that the responsibility for these essentially business matters would be turned over to someone else.

This impending administrative change and my lame duck position may have contributed to what happened next. At 8 A.M. on January 5, 1980, Charlie Halgrimson and I had a new year (and new decade) meeting with Dean Schwarz, who announced his decision to fire two of my surgical division chiefs. He had prepared a letter to one of these men on a sheet of light green paper and indicated that he had reviewed it with the university attorney. He asked me to retype the letter on departmental stationary and sign it, which I declined to do. Halgrimson and I remonstrated for an hour that the grounds for dismissal in both cases were not established or were insufficient. I asked if this decision had been cleared with the chancellor, John Cowee, and the governing board of regents of the university. The answer was affirmative. Nearly a year later on the day I left Denver, Cowee told me that this was not true. How such a misunderstanding could have occurred was never explained.

At 9 A.M., Dean Schwarz announced that he had to catch a plane to Grand Junction and that he considered the matter settled. I walked back to my office, wrote a letter of resignation from the chairmanship, and carried it back to the dean's office. Then I found the division chiefs in question and explained to them that they had been fired. Both were Jews. They reacted with the dignity that two thousand years of history had taught them.

My own plans to stay at the university were not yet irreversibly altered, because neither of the discharged division chiefs had any interactions with the transplantation service. However, within a few more days, there were two more firings that destroyed the substructure on which transplantation depended. The first to be dismissed was Jack Franks, the director of the Clinical Research Center where we did our clinical liver transplantations. A few days after this, Tony Aldrete, now chair of anesthesia, received a letter from the dean accepting a resignation which Aldrete, a Chicano, claimed had not been tendered. All four dismissals ended up in the law courts.

These events, added to the university-instigated letter of January 7, 1980, to the nephrology society (see chapter 19), meant to me that the university was no longer interested in transplantation research and that the definitive cyclosporine trials should not (or could not) be conducted in Colorado. I wrote to the dean resigning from the university, effective by the end of the year. I had no place to go. I only knew where not to be.

On January 24, 1980, I was scheduled to give a lecture to the Los Angeles Academy of Medicine entitled "Recent Developments in Transplantation." Jim Maloney was my host. I told him what had happened, and we made a gentlemen's agreement that I would join his department as soon as I could see a logical place to interrupt the Colorado cyclosporine trials and fulfill other obligations. There were no negotiations of any kind regarding space, salary, or resources. He promised only to create the best environment for creative work of which he was capable. My promise was to do the best I could. It did not work out as planned, but no one ever tried harder than we did.

By the time of my return from Los Angeles, the dean's office had released an announcement of my resignation. Rumors circulated about the reasons, and because there was no simple or single explanation, I said nothing. An innocent response to a journalist's question made things worse. When someone inquired about a purported battle within the university between titans, I asked, "Who is the other titan?" not meaning to imply that I claimed that status. Those who did took offense.

Leaving Colorado was a difficult decision. Few people knew that the balance was tipped by the lady in Dallas who did not know what was going on, but without whom the rest of my story would have been different. If it had not been for Joy, I would have stayed in Colorado in spite of what had been done to the program. Jim Maloney knew the key to the mystery because I told him. The others would not have believed the truth anyway, except for a reporter named Bill Simon from the Denver *Post* who had been assigned the task of finding out. Instead of exploring the devious pathways of the new breed of investigative reporters, he tried the simpler expedient of asking me. I asked him to consider our conversation private, which he did.

The responsibility remained to finish at least the first phase of the cyclosporine trials. The Colorado transplant team would be intact for a few more months. Like the notes from an exhausted musical toy, its sounds came slower, week by week, as the Rocky Mountain spring chased out the winter. But there was no mistaking the tune.

» «

The surrealism of my last days in Colorado was epitomized by the eighth floor Clinical Research Center at the Colorado General Hospital. At the entrance of its ten-year-old transplantation wing was a plaque inscribed with the date of the ribbon-cutting ceremony that was to launch a new day for transplantation. This special ward had been built with private and state legislative donations raised by Bill Waddell while he was surgical chair. Now, the maintenance workers arrived with screwdrivers to take the plaque down. They came away red-faced. The death grip of the bolts was too strong for simple extraction. When the bolts were cut, Waddell's request for the souvenir went unheeded. The worthless piece of bronze was thrown away.

Beyond the CRC entrance, the ten beds were still filled with patients and would be through midsummer. Among these were the first liver recipients treated in Colorado with cyclosporine. No one except those caring for them seemed to realize that they were unique. They competed for space with architects and administrators who were dividing up the rooms, or planning how to. The changing of the guard was scheduled for November 1, 1980. By then, conversion of this historic place to administrative offices must begin.

By March 1980, after more than twenty kidney recipients had been treated with cyclosporine, the liver trials began. Twelve patients were entered between March 6 and September 28, 1980. Eleven of the twelve lived for a year or longer. The single patient who did not survive was the one best remembered. It always was that way. The recipient was an eight-year-old child named Traci Pagel. She had a poorly understood disease (Byler's syndrome) which runs in families and causes slow destruction of the liver. The donor, a victim of a domestic accident that had caused brain death, was in a Chicago hospital. After being up all night obtaining the liver, I performed in the Pagel child what I thought was a perfect operation. A few days later, the main liver artery (hepatic artery) clotted. The child lived for twenty days, during which no other donor could be found for an attempt at a second transplantation.

Traci's parents had another child named Mark with the same condition. They put off transplantation for as long as they could, but eventually this was done in April 1983 at Children's Hospital in Pittsburgh. The same complication cost the life of the second child. A year or so after this, Mr. Pagel (the father) was found dead at home. He had taken an overdose of antidepressant drugs. It was another example of the silent mortality in transplantation. The mother still writes to me. Eight years later, in 1990, she remarried.

To dwell on the one failure and ignore the eleven successful cases would be a distortion. For the first time, it looked as if liver replacement might be more than a curiosity and a subject for ethical debate. I thought that this should be said at the biennial congress of the Transplantation Society which was held in Boston in 1980 over the Fourth of July holiday. My assignment, as it had been in previous society meetings since 1968, was to summarize progress in liver transplantation. These always had been dreary recitations of problems and failures, with a few spectacular successes that justified expressions of hope. This year it was different.

I began by paying homage to Roy Calne, who was sitting in the front row. His courage and persistence had made possible what I wanted to say. Then I explained what had happened with our recent cadaver kidney recipients, whose course of recovery bore little relation to the complicated and unfavorable picture described from other centers in a symposium on cyclosporine earlier in the same meeting. The difference was due to our systematic combination of cyclosporine with steroids.

Finally, I described the fresh batch of liver recipients treated with cyclosporine, whose follow-up was only one to four months, much too short to allow triumphant claims. Still, they were all alive and well. We had never seen so little trouble before in eight consecutive liver recipients. This, plus the supporting observations in the much larger series of kidney recipients, meant that we were at the beginning of a new phase in transplantation which I predicted would be called the cyclosporine era. This came to pass. One year later, a more complete account of our liver experience was published in the *New England Journal of Medicine*, and the stampede began for the development of other liver transplant centers.[1]

» «

After coming back from the Transplantation Society congress, we needed to make our final plans for the move to UCLA. Returning to Los Angeles had never been far from my mind after living there in 1951. It was possible for ten cents back then to take a streetcar to the beach from most parts of the city. The freeway system was still on the drawing board or under construction, except for a stretch from Pasadena to Long Beach. If there was smog, I did not notice it. There was an outdoor restaurant on every street corner, and in Hollywood, a star or starlet was behind every stop sign—or so they claimed. The inner city never slept. Driving north to Santa Barbara one heard the sound of a background symphony played by the waves of the Pacific Ocean. To the south were Laguna Beach, Balboa Island, San Diego, and Mexico. This was heaven to someone from a small town in Iowa whose only big city experience by 1951 had been in Chicago.

For my Colorado colleague, Shun Iwatsuki, the lure of California was even greater. Although classified as a fellow in training, the title belied Iwatsuki's credentials. After graduating from the medical school of Nagoya University in Japan, he had acquired thirteen years of further training, most of it in the United States and

directed to transplantation or to the understanding and treatment
of liver disease. He held a transplant fellowship in Colorado in 1971–
73 and had returned for a refresher year beginning in July 1979.
Along the way, he had married an English woman whose identical
twin sister lived in Southern California. Iwatsuki not only wanted
to be considered for a move to UCLA if one occurred, he insisted
upon it.

Jim Maloney, the surgical chair at UCLA, had a long-standing
love affair with his university, where he had worked for more than
twenty-five years. He said that it was an institution built by
geniuses so cleverly that it could be run without effort by idiots. If
anyone could make such a judgment, it was he. He had an uncanny
grasp of biomedical science, applied physics, and mathematics.
Precision in all of these disciplines was reflected in his administrative practices.

Nothing about Maloney had changed in the nearly thirty years
since we were roommates at the Johns Hopkins Hospital. It was he
who was a genius, not some unnamed university founder in the
background shadows. In 1954, Maloney had gone from Hopkins to
the faculty of UCLA to be in the department of Bill Longmire, the
first surgical chair of this new medical school. Together, they
helped make UCLA the crown jewel of state universities, competi-
tive from the first day with the established prestige centers in the
east. A natural leader, Maloney was selected as chair in 1975 when
Longmire retired.

Maloney's brilliance was only a plus, however. The most important thing was that he was a trusted friend and a model of probity.
His presence, not institutional mystique, was the attraction of
UCLA. He knew that our mission would be more than the conventional development of a university program. The evidence accumulat-
ing in Denver indicated that the day of liver transplantation had
arrived, made possible by cyclosporine, a drug that would improve the
transplantation of all organs. These Colorado-based developments
could not be interrupted. Their continuation would depend on a fit of
only three people—me, Iwatsuki, and the organ procurement coordinator, Paul Taylor—with existing UCLA faculty whom we would
recruit to the project. The fit would have to be perfect.

As the months went by, the three of us realized that an unresolvable problem had developed. There was no place to work. The Wadsworth Veterans Hospital on the UCLA campus was a prime location for a research laboratory and for the vitalization of the small clinical kidney transplant program that Will Goodwin had started there fifteen years earlier. Not long after Maloney and I made our handshake agreement, however, an epidemic of Legionnaire's disease, an infection that causes pneumonia, occurred at Wadsworth Hospital, precluding the admission of patients who were on antirejection treatment.

Loss of the VA facility had a domino effect. Beds and operating room time at the nearby University Hospital were at such a premium that a large new program could not be accommodated overnight. Other beds might be available at the UCLA Harbor Hospital thirty miles to the south or at the Sepulveda Veterans Hospital twenty-five miles to the north. With such a consortium of hospitals, each contributing a small number of beds, we calculated that it would be necessary to drive more than one hundred miles a day to see all the patients. By May 1980, we had decided to centralize the transplant activities at the Sepulveda VA Hospital.

Although the central office of the Veterans Administration was interested in going forward, it became obvious that the Sepulveda Hospital could be used in the foreseeable future only to accommodate kidney transplant recipients. The development of liver transplantation seemed out of the question. The intensive care facilities were limited, the necessary blood bank support was not identifiable, and the anesthesiology department was opposed to even trying. In addition, I had heard rumors during the summer, which I now confirmed, that a minority clique of the surgery faculty had made an unsuccessful effort in the spring to block my appointment. Some of this group were old acquaintances who had pretended to welcome my arrival and upon whose help I was counting. They had their own plans for developing portions of the total package we were bringing, which had many composite parts. It was a turf issue. The prodigious amount of work that we were proposing would have to be done under siege.

In early September, on the eve of the irrevocable final step in the move to California, Iwatsuki, Taylor, and I were in Los Angeles. We sat up all night in our hotel room discussing the ethics of bringing a crucial experimental trial of cyclosporine-steroid therapy and the still controversial operation of liver transplantation into a medical center and surgery department which had such divided purposes. If the slightest thing went wrong, it would be a death blow to a lifetime of work and also a potential professional disaster for Jim Maloney.

The next morning, I canceled our plans to go to UCLA at a meeting with Jim Maloney and Wiley Barker, the chief of staff at the Sepulveda VA. We were in Barker's office. The meeting was preparatory to the visit of an outside review group which would arrive later in the day to decide how much of the requested $4 million of VA funding should be given as start-up funding. I hardly listened to what was being said during the first hour or so. Then I stood up and announced that I would not be coming.

After they were convinced that the decision was final, I told Jim Maloney that I wanted to spend the afternoon on the beach with my friends, Iwatsuki and Taylor. Jim said, "I thought that I was your friend," and I answered, "That is why I cannot come." Most of the site visitors were waved off and spared the trip to California. Eli Friedman, a kidney specialist from Downstate Medical Center, Brooklyn, already was in the air and was sent back home from the Los Angeles Airport. Several years later he told me that it was the most profoundly unproductive day of his life.

Following our walk on the beach and dinner at the Maloney house, we took the midnight flight back to Denver. On the way, Paul Taylor said he was going to try to repair some fences. He had two boys who would have to be supported through college. He could not afford to be out of a job. Iwatsuki's English was not as fluent as it is now, and therefore more direct. When I told him that we probably would be ruined by what I had done, he said, "Wherever you go, I come too!" Iwatsuki already was one of the best surgeons in the world. Within less than three years, he also would be one of the best known.

» «

Leaving Colorado and then not going to California were professionally the hardest and most dangerous decisions of my life and perhaps the most important. The following afternoon, I called Hank Bahnson in Pittsburgh and told him what had happened. He asked if I would mind if he talked to Jim Maloney, which I did not. The day after that, I flew to Pittsburgh and spent a day talking to key members of the hospital's small transplantation group. As usual with my moves, there were no discussions of salary, space, faculty rank, or prerequisites. Bahnson and I discussed a position for Iwatsuki, our fit with the existing kidney transplantation program (which was in urology), cyclosporine, the development of liver and heart programs, and Joy. If there was anything more than this, I cannot remember it. The starting date in Pittsburgh would be January 1, 1981.

Pittsburgh's kidney transplant program had been started in 1964 by a general surgeon named Bernard Fisher during the proliferation of centers that followed the discovery of combined Imuran-prednisone immunosuppression (see chapter 10). Because Fisher's interest was in cancer research, the transplant program was passed on to other general surgeons over the ensuing years. In 1976, it was given by Hank Bahnson to Thomas Hakala as an inducement for Hakala's recruitment to be chief of the Division of Urology, but with the proviso that it would be shared equally with a general surgeon interested in kidney transplantation when such a person could be found by Bahnson. Bahnson himself was interested in the field and had performed some of the earliest heart transplantations in the United States in 1968. He knew that antirejection treatment was not good enough to warrant continuation of these efforts except in research centers such as Stanford, but he was ready for the next phase if the time came. He realized that an advance which would make this possible would be made with the kidney transplant procedure, and he believed me when I told him that we already had accomplished this in Denver.

I did not know Hakala or even of him until we met during my one-day visit to Pittsburgh in mid-September, 1980. However, it was obvious that he was a skilled and forceful person. His office in Presbyterian University Hospital was the center of his life. On one side of the room was a large sofa with cushions that had been flattened and frayed during the fitful naps that substituted for sleep during the nights when kidney transplantation operations or donor procurement activities were going on. He looked exhausted. His naturally round face was swollen after an all-night transplant operation, followed by a full day of scheduled urology procedures. At one end of the sofa was a pile of operating room scrub suits. He had just changed and was wearing a fresh one, covered with a white lab coat. This was a man with commitment.

Hakala had much on his mind that day. The unwelcome news of my visit had caught him by surprise. He explained to me how, after taking over the transplant program, he had developed an effective apparatus to screen prospective kidney recipients and find cadaveric donors for them. The apparatus included two key people. One was Donald Denny, a former social worker who previously had worked in organ procurement in Philadelphia and now had the title of director of the Transplant Organ Procurement Foundation (TOPF). TOPF was incorporated as a private foundation about two years before my arrival, with a three-man board. Hakala was president. The other two members were Bahnson and a university urologist who worked under Hakala in his division. There had been no meetings of the directorship. It would be another five years before the first board meeting was convened in November 1985, when TOPF was reorganized in compliance with the new federal legislation known as the Gore Bill.

The other key person in the apparatus was a clever nurse named Mary Ann Palumbi with exceptional organizational abilities. Her principal job was to keep track of kidney transplant candidates and to select from them the ones who would receive cadaver kidneys from TOPF. However, she also worked at organ procurement and was not only skilled technically but also a persuasive lecturer and spokesperson for the recruitment of cadaver donors. She understood how hospitals functioned. Because she had several years of job experience in an intensive care unit, she argued that her medical knowledge rivaled that of most physicians if not all.

Hakala had chosen well. These were determined people who gave him their undivided loyalty in return for autonomy in running the kidney business. This was *their* business. They recruited a network of underlings who answered *to them*. The apparatus was inextricably woven into the affairs and support of the urology division. Hakala had announced his intention to solicit independent departmental status for urology, and if this was successful, he planned to take the transplant organization with him and to use it as the economic base of his new department. Bringing me in as the director of transplantation overall was a direct affront to these plans and in his opinion a violation of the spirit of his understanding with Bahnson.

As to the transplantation practices, he explained that he was using the double drug therapy I had introduced in 1963. He had my 1964 book on kidney transplantation in his office and said that it was his bible. Hakala used Imuran and prednisone intelligently and had a one-year kidney graft and patient survival which was in line with national standards. The results reflected what could be accomplished elsewhere, using Imuran and prednisone without ALG.

He told me to stay away from Pittsburgh. This is a small program, he said, in a mediocre school. No one knew or cared what went on in this little corner of the world, and he preferred it that way. He realized that his program could never compete with the large centers. No one from his team had gone to the Transplantation Society meeting in Boston ten weeks earlier or knew anything but rumors about cyclosporine. In defending what he regarded as his turf, he reminded me that all was fair in love and war.

I liked him enormously. This was someone who could be believed if you asked a direct question. It was important to have this conviction later when it became my responsibility to decide on changes, including those involving him. For the moment, I thanked him and told him that I would not be around long if we could not do better than what he had just described. Before I went back to Denver, I told Hank Bahnson that I could work with Hakala, whose soliloquy may have been the most honest one I have ever heard.

» «

I had hoped that the final year in Colorado would be my last great conflict. If the Armageddon had to continue, at least there was a time out during the last three months of 1980. There were places to see and teaching debts to pay. I started in October with a tour of medical schools in Japan and continued in November with a stop in Quatar to arrange the first dialysis facility in that country, a pause in Khartoum to see the union of the Blue and White Nile rivers, visits to the museums in Luxor and Cairo, and a reunion with the Italians Mazzoni and Francavilla. The odyssey ended in December with a visiting professorship at San Marcos University in Lima, the oldest medical school in the Americas.

Joy went with me. Her existence was known to a group in Pittsburgh who now opposed my faculty appointment. For political purposes, her dark skin was a certifiable sin, but the storm clouds and thunder in Pittsburgh were too distant to be seen or heard in South America. My old Johns Hopkins friends would take care of the details. In Pittsburgh, there was Hank Bahnson who had been my best man in the distant past, and in California there was my old roommate, Jim Maloney.

Jim Maloney did more than release me from my promise to him. He protected me. The story gleefully was floated in inimical quarters that the UCLA appointment had been withdrawn. Maloney corrected this. My professorial appointment at UCLA had been in effect since July 1980. To help Hank Bahnson, Maloney gathered my UCLA dossier and letters of support and sent them to the University of Pittsburgh. With the precision of a scientist and the conscience of a priest, he unfolded the paper trail.

Two years later, Maloney called me in Pittsburgh about a young protégé named Ronald Busuttil who wanted to start a liver transplant program. UCLA was ready now with room at the University Hospital in Westwood. Could Busuttil spend a sabbatical in Pittsburgh to be trained? If there had been a better way to thank Jim Maloney, I would have done it, but this was a start. Before long, UCLA had one of the premier liver transplant centers in the world. Later, the UCLA kidney transplant program was taken over by Thomas Rosenthal, one of the young Pittsburgh urologists whose career was based on the Pittsburgh cyclosporine trials of 1981. By then, Maloney had moved on from the surgical chairmanship to be associate dean.

» «

By the time the fat lady sang in Colorado, the audience was gone and so was the theater. The cyclosporine trials ended in September 1980, and a few weeks later the Clinical Research Center for Transplantation closed down for its conversion to administrative space. Ten years later, I visited it. The reader may imagine the amount of business that can be transacted there in the complex of administrative offices that had replaced the patient rooms.

In July 1988, the Colorado liver program was reborn when Alden Harken, the new chair of the Colorado Department of Surgery, decided to resume these efforts. We sent him Igal Kam, a talented Israeli surgeon who had trained with us in Pittsburgh for two years. Kam was joined by Fritz Karrer and Roberta Hall, two other products of our Pittsburgh fellowship. A new pearl would grow from this perfect nidus. With it, my commitment to my university haven for nineteen years was fulfilled. A liver transplant program belonged at the University of Colorado of all places in the world.

» «

The day I arrived in Pittsburgh, December 31, 1980, was the city's coldest New Year's Eve in 100 years. The three others from the Denver transplant team had come a few days earlier. Shun Iwatsuki was appointed assistant professor of surgery. There also were two fellows who would complete their training and leave in four months, Goran Klintmalm of Stockholm and Carlos Fernandez-Bueno of Puerto Rico. No administrative support structure awaited us, not even an office. For organ procurement and for kidney transplantation, we would use the administrative apparatus build by Tom Hakala and administered by Don Denny.

This was not an invading army of people. What we brought in bulk was opportunity. The Colorado trials had gained us an IOU from Dave Winter of the Sandoz Corporation. Cyclosporine in early 1981 still was available for kidney transplantation in only four American cities. Boston remained of the original two, and Pittsburgh now replaced Denver. The others were the universities of Minnesota and Houston.

The consequent growth of the Pittsburgh kidney program was phenomenal. Throughout 1981, 106 kidney transplantations were performed, three times the number in any previous year. Candidates swarmed to western Pennsylvania. The newly arrived Colorado team was a collective teaching machine, conveying what had been learned in Denver and converting information to therapeutic recipes that could be used in Pittsburgh and then exported around the country and world.

21

Letter in a Birmingham Jail

A standard dictionary definition of a minority is: "the smaller in number of two groups constituting a whole; a group having less than the number of votes necessary for control; a part of a population differing from others in some characteristics and often subjected to differential treatment."[1] Most minority groups are peace loving, or begin that way. Nevertheless, a minority revolt occurred in Pittsburgh in 1981. The uprising was of the renal transplant population and the surgeons and physicians who were treating them.

In his *Letter from Birmingham Jail* (April 16, 1963), Martin Luther King addressed the benevolent master class that ruled his disenfranchised minority with the avuncular wisdom that comes with presumed superior knowledge and wisdom: "as Reinhold Niebuhr has reminded us, groups are more immoral than individuals. . . . We know through painful experience that freedom . . . must be demanded by the oppressed. . . . An unjust law is a code that a majority inflicts on a minority that is not binding on itself."[2]

What has this to do with transplantation? It requires no imagination to appreciate that patients with chronic illness make up a collective minority. They must compete with the majority who do not have the burden of disease. To the extent they are invalided, they can become the subjects or even the captives of the doctors, nurses, and institutional employees who care for them. Nowhere is this more obvious than in evolving fields like transplantation. The patients on one hand can be deceived about the validity of unproved claims, or on the other stripped of all input into decision making about their own care. Either way, the result can be decay of public trust in our medical institutions and atrophy of the souls of those who work there.

» «

By the end of 1980, the superiority of cyclosporine-steroid treatment had been well established in Denver for both kidney and liver transplantation, and it was assumed that this advance would apply to the heart as well. Getting this far had not been simple. When we first used cyclosporine in patients, we encountered multiple unanticipated management problems. Effective management schemes evolved only after some fifty pilot cases. The best of these required a combination of cyclosporine and prednisone.

By the end of the learning process, there appeared to be little justification to resume the Imuran-prednisone treatment, which gave inferior results. This would be particularly indefensible with liver or heart transplantation where the penalty for failure to control rejection was death. Although patient and graft survival after liver transplantation appeared to have been doubled in the Denver pilot trial, there was nearly continuous pressure to conduct a randomized trial.

In a randomized trial, patients selected by lot receive either conventional treatment with drugs that are certified by the Food and Drug Administration (FDA) or the so-called experimental treatment. The conventional drugs can be prescribed and bought at drug stores, whereas the experimental drugs are unavailable through commercial channels. The lottery, once started, is expected to involve a predetermined and equal number of patients in both treatment arms, the exact number being determined by a statistical calculation called a "power" number.

It seemed to us that randomization between a superior versus less effective drug regimen would create a profound inequity in the recipient population. In our opinion, a randomized clinical trial, if it was to be ethical, should be done only if we were uncertain that there was a treatment difference. This is referred to as a null hypothesis. The instruction to carry out a trial in spite of our conviction that a null hypothesis no longer existed came from the Institutional Review Board (IRB) of the University of Pittsburgh.

There was bitter resistance to a randomized trial for liver and heart transplantation, and the order eventually was rescinded. However, the IRB was implacable in its insistence upon a randomized trial for patients receiving their first cadaver kidneys, and this was conducted for most of 1981. The patients who entered the kidney trial had no option other than to refuse participation in the experiment. If they refused, they were consigned to old-style therapy. If they accepted, at least they had a fifty-fifty chance of obtaining the new treatment, which by now was increasingly conceded to be superior. They then had to sign an elaborate document, several pages in length, which explained in detail the risks and benefits of the new treatment. This was known as informed consent.

No one who drew the long straw (actually a sealed envelope) ever asked for the conventional therapy. Those who drew the short straw that meant consignment to the older therapy were angry. They had lost their chance to obtain the drug that had brought many of them to Pittsburgh. Their anger deepened when they began to see the actual results in cyclosporine-treated patients with whom they shared the hospital ward. Not only was graft survival better with cyclosporine, but the doses of prednisone needed were lower. They came to understand that they were part of a human experiment comparing two methods of treatment in which the answer already was known.

The randomized trial was abandoned only after nearly one hundred patients were entered. What was the IRB—the board that had ordered this trial? It was not some cruel and disembodied group lusting for information no matter what the cost. It was a collection of human beings who had assumed the authority and responsibility of protecting patients' rights. Their charges were simple: to prevent unwarranted human experimentation and to make sure that the subjects, as the patients were called, knew what they were agreeing to when they signed the permission forms. On the board sat respected members of the university medical faculty, faculty from other branches of the university, clergymen, lawyers, ethicists, and community representatives. My respect knew no bounds for those who were willing to accept this difficult assignment. Yet my differences with them were irreconcilable.

» «

The guidelines for clinical investigation had seemed clear in the early days of transplantation. The essentials were self- imposed restraint, insistence upon an experimental research basis for clinical application, nonconcealment of results, and above all, maintenance of the doctor's responsibility for the welfare of each individual patient. In those days, transplantation was conceived as an innovative form of treatment in which the risk was borne by the patient—who also received the benefit, if any. This had been the credo of physicians and surgeons since the dawn of medicine, and it was the fundamental background for each of the great advances in transplantation.

Francis Moore of Harvard may have been the first to sense a change. When I reported the first successful cases of human liver transplantation at the American Surgical Association in 1968, Moore's discussion was prophetic. In commending the four-year pause that followed our unsuccessful efforts with this procedure in 1963, he pointed out that the moratorium was imposed by the transplant surgeons themselves without a need for consultant boards. He concluded:

> There has recently been a statement issued by a committee in Washington that attempts to deal with these matters as applied to the heart [transplantation]. As nearly as I can see, none of the authors of this document has busied himself with the transplant problem over these last 15 years. . . . Nor does it [the document] make reference to the fact that the moral security of the next 25 years of American surgery, in exploring this new field, will rest secure just where it has in the past 20 years . . . free and untrammeled . . . [in the hands of] those departments and individuals that are willing to take the time and trouble to develop both the immunological and surgical aspects of organ transplantation, as Dr. Starzl has demonstrated today with a project that was held in abeyance until the fundamentally ethical nature of science itself indicated that it was time again to move ahead.[3]

Movement away from Moore's principles for the transfer of therapy from the laboratories to the clinic occurred so slowly that it went almost unnoticed until it was complete. The change was not a phenomenon unique to Pittsburgh, where the historical record was fierce defense of patients' rights. It was a worldwide trend for which the leadership came from the least likely source. It was from a U.S. government policy which actually was designed to protect patients from unwarranted human experimentation.

Notwithstanding the purpose, the result of this policy in many cases was a conflict of ideologies and objectives that distorted the bond between physician and patient. There also was an unspoken disenfranchisement of patients. This minority population of ill people—for whose benefit the health care system existed—lost their vote and even the right to protest. Starting with safeguards against potential abuses in clinical experimentation, other changes occurred that had the potential of even graver abuses. This was the institutionalization of human experimentation by the most trusted of social instruments—universities, hospitals, and government agencies.

A movement so momentous must have an origin, and this one did. Its seed, the National Research Act (Public Law 93-348), was of such purity that it is difficult to see how a crooked tree could grow from it. The bill, signed by President Gerald Ford on July 12, 1974, created the National Commission for the Protection of Human Subjects of Biomedical and Behavioral Research. The charges to the commission were "to identify the basic ethical principles that should underlie the conduct of biomedical and behavioral research involving human subjects and to develop guidelines which should be followed to assure that such research is conducted in accordance with those principles."[4]

The commission was made up of eleven people: three physicians, three lawyers, two psychologists, one Christian theologian, one ethicist, and the president of the National Council of Negro Women. One of the members, David Louisell, professor of law at the University of California, Berkeley, had been at the Ciba Ethics Symposium in 1965 (see chapters 14 and 16). He and another lawyer died during preparation of the commission findings. The document was called the Belmont Report because many of the discussions took place at the Belmont Conference Center of the Smithsonian Institution in Washington, D.C.

The Belmont Report focused on defining boundaries between patient care (the practice of medicine) and clinical research. There was no ambiguity about the meaning of "practice." It involved "interventions that are designed solely to enhance the well-being of an individual. . . . The fact that some forms of practice have elements other than immediate benefit to the individual . . . should not confuse the general distinction between research and practice. . . . an intervention may have the dual purpose of enhancing the well being of a particular individual, and, at the same time, providing some benefit to others" (p. 3 and n. 2).

The three ethical principles mandated for clinical research were stated with equal clarity. First was *respect for persons*, which meant acknowledgment of their autonomy and respect for those with diminished autonomy. The meaning was defined by negative example:

> To show lack of respect for an autonomous agent is to repudiate that person's considered judgments, to deny an individual the freedom to act on those considered judgments, or to withhold information necessary to make a considered judgment, when there are no compelling reasons to do so. . . .
>
> Some persons are in need of extensive protection, even to the point of excluding them from activities which may harm them; other persons require little protection beyond making sure they undertake activities freely and with awareness of possible adverse consequences. (P. 4)

The second principle was *beneficence*. The report read:

> The term "beneficence" is often understood to cover acts of kindness or charity that go beyond strict obligation. In this document, beneficence is understood in a stronger sense, as an obligation. Two general rules have been formulated as complementary expressions of beneficent actions in this sense: (1) do not harm and (2) maximize possible benefits and minimize possible harms.
>
> . . . However, even avoiding harm requires learning what is harmful; and, in the process of obtaining this information, persons may be exposed to risk of harm. Further the Hippocratic Oath requires physicians to benefit their patients "according to their best judgement." Learning what will in fact benefit may require exposing persons to risk. The problem posed by these imperatives is to decide when it is

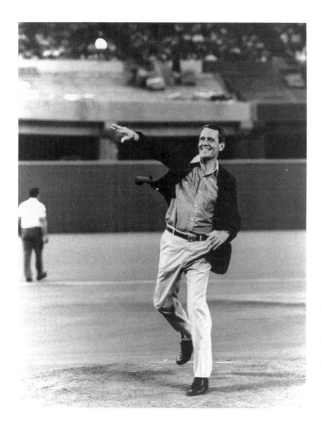

Throwing out the first ball at Three Rivers Stadium in Pittsburgh 1983. *Pittsburgh Post-Gazette*

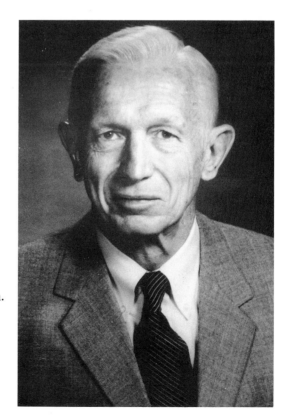

Henry T. Bahnson.

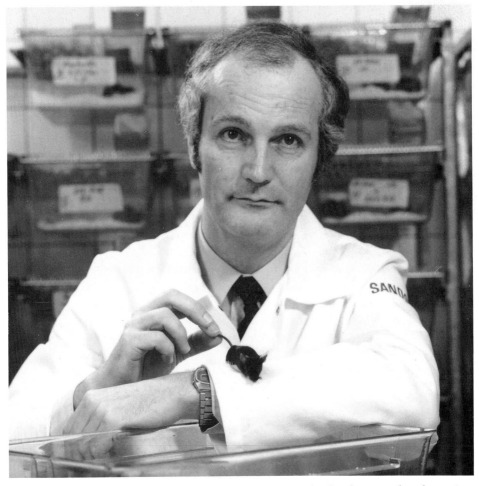

Jean Borel, who discovered cyclosporine.

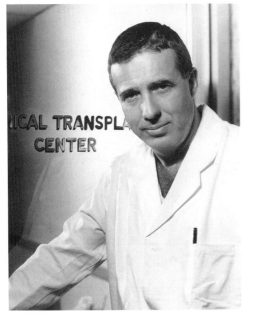

David Hume, about 1970. *George Miles Ryan Studios, Minneapolis*

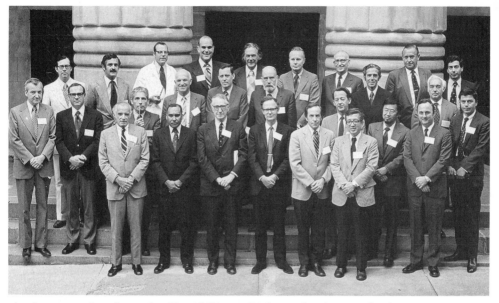

At the symposium honoring David Hume, Richmond 1974. In the front row (L to R) are John Merrill, Samuel Kountz, Francis D. Moore, and Kendrick A. Porter. Second row: I am between Joseph E. Murray and Don Thomas (Nobel Laureates, 1990); second from right is Paul I. Terasaki, and third from right is Folkert (Fred) Belzer. Third row: fourth from left is John Najarian; seventh from left is Jean Hamburger; and Roy Calne is at extreme right. The white-haired man in front of Calne is Rupert Billingham.

A break in the action, Denver 1978. In the background, Paul Taylor talks with Linda Yamamoto. *Photo by Carl Iwasaki*

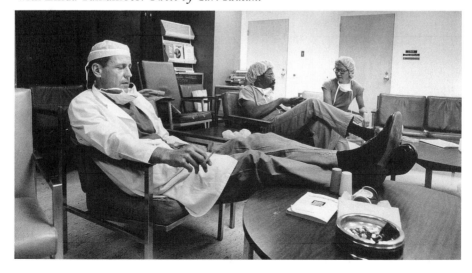

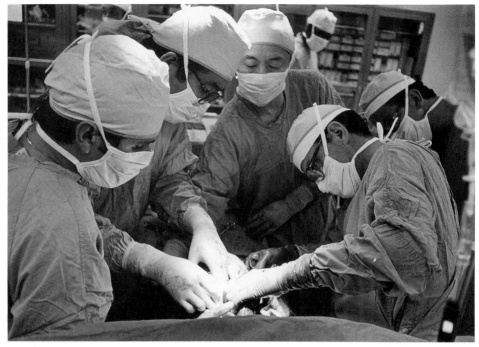

In surgery with (L to R) Hector Diliz-Perez, Shun Iwatsuki, and He-Qun Hong, Pittsburgh 1981. *University of Pittsburgh Medical Center*

With Adrian Casavilla (L) and Andreas (Andy) Tzakis (R), 1989. *University of Pittsburgh Medical Center*

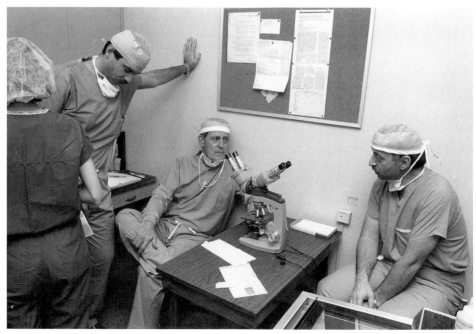

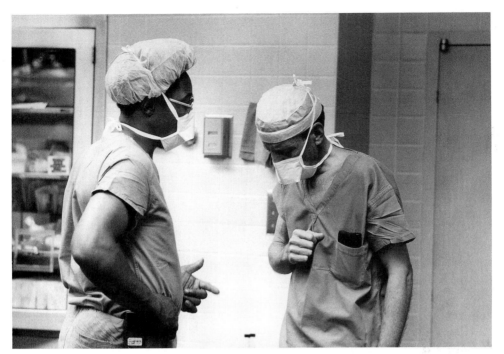

Obtaining information from Paul Taylor, Denver 1977. *Photo by Carl Iwasaki*

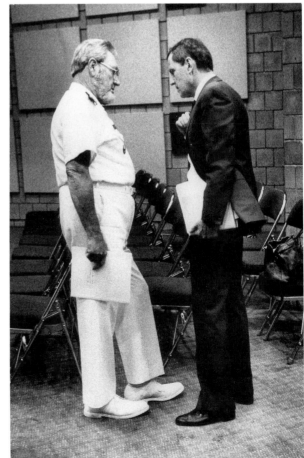

Discussing tactics with U.S. Surgeon General C. Everett Koop, September 1987. *Pittsburgh Press*

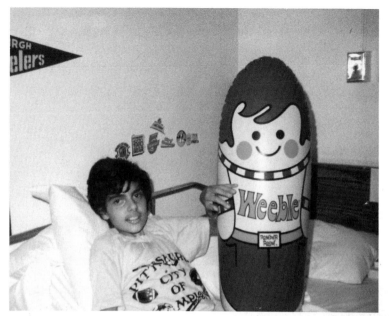

David Yomtoob. This picture was taken on November 27, 1981, two months after his liver transplant.

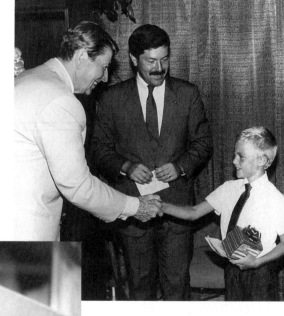

President Ronald Reagan with Austin Szegda, 1987. Austin received a new liver in January 1984. (Man in center is an unidentified White House aide.)

Stormie Jones. *Children's Hospital of Pittsburgh*

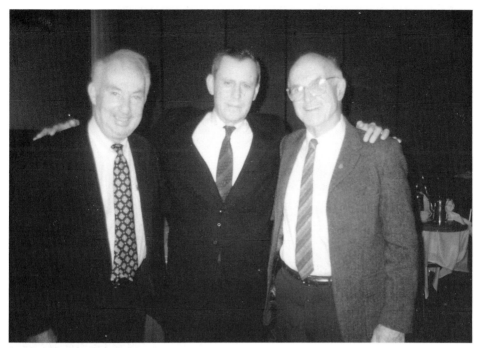

With Norman Shumway (L) and Joseph E. Murray (R) in Boston, November 1990.

With Noriko and Satoru Todo, Pittsburgh 1991. *Photo by Paul Taylor*

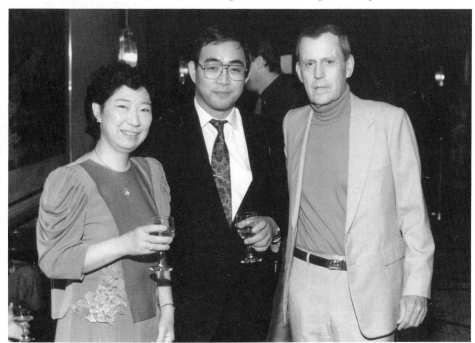

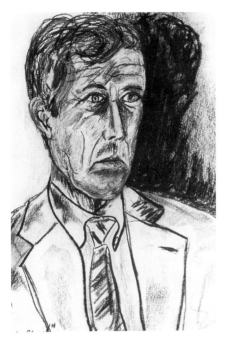

Portrait by Roy Calne, drawn in San Francisco, August 1990, one day before my coronary artery bypass.

Roy Calne speaking at a symposium marking twenty-five years of clinical transplantation, Pittsburgh 1987. Joy is on my right. *University of Pittsburgh Medical Center*

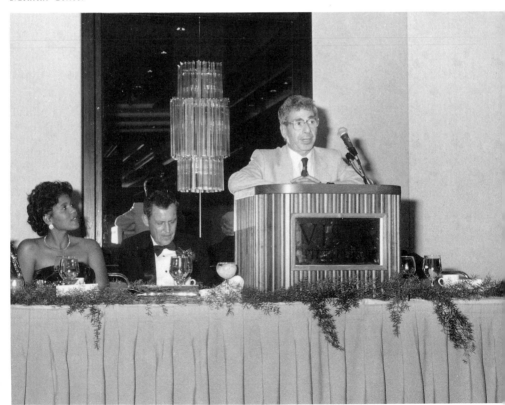

justifiable to seek certain benefits despite the risks involved, and when the benefits should be foregone because of the risks. (P. 4)

The third principle was *justice*. It also was defined by negative example:

An injustice occurs when some benefit to which a person is entitled is denied without good reason or when some burden is imposed unduly. Another way of conceiving the principle of justice is that equals ought to be treated equally.
. . . during the 19th and early 20th centuries the burdens of serving as research subjects fell largely upon poor ward patients, while the benefits of improved medical care flowed primarily to private patients. Subsequently, the exploitation of unwilling prisoners as research subjects in Nazi concentration camps was condemned as a particularly flagrant injustice. In this country, in the 1940's, the Tuskegee syphilis study used disadvantaged, rural black men to study the untreated course of a disease that is by no means confined to that population. These subjects were deprived of demonstrably effective treatment in order not to interrupt the project, long after such treatment became generally available.
. . . Finally, whenever research supported by public funds leads to the development of therapeutic devices and procedures, justice demands both that these not provide advantages only to those who can afford them and that such research should not unduly involve persons from groups unlikely to be among the beneficiaries of subsequent applications of the research. (P. 5)

The rest of the Belmont Report described in general terms how these principles could be fulfilled. This too was straightforward. It involved assurance of informed consent, assessment of risks and benefits, and selection of subjects. The document was acclaimed. It embraced all the tenets of the Nuremberg Code, the Helsinki Declaration, and the Ciba Symposium more clearly than ever before. Within 240 days after receipt of the commission report, and based on it, the secretary of the Department of Health Education and Welfare (HEW) was obligated to issue guidelines to all institutions receiving public funds. Failure to comply with the regulations would result in loss of these federal monies.

The secretary's derivative document, "Protection of Human

Subjects," mandated a watchdog Institutional Review Board (IRB) for each institution.[5] Places like the University of Colorado and the University of Pittsburgh already had such groups, commonly called ethics or oversight committees. Other hospitals and universities now scrambled to create them. An enormous and complicated bureaucracy arose overnight. The constituency, responsibilities, administrative structure, lines of reporting, and even the conditions for their meeting place were spelled out in the kind of detail that could confuse a member looking for the meaning of his or her role.

A federally mandated network now existed that would prevent the isolated but serious and highly publicized abuses of the past, such as the Tuskegee syphilis experiment. The law and its interpretation gave the local IRBs unprecedented autonomy, so great that they could block proposed work, or if they wished, formulate their own experiments.

Soon it would be asked if the spirit of the new code had been lost while the letter was being fulfilled. As the new system settled into place, another distinguished voice in the wilderness joined that of Franny Moore. This one belonged to Mark Ravitch, a seventy-year-old professor of surgery at the University of Pittsburgh and one of the founders of the specialty of pediatric surgery. He was president-elect of the American Surgical Association and the reigning surgical philosopher in the world. His defense of civil (and patient) rights stretched back fifty years through a career at the Johns Hopkins Hospital, in the U. S. Army in World War II, at Mount Sinai School of Medicine (surgical chair), the University of Chicago (chief of pediatric surgery), and the University of Pittsburgh (chief of surgery, Montefiore Hospital). He understood the past and had just written the history of the American Surgical Association.

Ravitch also was the conscience of the present. Now entering the last years of his life, he wrote an editorial about the new IRB system entitled "Colleagues Suborned" for the journal *Perspectives in Biology and Medicine*.

Any grade school teacher knows the way to get discipline is to involve the students, make the biggest boy a monitor. It is no secret that student councils impose harsher penalties on student offenders than faculty would dare to do. The authority of the governing body is only indirectly threatened by any insurrection when its will is imposed through an instrument. At the same time, the instruments, though chosen from the regulated group, presently identify with the ruling group. In the obscene, if all too understandable, example of the Kapos in the Nazi concentration camps, or the tragic example of the ghetto elders who chose who should be shipped out and who might stay yet awhile, there was also the double element of self-protection and of the argument that "we will do it more compassionately." Another force that operates with suborned or co-opted representatives of a group is the need to prove purity, and freedom from whatever guilt or taint is currently being attributed to the group. . . . set up a governing structure, allocate authority, and it will be surprising if the exercise of authority does not become a pleasurable end in itself. . . . with Human Use, or Human Experimentation, Committees . . . something has crept into the "game" of research which causes things to be done that have raised valid questions about ethics and morality, as well as scientific integrity. And perhaps such things can be prevented by committee procedures . . . [when] these procedures are in the hands of committees of our own colleagues, investigators themselves. But like all other examples of suborned, co-opted enforcers, our colleagues on these committees— and I hear this over the country, . . . become overzealous, righteous, bureaucratic. Forms multiply, hearings are held on phases of the proposed study which have nothing to do with any aspect of protection of the human subjects. . . . At times, the absurdity of it all brings a certain comic relief, as when a tissue committee ruled that portions of tumor specimens removed in the course of therapeutic operations could not be separately analyzed in a federally funded clinical research project without special approval of the human use committee. . . . The university in which this happened and the general picture in the United States are only symptomatic of what is going on the world over.[6]

To IRB-watchers like Ravitch, it was evident that each board developed its own personality. Individual members could construe their mission differently. For some it was to gauge the intention of the investigator, to judge the role of the investigator's ambition and enthusiasm in advancing the proposal, to identify unnecessary instrumentation and sample collection, and to guard against mis-representation to the patient of the risks and benefits. To others, the first priority was to ensure scientifically valid results. This re-quired the construction of perfect experiments. The placating explanation of many was that they were protecting the investigator and the institution from disgrace and liability.

The decision to become a member of the new power group of coopted enforcers called the IRB must not have been an easy one, or at least for those who read the document of intent, which was the Belmont Report. Once on duty, they found that they had a second submaster, the FDA, which is responsible for protecting the public from dangerous drugs and devices and against fraudulent claims by those who manufacture them. To meet these obligations, the FDA seeks unassailable evidence. The best scientific evidence is from randomized trials, and consequently such trials often become the final filter through which a new drug must go before it can be certified and sold. This sometimes required an unspoken collaboration between IRBs and the FDA which both are quick to deny.

For cyclosporine, the FDA considered randomization to be a desirable condition for clinical trials, but not a mandatory one for every center. The decision was thrown back to the local IRBs. In Pittsburgh, the IRB at Children's Hospital decided against a randomized trial. The IRB governing Presbyterian University Hospital voted for it, but only for patients receiving cadaver kidneys for the first time. Those receiving kidneys after previous grafts had failed could have cyclosporine and so could recipients of hearts and livers. These were the patients at high risk from transplant failure and death. Thus, the concession was a tacit admission of cyclosporine's superiority.

Jessica Lewis, a wise and gentle lady who was chair of the University of Pittsburgh IRB, was responsible for the compromise that gave the greatest weight to the surgeons' opinions that cyclosporine was superior. The compromise was designed to avoid deaths by limiting the randomization to good-risk kidney transplant recipients. If treatment failed and the graft was rejected, return to the artificial kidney and retransplantation under cyclosporine would be possible. Although the transplant surgeons were united against even this limited compromise, many others—whose role in patient care was less direct or nonexistent—held a different opinion. They pointed out that the randomized trials with all organs would be a gold mine for secondary investigations in which patient and transplant survival were not the primary concerns. The two populations defined by the treatment arms would allow controlled observations leading to articles on which professional careers would be built. One person who was lobbying for the randomized trial pointed out to me that publication of the results in prestigious journals would be impossible without controlled randomized trials. The *New England Journal of Medicine* (NEJM) was mentioned by name as an example of a journal that demanded this kind of precision in clinical reports.

Jessica Lewis's leadership prevented a large-scale tragedy. Randomized liver and heart transplant trials were never performed anywhere. Nevertheless, the kidney trials went forward. At the end of a one-year follow-up, the graft survival rate was nearly 90 percent in the cyclosporine-prednisone group and 50 percent in the control (conventional treatment) group.[7] The randomized trial had not been an instrument of discovery, but a validation of a conclusion already reached in previous patients and preceded by evidence in animals of cyclosporine superiority.[8]

» «

More than two years later in Capri, Italy, I received the Uremia Award of an international nephrology (kidney disease) society. It was to be shared with John Merrill of the Peter Bent Brigham Hospital (who was too ill to come) and Richard Glassock of UCLA (who did). Still haunted by the randomized trial, I gave an acceptance talk on September 4, 1983, entitled "Protecting the Patient's Interest." In it, I discussed the concept of patient populations, their loss of free choice, and the ethical disease which I called "randomized trialomania."[9]

The typed manuscript was delivered to the organizer at the meeting, but was not "received" until December 28, 1984. It finally was published in a supplement of the journal *Kidney International* in the autumn of 1985. By this time, most of the patients on the control limb of the randomized trial whose kidneys had been rejected had undergone retransplantation or had died. Like a smoldering virus, the disease of randomized trialomania slept, ready to strike again. When it came, those on the Pittsburgh IRB had changed, the lessons had been forgotten, and the cycle would begin again.

When it did, it was no longer possible to use the *New England Journal of Medicine* as a shield in such arguments. In 1990, the editorial policy of this journal was reviewed by one of its editors, Dr. Marcia Angell, under the title "The Nazi Hypothermia Experiments and Unethical Research Today." The message was clear:

> In my view the unethical research of today . . . stems largely from the desire to obtain scientifically unambiguous answers. . . . it is unethical when there is good reason to believe the treated group will fare better. . . . the most frequent types of unethical research occurring today involve obtaining informed consent as a legalism, without truly informing the subjects. . . . journal editors and peer reviewers sometimes encourage these practices by emphasizing scientific over ethical rigor.
>
> The *Journal* has taken the position that it will not publish reports of unethical research, regardless of their scientific merit. . . . the approval of the institutional review board . . . and the informed consent of the research subjects are necessary but not sufficient conditions. . . . Publication is an important part of the reward system in medical research, and investigators would not undertake unethical studies if they knew the results would not be published. . . . such studies may be easier to carry out and thus may give their practitioners a competitive edge. . . . refusal to publish unethical work serves notice to society at large that even scientists do not consider science the primary measure of a civilization. Knowledge, although important, may be less important to a decent society than the way it is obtained.[10]

22

The Liver Wars

The kidney transplantation trial with cyclosporine was the essential first step in Pittsburgh. This was the only kind of transplantation accepted as legitimate therapy by the medical establishment, and it was the only transplant procedure for which there was identifiable support for the costs of hospitalization. Dave Winter of the Sandoz Corporation had given us carte blanche for all other kinds of transplantation, creating the means to develop in our adopted new city a multiple organ transplant center of unprecedented variety and size. Bahnson reopened his long dormant heart program, which overnight became the largest one in the United States. It was the only heart transplantation center other than Stanford to have access to cyclosporine.

However, the fate of the Pittsburgh phoenix would rest with liver transplantation. This was inevitable because liver transplantation was a unique service, available only in Pittsburgh. The small Colorado series of successful liver transplantations under cyclosporine in 1980 had provided the first evidence that this operation could be made practical, but our first attempts in Pittsburgh raised the possibility that the Colorado successes had been a statistical artifact, or else a fraud. The first four patients treated at the Presbyterian-University Hospital died after four to twenty-two days, either because the organs used did not function properly, because of imperfections in the recipient operation, or because of rejection. The failures played out in a blinding glare of publicity.

Because I was too busy to look for a place to live, I had moved into a lower-level bedroom in Hank Bahnson's house in Fox Chapel, a suburb of Pittsburgh. One morning while driving in, I heard a phone survey on a local radio station. The audience was being asked if the liver transplant program should be closed down before more failures occurred. The vote was a close one. I cannot remember hearing which side won.

No one thought to ask what had brought Carl Groth of Sweden to Pittsburgh at this darkest moment, almost fourteen years after he had helped perform the first successful liver transplantation in Denver. Was Groth sent by some mysterious force from the twilight zone or was this one of those simple accidents of timing about which people later romanticize? A few hours before he arrived on May 8, 1981, I received a call from the University of Iowa that a twenty-five-month-old brain dead donor was in an Iowa City hospital.

That night, Groth and I flew in a small plane to Iowa and brought back a liver and a kidney. When we arrived with the liver at Children's Hospital, Shun Iwatsuki had started the recipient operation on a child named Todd McNeally, whose liver disease was biliary atresia. Groth and I joined Iwatsuki and within a few hours, the operation was finished. A few days later, Todd McNeally was seen on television, laughing and running like a normal child down the hospital corridors. Today, he is a teenager.

Without sleeping, Groth now helped me transplant the small kidney from the same donor into a college student sent to me from Washington, D.C. This patient had undergone several kidney transplantations over the previous seven years, using up the usual places to sew in the new organ. The small size of the cadaver kidney was an advantage because we could find a suitable pocket for it more easily in the midst of the scar tissue. The new kidney produced urine and still does more than ten years later. This patient has married since, has children, and runs a business.

Groth's visit lasted four days. On the day he came, the liver transplant program was in jeopardy. On the day he left, it was afloat. Before walking onto the airplane ramp to leave, Groth turned to me and said, "I had forgotten how skillful you are." I laughed and answered, "I had forgotten how magic you are."

Once the barrier was broken, the next twenty-two liver transplantations went much the same as in the smaller Colorado series of 1980. Nineteen had long survival. We treated twenty-six patients in 1981, far more than in any of the preceding eighteen years since liver transplantation was first tried in man. The number would be doubled again each year for the next five years. Also, normal life could resume for me. During a half year of camping at Bahnson's house, I had not unpacked. Now, I had to find a place to live because Joy soon would be arriving.

On August 1, 1981, we were married in Dallas. It was a small wedding with little fanfare. John Fordtran, who had taken the job of chief of medicine at Baylor University Hospital (Dallas) was the best man, accompanied by his son, Billy, upon whom I had performed the cadaver kidney transplantation ten years earlier. Burl Osborne, the kidney recipient from 1966 who had become publisher of the Dallas *Morning News*, sent a photographer who took hundreds of the best wedding pictures I have ever seen. They were Osborne's present. My three children, who now were on their own, already were Joy's great friends and admirers. Their anxieties about her welfare in this strange new world faded as they slowly realized how well she was able to cope.

In November 1981, a delegation came to see me in the chemistry laboratory which Iwatsuki and I still were borrowing for an office. I had been selected Pittsburgh Man of the Year in Science and Medicine. The exciting thing was that Willie Stargell of the Pittsburgh Pirates and Franco Harris of the Steelers were receiving awards in other categories. At the banquet, Joy and I would get their autographs. Anxious at first about her reception, she need not have worried. In a steel town, people are judged by what they do, not the color of their skin. When she walked down the center aisle in an orange and yellow gown, there was silence and then a thunderous ovation. We were in the right city.

Dave Winter was like a mother hen throughout this time and until cyclosporine finished its long journey through the FDA at the end of 1983. The liver trials offered even more persuasive testimony for cyclosporine than those with the kidney, and soon the evidence from Bahnson's and Shumway's heart trials would follow. From time to time, I see Winter. He still calls us "moonwalkers," a complimentary term which he first applied to Roy Calne. Being a modest man, it never dawned on him that he was one also.

» «

To make transplantation work, surgeons must form coalitions with the physicians whose specialties are defined by organs: kidney (surgery and nephrology), liver (surgery and hepatology), heart (surgery and cardiology), and others (always involving surgery). At Pittsburgh, the most powerful liaison was with hepatology and its chief, David Van Thiel. It was a fortunate marriage for liver transplantation.

Van Thiel's special knowledge was of the gut and of the liver. That he understood food and how the body used it did not seem particularly inappropriate. To call him portly would be an extreme example of verbal discretion. When I met him in the first week of 1981, he explained that he was practicing dietary restraint which had not yet taken effect. He was five feet ten inches tall and weighed 320 pounds.

In November 1979, Van Thiel had been made chief of the Gastroenterology (Digestive) Division of the Department of Medicine. The appointment was made by Gerald Levey, the new departmental chair who recently had come to the University of Pittsburgh from the University of Miami. Levey, a specialist in endocrine diseases (such as diabetes and goiter) had done a masterful job of reorganizing a department that had been leaderless for several previous years. Most of his numerous specialty division chiefships were filled by recruitment from other universities, but Van Thiel was an inside appointment. Although his gastroenterology division was a small one, it was highly productive in terms of scientific creativity and also in terms of money earned from seeing patients.

At first Van Thiel's role in the still nonexistent liver transplantation program was unclear, for one reason because the survival of the program was highly questionable. However, the need for liver replacement, if it could be made to work, was overwhelming. The hospital beds which had not been fully occupied at Presbyterian University Hospital and the Children's Hospital of Pittsburgh during the preceding several years began to fill up with desperately ill patients seeking liver transplantation which they had heard was available in Pittsburgh. Coming from all over the world, the adults were admitted to Van Thiel's medical service. Their sheer numbers, as well as the complexity of their care, was completely unexpected and soon unwelcome to the medical residents and interns in training. Scattered through the medical wards of the hospital were these deathly ill patients whose bloated bellies, spindly arms and legs, and yellow eyes and skin tended to make them all look the same. On June 30, 1981, the fifty-four medical residents and interns unanimously signed a resolution and brought it to Levey, denouncing liver transplantation as an unrealistic objective, and possibly an unethical pursuit. The interface between medicine and surgery had been ruined.

On the surgical side, Hank Bahnson already had adjusted to the increased work load by opening another operating room and creating a surgical liver transplant service to which two surgical residents were assigned. Shun Iwatsuki and I were the only faculty members. When Levey delivered the petition to Bahnson, it was a potential death blow, and I responded formally on July 9, 1981, with the only "Dear Dr. Bahnson" letter I had ever written:

Thank you for showing me the petition. The document was mercifully brief and I will answer in the same vein.

Since January 1981, I have deflected all referrals for consideration of liver transplantation to the medical services, where evaluations, selection for candidacy, discussions leading to informed consent, and preoperative care have been supervised by senior faculty members of the Department of Medicine. Every case has been discussed at an Interdisciplinary Conference held weekly on Tuesdays at 1:30 P.M. Taped records of all these meetings are available.

My principal collaborator in these efforts has been David Van Thiel. The spirit of interdisciplinary cooperation and purpose has been outstanding. However, I have been aware that there have been stresses within the medical service for reasons which I see no reason to try to decipher.

Instead, I have concluded that these patients should *not* be admitted to the General Medical Service. In the future, I will send them to the C - Surgical Service which has the highly focused objective of providing transplantation expertise. The cherished collaboration with Dr. Van Thiel will be assiduously protected.

Sincerely,

cc: Donald Leon, M.D., (Dean), Gerald Levey, M.D. (Chairman, Department of Medicine), Jessica Lewis, M.D. (Chairman, Institutional Review Board), Mr. Daniel Stickler (Hospital Director).

To continue working with us, Van Thiel broke ranks with those in his department who opposed the program. Soon, his interest changed to a passion. Long a student of liver disease, Van Thiel had watched for many years the gradual decline of these patients, always fighting a rear guard battle with no hope of victory. The only possibility was to delay death, and even this was more an exercise in the prolongation of misery. The first time he saw someone return from the last moments of life to complete health after transplantation, he found a new vision of what he was meant to do. This was to be a liver transplant physician, and as it turned out, he became the most remarkable one the world had produced.

It may have been a man named Richard Smith who made Van Thiel's conversion complete. Smith came to Pittsburgh from Jamestown, North Dakota, where he was a professor of music at Jamestown College and the director of the famed Jamestown Choir, which he led on tours to Europe and elsewhere every year. He knew that this would be his last hospitalization. He was not only prepared to play his final card, he demanded the right to do so. He realized day by day that a gray fog was descending over his brain. The notes of Mozart were in the distance, but the movements and harmony were gone. Subtracting 7 from 100 gave him an answer of 78. His hands moved in a rhythmic beat, as regularly as a metronome, in what is known as a "liver flap." Then his kidneys began to fail. Before he became unconscious, he sat on a chair, outside the elevator on the eighth floor of Presbyterian University Hospital, grasping the white coats of startled physicians or nurses as they came out when the doors opened. He demanded of them a liver.

An organ was found in October 1981. By this time, Smith was so ill that sewing it in was an act of seeming folly. All night long, the surgical team worked in a desperate fury to control the bleeding that would never stop unless the new liver could be installed and then only if it would begin to make the substances necessary to allow blood to clot. By dawn, the job was done. John Sassano, the anesthesiologist, had given almost two hundred bottles of blood, all of it with a hand pump.

White-faced, Sassano buried his head in his hands and sobbed, not from sorrow as had been the case with Bennie Solis, but from joy—and also from the pain in his cramped arms and hands. Mr. Smith would live, and Sassano would never go through this experience again. By the next case, he had invented a rapid infusion pump which could keep up with any amount of blood loss by pushing a button and turning a dial. The Sassano pump became commercially available and now is a piece of standard operating room equipment everywhere.

But would this be only a prolongation of dying, as Van Thiel had seen before in his patients with end-stage liver disease? For six weeks, Smith lay in the intensive care unit, attached to a breathing machine. His incision was open because of an infection inside the abdomen. Every six hours, the exposed intestines and the new liver were washed with sterile fluid. Was it ethical to continue treating him, asked some of the intensive care physicians who had never seen anyone recover from an illness so severe. Staked out by restraints on his hands and feet like Christ on the cross, he heard Mozart's notes again, but this time in perfect sequence and with glorious harmony. Faint at first, the music came closer every day.

By Christmas time, Smith went home, too early we thought, but he insisted. In late January 1982, I was surprised to receive a notice that he had been guest conductor for the St. Paul Chamber Orchestra. In 1983, he became academic dean of Jamestown College. Almost ten years after his liver transplantation, he wrote to me and Dr. Van Thiel, "When I came to you in 1981, many were saying that the transplant program would fail because you could not keep up your frenetic pace and train other surgeons to do the difficult things which you were doing. You have, of course, proved them wrong. . . . When you are sometimes discouraged or wondering about the wisdom of the choices you have made and the energy you have put into your work, be assured that many like me remember you with thanks every day."

Van Thiel's prodigious contributions to the transplantation program made him famous, and his management policies became the original from which copies were struck as other programs of liver transplantation opened in all the inhabited continents. Each new team built in a medical arm, often with more physicians for this specific purpose than in Van Thiel's entire division. He struggled doggedly to keep up with the load of patients who soon occupied more than one hundred hospital beds, waiting for liver transplantation or recovering afterward. He knew them all, even when the number of transplantations rose to more than five hundred per year.

Van Thiel merely lengthened his days, now starting at 4:00 A.M. and ending at midnight. Gone was his country house in favor of a small townhouse near the hospital. It had become too dangerous to risk falling asleep while driving the twenty miles to and from work. He became desperate at first and later militant as the fatigue lines deepened on his leonine face and his hair turned silver. What he had done and was doing was to rewrite the rules on the care of patients with end-stage liver disease.

To meet his new as well as preexisting obligations, articles poured from Van Thiel's pen. In 1989 he was accused of plagiarism in the preparation of a chapter for a general medical textbook on a nontransplant subject. His life was in ruins as he awaited punishment. Old enemies swarmed to the attack. Many who were the beneficiaries of his past generosity turned from him or buried their long concealed knives in him even as he forgave them.

Catching a large lion, wounded and in free fall, is not an easy matter in an academic community that purports to place ritualistic integrity above all other virtues. That Van Thiel could now relinquish all other responsibilities and become physician-in-chief of the liver transplant services, supported by an adequate staff which allows him time to sleep and think, means that this was possible. From the new arrangement came a multidisciplinary service that blurred the artificial lines separating medicine and surgical specialties or sequestering basic scientists from those who practice clinical medicine.

» «

By the end of 1981, we had reached two conclusions. First, the quality and safety of antirejection treatment with drug cocktails that contained cyclosporine and prednisone were superior to anything previously available. Improvements would be possible for all kinds of organ transplantation. Second, there was no way, because of administrative roadblocks, to systematically apply this great scientific advance for organs other than the kidney. The reason for this was that transplantation of the liver, heart, lungs, pancreas, and all organs other than the kidney was classified as "experimental."

This designation had been used by government agencies to describe liver and heart transplantation for more than a decade with the ostensible justification that the results were too poor to be considered a "service." Behind the scenes, this was a tactic to avoid financial responsibility. Liver and heart transplantation were known to be expensive, and no one wanted to underwrite the hospital bills. Just before Christmas in 1981, I took the problem to C. Everett (Chick) Koop, the acting surgeon general of the United States.

Koop recently had retired from his position as surgeon-in-chief of the Children's Hospital of Philadelphia in order to work in government service. He still was in an "acting" capacity and had a complex title because his designation by Ronald Reagan as surgeon general awaited confirmation by the U.S. Senate. The outcome was uncertain because of Koop's strong feelings about the sanctity of life (pro-life and anti-abortion), smoking and self-abuse generally, pornography, and other controversial matters. His intelligence, rectitude, and sincerity broke through all political barriers. Opposing him was like fighting a very smart bear, which he resembled with his large build and grizzly white beard. When he left office eight years later, those qualified to judge pronounced him the greatest surgeon general this nation had produced. I agree with them.

When we arrived at Koop's office, I was surprised to find that he had put aside most of the morning for us. Also in attendance were the mother of a child who had biliary atresia and a physician from Allentown, Pennsylvania, whose wife was nearing the need for liver transplantation. We sat around an oversized rectangular table.

Almost all the conversation was between Koop and me. By letter, he had asked for all available information about cyclosporine, including its use in kidney and liver transplantation. For him, biliary atresia had been a lifetime frustration. He had seen almost every child with this disease in Philadelphia over a period of more than thirty years. The possibility of truly helping these children was almost too good to believe.

Patiently, he heard the evidence while the others dozed. Slide after projection slide flashed onto the screen as I talked, interrupted by him for clarification or for more detail. I described the tactic of avoidance by insurance carriers, in which the government itself played a pivotal collaborating role. By defining liver and heart transplantation as "experimental," the federal bureaucracy (Medicare was the most important example) constructed a shield behind which private insurance companies took refuge. The argument was always the same: if Medicare, the government's most powerful and pervasive health care provider, had determined these operations to be experimental and therefore nonreimbursable for costs, why should a private company take any other position? The logic was unassailable.

I explained that there were numerous exceptions and that the majority of the most prestigious insurance companies had abandoned this tactic. For example, the Western Pennsylvania Blue Cross Association had decided to fund hospitalization costs for liver and heart recipients. In New York, the commissioner of health, Dr. David Axelrod, announced that no New York resident who was indigent would be disallowed liver transplant care for that reason alone. Consequently, numerous indigent patients who were screened by strict medical criteria in New York and found to be bona fide liver candidates were being sent to us across the state line.

Koop was sympathetic. Before we left his office, he outlined a strategy that he thought might break the impasse. It was to submit liver transplantation to a process which I had never heard of called Consensus Development Review. In essence, it consisted of a trial by jury of new forms of medical treatment. During the trial, which would be public, all evidence about liver transplantation would be presented by those who advocated its acceptance and by those who opposed it. The jury hearing the arguments would consist of about fifteen wise men and women, carefully selected to avoid bias for or against the proposition under discussion. At the end, the jury would retire and render a verdict. During their period of deliberation, they would be in continuous confinement under the same general conditions as in a court case. They would produce a verdict and a document supporting it, which would be made public. This was expected to define national policy for the United States and to have a ripple effect worldwide.

Koop emphasized the risk, explaining that he could not predict the outcome if this is what I decided to do. A negative judgment after a process so formal and public would put off general acceptance of liver transplantation for one or more generations and could bring discredit to its advocates. On the other hand, success would destroy the artifice which had arrested its growth. I did not hesitate. I decided to go forward.

From Koop's office, we walked to the White House. There, the president's physician, Daniel Ruge, met us for another conversation on the same subject. Many years earlier when I was a medical student at Northwestern, Ruge had been a member of Loyal Davis's neurosurgery group. He had known Nancy Reagan, Davis's daughter, from the time she was a young woman and was fond of her as well as of the president. I knew Ruge well. He promised to help if the opportunity arose.

He saw President Reagan frequently and had great respect for him. Their conversations tended to be nonpolitical, particularly after the assassination attempt in March 1981 when Ruge played a major role in organizing the care given to Mr. Reagan and to Jim Brady. I learned for the first time how life-threatening Reagan's injuries actually had been. Ruge said that he would bring up the issue of transplantation if the opportunity arose. Whether he did, I do not know, but Mr. Reagan's public support of this field was always powerful and highly public thereafter.

Koop was as good as his word. In June 1982, I went to a Consensus Development planning session in Bethesda to which Roy Calne of Cambridge also was invited. Koop was there. The Consensus Development Conference was to be sponsored by the

National Institutes of Health (NIH); the Health Care Finance Administration (HCFA), which paid the bills for the End-Stage Renal Disease program; the Veterans Administration; and the surgeon general's office. The hearing, at which I would be allowed to testify, would take place June 20–23, 1983, in Bethesda. Koop's countdown had started.

» «

Two days before the Consensus Development Conference began, a group of children who had survived after liver transplantation in Denver or Pittsburgh had a reunion in Pittsburgh at the Greentree Marriot Hotel, near the airport. Now there were many examples of success. Kim Hudson, the child with biliary atresia whose operation in Denver was in January 1970, had lived for thirteen and a half years, and seven more of the children had survived for more than ten years.

A more recent patient, David Yomtoob, also came. He had played a special role in the acceptance of transplantation by the medical community. An inherited disorder known as Wilson's disease was responsible for his nearly fatal original illness in 1981. With Wilson's disease, there is an accumulation of copper in all the body tissues, causing damage of the liver and brain. The exact explanation for Wilson's disease still is not known. Because we had shown in the 1960s that the copper deposition stops and is reversed by liver transplantation, it was certain that the fundamental defect in metabolism involved the liver.

Young Yomtoob's first eleven years were not unusual except for a brilliant academic record. He played on the soccer team and was normal in every way. Then came his illness, subtle at first, but quickly evolving to catastrophe as he moved from his local hospital in Michigan to Children's Memorial Hospital in Chicago, and to the court of last appeal at Children's Hospital in Pittsburgh at the end of August 1981. Now his skin, into which he bled with the slightest contact, was deep yellow with islands of purple from the hemorrhages. His eyes were sunken from dryness, and his belly and legs were swollen with fluid. As happens with liver disease, water was in the wrong places. His mind wandered and as the decay deepened, his kidneys failed. He became paralyzed, arms and legs, and soon he was unable to breath. A metal tube was placed into his windpipe and, by attaching it to a breathing machine, the instrument drove his lungs. It seemed too late. Or was it?

Another child with a fatal brain injury lay in a bed thirty feet away. What could Yomtoob's mother do? She prayed to God for the life of both children, believing that there was no hope for either but knowing that the other patient already had been pronounced brain dead.[1] That night, September 26, 1981, the second child's liver was used to replace that of her son, who turned back from shadows so deep that no one had been there before and returned. Now, he had a perfect liver in his functionless body. In a few weeks, the kidneys began to make urine, but there was no movement except of his eyes. Deviated to one side, his gaze was interrupted by the rhythmic movement (called nystagmus) of his eyeballs as if they were transmitting distress signals from his soul.

A month later, David could be transported to a large mat in the Physical Medicine Department. Unable to control his body, he lay there in a contorted position, incapable of rolling over. In an accidental movement, his face turned toward a video camera that was recording his progress. It showed a mask of hatred. If only he could have died. When they showed it to me, I cried. I told them never to let his mother see it. If he had been a wounded animal, I would have known what to do. What was this terrible crime which we had committed in the name of healing?

By Thanksgiving, something had changed. His shoulders moved. When he was placed on the mat, he could roll over. Sometimes he seemed to smile, or at least to grimace. When Christmas came, his parents carried him home in their arms. In March 1982, he walked into my office, dapper in his blue and white soccer jacket. Full of life, he shuffled slightly, but otherwise this was a normal boy. Perhaps I had been wrong when I looked at the video before. Where was it? When I found it, it was the same. It was David who had changed, as if he had been visited by an angel.

In the first week of November 1982, thirteen and a half months after his liver transplantation, David Yomtoob made another appearance, but this time in front of several thousand people. I was to give an address on progress in liver transplantation for the annual meeting of the American Association for the Study of Liver Disease. My talk was as dry and boring as these lectures tend to be, complete with slides of tissues, slides of chemical information, and graphs showing survival curves. It was all so mathematical and scientific as befitted the occasion. However, at the end, I showed the awful video and mentioned that the patient was in the back of the room. His parents had brought him to Chicago for the meeting.

He came running down the aisle, soccer ball in hand, every step a symphony of coordinated motion. Those in the crowd rose to their feet to acclaim him. Averting my eyes, I pretended not to notice. But I know that not many who were there would forget what they had seen. Nor would David. Like a child of destiny he grew up. In 1991 he is a graduate student in college, an airplane pilot, a soccer player, and probably many more things which he will keep to himself. Only those who have known complete despair can understand the full meaning of jubilation. It is their delicious secret.

After the reunion, the caravan of children led by young Yomtoob moved on to Bethesda to be observed and to be witnesses for liver transplantation, mute but eloquent by their mere presence. As the proceedings droned on, I thought that we had failed. Some of the presentations and discussions were pessimistic or hostile and others were irrelevant. The chair of the judgment panel was Rudi Schmid, dean of the school of medicine of the University of California, San Francisco. As one of the world's leading liver specialists, his opinion would be critical to the outcome, but he was careful not to reveal it. Late on the second day, Dame Sheila Sherlock of the Royal Free Hospital, London, Schmid's European equal in stature, suggested to the children that they leave their seats in the auditorium and go out and play in the sunshine. Dismayed at what I thought was a negative sign, I remarked that the time had come for all of us to enjoy the sun.

It was only an expression of Dame Sherlock's maternal instinct. After an all-night session, the jury came in. Their conclusion was that liver transplantation was a service, not an experimental operation. They had a list of liver diseases that should be susceptible to cure with liver replacement. These were the diseases we had already treated. There were very few exclusions, and even these were not absolute. Then followed a sweeping mandate to go forward with development of this field. The full report was to be published in the liver journal, *Hepatology*.[2] Long before it came out the gold rush was on.

» «

It was uncanny how much the liver transplant gold rush of 1984 resembled that of kidney transplantation twenty years earlier. As before, there was a shortage of gold miners. Eager surgeons or surgical teams descended on Pittsburgh. They came like flocks of swallows watching intently, scribbling notes, and taking photographs before moving on to start their own programs. Familiar faces reappeared. These were transplant fellows from older days who came to find out why achievements were now possible which then had been at their fingertips, but no closer. And there were the hard core new fellows who invested one to three years of their young lives to learn the secrets that had been bought and paid for by the sorrow of the preceding generations. Their brittle self-protective shells had yet to feel the gentle impact of the tears which soften all they touch.

No past mistakes would be repeated, or so we hoped. How to avoid them was a mania. The fresh crop of youthful men and women inherited the earth, or at least that part of it where they landed and staked their claims, hard-eyed now and determined to limit the numbers of new intruders who came close behind. They were like high-priced football players whose presence would be the nucleus of new transplant franchises or the salvation of old ones throughout the United States and the world.

Training of the new army of surgeons was helped by resurrecting a forgotten first principle which had made liver transplantation feasible in the dogs of 1958 (see chapter 6). While the diseased liver is being removed and the new one sewed in, the great vein returning blood to the heart from the legs, trunk, and kidneys (inferior vena cava) and the vein draining the intestines, pancreas, and stomach (portal vein) must be temporarily blocked. External venous bypasses to reroute the dammed-up blood to the upper part of the body were essential for success in the animals. However, it was found in the first human trials that patients could tolerate this insult better than the dogs. For the next twenty years, the bypasses were not used.

The time during which the vein blockage could be permitted was short, sometimes as brief as thirty to sixty minutes. This meant that the human operations were carried out in a crisis atmosphere, especially in adults. No matter how short the period of the great vein blockage, there was a price for the patient to pay—with variable injury of the bowel or kidney, blood loss, and shock. The price for the surgeon and anesthesiologist was stress. It was impossible to systematically train new generations of surgeons to do an operation which required a virtuoso performance and even then resulted in the death of 5 to 10 percent of patients in the operating room or shortly afterward. What good was it to develop a procedure if less than five or six people in the world were capable of performing it?

This all changed following a tragedy that utterly demoralized the Pittsburgh transplant team on May 13, 1982. A teenaged hemophiliac boy whose own liver had been destroyed by hepatitis died on the operating table while the new liver was being sewed in. His mother's grief was above description and beyond relief by members of the transplant team who spent the night with her. She moaned and sobbed, making animal-like sounds as she rocked in her chair in the waiting room near the operating theater.

I closed the program for more than a month until the middle of June. No one wanted to work. In the middle of the afternoon on June 15, I went to the office of Hank Bahnson and explained the problem to him. I asked him to set up a venous bypass for the next case. He agreed immediately, and that night we replaced a liver in a six-year-old child with biliary atresia, using a pump-driven veno-venous bypass after administering a drug called heparin to prevent clotting in the bypass tubing. After the new liver was in, the anticlotting effect of heparin was easily reversed with another drug. All those who were there that night were ecstatic about the ease and nonstressful nature of the transplantation under bypass conditions.

The solution to the problem created some problems of its own. In further trials, it was found that the anticlotting effect of heparin could not be easily reversed in some patients. Two adults bled to death when clotting could never be restored. Bart Griffith, a young cardiac surgeon who had just completed his training under Bahnson, proposed that a bypass system be used without anticlotting drugs, a suggestion which first was considered heretical by Bahnson, but later accepted when it was shown to be feasible in animals by a surgery resident named Scott Denmark working with Griffith and Byers (Bud) Shaw, Jr., the fellow in transplantation at the time.

By early 1983, all liver transplantations in adults were performed with the veno-venous bypass. It was obvious that from this moment forward liver transplantation would be a far easier procedure, well within the capability of most general and vascular surgeons, and that it could be taught to surgeons-in-training in a systematic way. An esoteric undertaking suddenly became routine. When the question was raised at the June 1983 Consensus Development Conference about the inability to train surgeons who could offer liver transplant services, we were ready with the answer.

The final practical questions for the Consensus Development panel concerned the technology of organ procurement. Until the early 1980s, it was assumed throughout most of the country that the removal of the liver, heart, or other organs from cadaver donors would jeopardize the quality of the cadaver kidneys. Only in Colorado, and later in Pittsburgh, were multiple organ donations a routine. Some predicted that there would be a turf war between kidney transplant surgeons and those who were trying to find livers or hearts.

An answer to this concern also was presented at the Consensus Development Conference. We had practiced multiple organ procurement in Colorado since the 1960s and had described it briefly as part of more general reports. The first procurement of all the major organs (kidneys, liver, and heart) was by a Colorado team working with the University of Minnesota team in Minneapolis on April 16, 1978. In the early 1980s, the same Colorado surgeons who now had relocated in Pittsburgh traveled throughout the eastern half of the United States and Canada, teaching the new method. The surgeon general, Koop, whose preoccupation had turned to organ donation, wanted the operation to be standardized. He requested us to provide a complete description.

To do this properly, a medical artist was needed—someone with creative skills combined with a deep knowledge of anatomy. The foremost candidate was a woman named Jean McConnell who was in retirement in Northfield, Illinois, outside Chicago. Her drawings in my earlier books on kidney and liver transplantation already were in the Smithsonian Institution. Suffering from diabetes, she had put down her drawing pen for the last time several years earlier and had no intention of picking it up.

Just before the Consensus Development meeting, I flew to Chicago, drove to her home, and asked her to take on this last great project of her life. As we talked, my thoughts went back thirty-five years to when we first worked together. Then, her slender and graceful hands were those of a young woman. Now, they shook and were gnarled with arthritis. I pled with her anyway and she finally agreed. She started slowly. During the next several months, the sketches came one by one through the mail, and then the finished pictures of human anatomy in brilliant color. If she trembled as she drew, there was no trace in the marks she made. What she depicted through her artistry became standard procedure for the United States and before long for the world.[3] These drawings will join her others at the Smithsonian.

» «

The University of Pittsburgh Hospitals in the early and mid 1980s resembled a progressively more congested beehive as the remarkable improvement there in liver and heart transplantation became public knowledge. The organs used for these operations could be preserved only for short periods—six or eight hours for the liver and four hours for the heart. On the way to their mission, the donor teams sauntered. Coming back, they piled out of squad cars with blinking lights and screaming sirens or jumped off choppers onto the helipad atop the Health Science Center—running, always running, with the refrigerated coolers and organs inside carried by the strongest and fastest of the group. Every minute could be the difference between success or failure for the recipient in the operating room.

The number of patients far outnumbered the donors available in western Pennsylvania. A few days after arriving in Pittsburgh, I contacted transplant surgeons out to a limit of one thousand miles in the eastern half of the United States and Canada who had trained with me in Colorado and now were running their own programs. Although their transplant practices were confined to the kidney, many still were interested in supporting trials with other organs. They pledged help in obtaining permission for us to remove the unused livers and hearts from their own cadaver kidney donors. Led by Don Denny, the Pittsburgh organ procurement coordinators systematically made similar contacts with their counterparts around the country. I also obtained the support of Gene Pierce, the director of an existing regional kidney-sharing network called the Southeastern Organ Procurement Foundation (SEOPF).

Reaching the donor sites and returning at all hours of the day and night depended on a special arrangement which may have been feasible on a large scale only in Pittsburgh. In January 1981, I met with Jack Christin, an executive of Rockwell Corporation, and his assistant, Richard Spence, about lending us the company's private jet (and pilot) for donor runs. The proposal was tabled temporarily by Rockwell's board of directors but in the meanwhile Mr. Spence had helped recruit an additional eight or ten large Pittsburgh corporations led by U.S. Steel, ALCOA, and Westinghouse.

Overnight, we had a "University of Pittsburgh Air Force." Later, when funds became available, these volunteer duties largely were taken over by a private company called Corporate Jets, Inc., and a smaller charter airline company called Air Charter, Inc., that exclusively used prop planes for shorter flights. They flew from Allegheny County Airport, located about thirty miles from the international airport and about ten miles from Presbyterian University Hospital. For the first year, I did all the liver procurements and then joined or started the recipient operation immediately after returning. After this, the trained donor surgeons took turns.

The skill and commitment of the private pilots were equal to the challenges—which sometimes were unexpected. One morning (June 8, 1986), I left Pittsburgh on an emergency donor flight to Halifax, Nova Scotia, with the surgeons Leonard Makowka (a Canadian), Michael Henderson (American), and François Mosimann (Swiss). Our purpose was to bring back a liver for a recipient whose first transplant had failed and ruptured, necessitating its removal a few minutes before our Lear jet took off. Our patient was in the operating room at Presbyterian University Hospital—being kept alive by an assortment of breathing machines, venous blood pumps, and an artificial kidney. The flight time each way was two and a half hours, and the predicted down time in Halifax was 120 minutes, including a wild ambulance ride to and from the donor location at the Dalhousie University Hospital.

Ten or fifteen minutes before landing, we looked down from 20,000 feet on the unbroken forests of Nova Scotia. Suddenly, the front and side panes of the cockpit were partly covered with an oily fluid. The hydraulic fluid system had ruptured with loss of control of the flaps, hydraulic brakes, landing gear, and the "spoilers" on the wings that are used to reduce air speed. I was sitting crossways three feet behind Richard Ryan, a former navy pilot (1967–72) and his copilot. They appeared calm. Opposite me were Mosimann, who was anything but composed, and Henderson, who quickly searched his wallet and found his tiny St. Christopher medal inside. Further back in the plane, Makowka sat silent and pale, his eyes closed.

I continued writing an article which was overdue for one of the medical journals. Half joking, I said to Mosimann and Henderson, "I always suspected that it would end this way." When I realized how this upset them, I advised them to find some work of their own. No one did. In the meanwhile, Ryan made a pass over the airport tower for visual confirmation that the landing gear hatch had been opened by the back-up manual procedure. The anxious observers in the tower who were eyes for the aircraft reported that the two main landing wheels under the body had dropped. The nose wheel was still up and remained so.

The Halifax airport recently had opened an extra long runway for impending supersonic (Concorde) flights from Europe. Captain Ryan touched down his crippled jet on the near end of this runway at high speed, as if he had come in too low on a strafing mission; then he worked desperately with hand brakes to stop the runaway plane without tipping it onto the unprotected nose. It skimmed straight as an arrow across the airport expanse, and seconds later, just beyond the far end of the exhausted runway, turned right and shuddered to a stop. We jumped out to find ourselves surrounded by fire trucks and an ambulance. Covered with an oily fluid and smoking, the plane would fly no more that day or for a long time. The first thing I asked was, "How are we going to get back?" Someone answered, "You're lucky you got here."

Within two hours, we went with a police escort to the hospital in Halifax city, removed the liver, and returned to the airport. The liverless patient in Pittsburgh was still alive, but when I called, the nurse who answered already had heard a false rumor that there had been an accident with no survivors. Instead, three planes were streaking toward Halifax—one each from Montreal, Boston, and New York. The winner (New York) would fly us back two hours later than originally planned. When we arrived home, nine hours after leaving, the recipient patient, who was near death, was given the liver and survived. Some claimed that the first of Makowka's gray hairs were seen the next day.[4]

The determination of the Pittsburgh pilots must have been like that of the pioneers of aviation. They found holes in the sky to come through when no one else was in the air, driven by the knowledge that the small white coolers stashed in the hold or gripped with a leg vice by the surgeons contained the essence of life which was slipping away with each tick of the clock. Ironically, the weather was perfect when tragedy struck on the morning of May 12, 1987. The donor team had just returned from Dallas, and the liver which they brought back already had been delivered to the operating room of Presbyterian University Hospital.

The pilots for the trip went home and were replaced by Al Stretavski and Walter Troy, who took the plane back up to perform simulated emergency exercises by taking off and landing using only one of the two engines. No one will ever know why the plane went out of control after they had reached the point of no return on their takeoff with the single functioning engine. The craft crashed and burned on the hillside opposite the air field, between nearby houses as if put in an open space by intention. Gone were our heroes and friends. They were forty-four and thirty-nine years old at the time. Stretavski was a born teacher and had been personally responsible for much of the training and professional development of Captain Ryan, the pilot who had saved us in Halifax. Today, Richard M. Ryan is president of Corporate Jets, Inc.

» «

Only four months after their death, the crisis atmosphere of liver procurement changed. This was made possible by the work of Folkert (Fred) Belzer, another senior figure in transplantation, recycled from an earlier generation. Belzer, a Dutch emigrant who came to the United States in 1951 at the age of twenty, became a physician, then a surgeon, and finally a transplant surgeon at the University of California (San Francisco). In 1966 he developed a preservation technique that allowed cadaver kidneys to be kept alive with a continuous artificial circulation for several days before transplantation. His reputation was made and his place in history secure. He moved to the University of Wisconsin (Madison) as chair of the Department of Surgery.

Not yet satisfied, Belzer and a long-time colleague, J. H. Southard, decided to work on the simpler method of refrigerating organs without an artificial circulation after chilling them to just above freezing temperature with a brief infusion of cold fluid. This was the method used when liver transplantation was first tried in animals (see chapter 6) and used routinely in humans. Patiently they experimented with different infusion fluids, testing the quality of preserved pancreases or other organs after the addition or subtraction of nearly a dozen ingredients. Years went by before the final formulation was ready for use with livers.

The testing was done in Madison by three surgeons. Two of them previously had been our transplant fellows in Pittsburgh: an Englishman, Neville Jamieson, who now was a junior member of Roy Calne's Cambridge team, and Munci Kalayoglu, a Turkish surgeon who had gone on to become chief of the Wisconsin liver transplantation section. The third surgeon was Ralf Sundberg of Stockholm, one of Carl Groth's protégés who soon would come to the University of Pittsburgh for his fellowship. Using the University of Wisconsin solution, they could successfully preserve dog livers for three times as long as had been possible with previously available solutions. Instead of having a safe time limit of six or eight hours, they would be able, they thought, to extend this ceiling in human livers to a day.

The work was presented by Jamieson without preliminary fanfare in early September 1987 at an international transplantation conference held in Pittsburgh.[5] The audience was large. When Jamieson finished, harsh questions were directed to him by incredulous transplant surgeons. Outraged at these questions, Kalayoglu rose to the defense of his English colleague.

Appealing directly to me, Kalayoglu spoke as if we were engaged in a private conversation instead of being in a room with a thousand people. He described the appearance of the livers before and after their blood supply was restored during transplantation and their function after stipulated periods of time in the refrigerator. I realized at once that he was talking about *human* livers, not those in the dog experiments. They had moved on to patients. Kalayoglu had worked on our Pittsburgh team for two years in 1981–83 and was a trusted expert. My response was simple: I said, "I believe you, Munci."

Kalayoglu gave me the names of the suppliers of the chemical ingredients of the University of Wisconsin solution, and we began to manufacture it within two weeks. After confirming the animal experiments, we began using it for patients at the end of September 1987. By Christmas, more than one hundred human livers had been transplanted with the improved method. The advance would change the strategy of liver transplantation.

Now, all parts of the United States and Canada could be interconnected in a liver-sharing network, and plans could be laid for sharing between continents. For policy planning, the difference between the previous time limit of six hours and the new one of nearly a day was like an eternity. There was no reason why a national pool of recipient candidates could not be created and provided with livers from the most distant parts of the country.

I met with Belzer in Rome a year or so later. He was happy, but far from being satisfied, he was hatching plans to approach the next unsolvable problem. Somehow, he looked younger than I remembered him. In the autumn of his life, he had breathed the air beyond the reach of those below who gazed up with awe and envy. How could he have found the trail when others failed? Was it genius, luck, or hard work?

It did not seem to matter anymore. With equanimity, Belzer accepted the admiration, the honors, and the criticisms and modifications that always follow the statement of a stark new principle or advance. He was an inventor and had been here before.

23

Politics

A few years ago, I went to the National Museum in Madrid (the Prado) to look again at a painting by Goya which had filled me with dread the first time I saw it in 1970. Entitled *Duel with Cudgels*, it shows two peasant gladiators in the countryside fighting to the death. They are flailing at each other with deadly weighted slings. The inhumanity in their faces can be seen by the lack of features, not by lines of cruelty or passion. With their feet and legs buried and transfixed in the ground, there is no escape. A small crowd stands by. The scene symbolized for me the political wars that have been set in motion by transplantation.

The most bitter of these struggles occur in medical universities and hospitals, for stakes which cannot be divulged because they are too ignoble to admit. Who wants to concede that money, academic territory, vanity, or control of the talents and ideas of one's colleagues is the reason for conflict? These motives are painted over and presented as generosity, virtue, morality, humility, institutional purpose, and concern for society in general. If one intends to permanently remove an adversary from the field of endeavor, one must do so secretly so as to avoid being accused of administrative murder—the termination of someone's professional career.

A turf war in Pittsburgh over who would provide kidney transplant services was discreetly deferred until the programs for the transplantation of the liver, heart, and other organs could be developed. The Colorado team that arrived in early 1981 had its own way of surviving and thriving in the midst of the kidney controversy. It was to decline battle. A scientific revolution was occurring in transplantation, and its epicenter was brought to Pittsburgh in an envelope of ingenuousness.

Inside was a world of ideas, not commerce or turf. Anyone who wanted to join was welcome, and even then there would be too few people to do the work. I had been right about Hakala. He stayed and shared the kidney transplant service with me and my associates in general surgery. By adopting the imported ideas, he brought his specialty of urology to a new level of skill and performance. Others who wanted to balkanize the rapidly growing transplant programs along conventional specialty lines exhausted themselves and moved to the sidelines. However, there were exceptions who stayed to fight.

The most notable was Don Denny, the social worker who directed the organ procurement agency. My greatest failure in Pittsburgh was my inability to win him over. Denny's most admirable trait of loyalty may have been the reason. He had been hired by Hakala and he recognized no other boss or even source of advice. As long as I performed kidney transplant operations on the general surgery service I was an intolerable intrusion and an open threat to Hakala's plans. It was a black-and-white issue from which all else derived. The resulting conflict eventually caused Denny to leave transplantation of his own volition. Before this, it committed him to activities which he would have deplored if he could have seen them through the eyes of a third person.

Although Denny started with no formal medical training, his intelligence more than made up for this during his organ procurement apprenticeship in Philadelphia. He became a skilled executive and an effective teacher of the new procurement coordinators he recruited. From them, he expected absolute loyalty to himself and to Hakala. Because Hakala was busy, and because Denny had the ability, he became an independent policy maker.

Above all, Denny knew how to relate to the communications media. Here also, he functioned autonomously. Working through the newspapers, radio, and television, he aroused public interest in organ donation. The information that he released openly or covertly to the reporters was newsworthy. If a reporter crossed him, his displeasure was monumental, painful to watch, and certain to lead to a news embargo. Those news people who pleased him and promulgated his views got preferential treatment, including scoops and interviews which he would orchestrate with donor families or with transplant team personnel. Growing community awareness of transplantation was the result.

This was a man with an important mission and a bright future. He was in his late forties, old for an organ procurement coordinator, but wiry and energetic to the point of being perpetually tense. He had a special knack of communicating with the bereaved families whose consent he needed for organ donation. It was as if something in his past life gave him a special understanding of their sorrow. Perhaps this was true, but if so he was too private to reveal any of it.

He dressed impeccably, although the sameness of his tweed sports jackets and his blue shirts with Oxford collars gave the impression that he owned only one of each. This is not an idle description of a minor figure who came and quickly went. Denny poured nearly eight turbulent years of his life into the Pittsburgh transplantation program. Eventually he became a political figure, because of his appointment to a presidential task force, and a spokesman at a high government level for a group whose views he failed to represent.

» «

Until the early 1980s, the word *transplantation* in political circles meant kidney transplantation. Intense pressure in 1972 had created the entrepreneurial End-Stage Renal Disease (ESRD) program which funded the organ procurement agency managed by Denny. The law pacified most of those who complained about government indifference to kidney disease. Its legislative provisions were assimilated into the existing American medical system, which has become an uneasy marriage of private enterprise and government support. After this, transplantation lapsed back into a decade of torpor, until the results of the Consensus Development Conference on liver transplantation set bells ringing again through the nation's capitol. In addition, the improved results with transplantation of other kinds of grafts became known as a result of the Pittsburgh liver and heart trials with cyclosporine.

However, the inability of people who needed these organs to find or afford them was a cause for outrage. Symbolic was the nightly pleading on television by the parents of desperate yellow-skinned children with liver disease, abandoned by the health care system because of lack of money or the alleged absence of a cadaver organ procurement system. The legislative (mostly Democrats) and executive (mostly Republicans) branches of government became activists in resolving the problem. However, they parted company on what to do, and so did workers in transplantation.

Congressional hearings on transplantation were convened in the autumn of 1983 by Albert Gore (Tennessee), Henry Waxman (California), and Doug Walgren (Pennsylvania). All were Democrats. Their proposed legislation (commonly called the Gore Bill) had three objectives. One was to increase the supply of organs through a small grants program that would strengthen organ procurement agencies already in existence or stimulate the development of new programs. An almost unnoticed proviso was the establishment of a national network for organ distribution. The second objective was to pay for expensive medicines such as cyclosporine. Cyclosporine had not yet been released by the FDA and could not yet be sold, but it was predicted to be too costly for many patients to afford. The third issue was a prohibition on the buying and selling of organs. This was a specific response to an unpopular proposal by a Virginia physician that a kidney brokerage business be established through which recipients could negotiate with living donors on a commercial basis.

Most transplant physicians and surgeons were in favor of the bill. Support was organized by the urologist Oscar Salvatierra of San Francisco. Those who testified for the bill in Washington included officers of the American Society of Transplant Surgeons, the heart transplant pioneer Norman Shumway on behalf of the thoracic surgeons, and me. I spoke for the University of Pittsburgh, although not all of our team was of one mind.

Hakala opposed the Gore Bill, although not passionately. Denny saw it as a death knell. It was certain to erode his authority and autonomy because it spelled out the governance and function of organ procurement agencies for the first time. In addition, Denny feared that a personal enemy named Gene Pierce, director of the Southeastern Organ Procurement Foundation, the Richmond-based consortium of voluntarily cooperating regional transplant centers, would become the national director if the bill passed and thus his superior at the final executive level. This is what eventually happened, but not before a remarkable campaign of vilification and media manipulation directed against Pierce that lasted for several years.

Denny worked furiously to prevent passage of the Gore Bill, directing his efforts at a recently formed nonphysician group called the National Association of Transplant Coordinators (NATCO). The members were of diverse background—nurses, technicians, social workers, laboratory technologists—but they had one thing in common. They had a powerful commitment to patients. Over Denny's objections, they lined up behind the bill.

Opposition to the bill was led by a number of powerful groups, such as the American Medical Association and the American College of Surgeons. To these conservative professional organizations, the Gore Bill represented an incursion into the private practice of medicine and the imposition of controls that inevitably would permeate other aspects of medical care. By coincidence, Hank Bahnson of Pittsburgh was president of the American College of Surgeons at the same time as the majority of University of Pittsburgh transplant physicians and surgeons (and Bahnson himself privately) supported the bill's passage.

There also was resistance to the proposed legislation from the Republican-dominated executive branch of the government. Its spokespersons argued that the most critical steps to relieve the crisis already had been taken by Surgeon General Koop, a member of their own administration. Koop's initiatives were to standardize and disseminate the new technology in transplantation, and above all to remove the impediments to private funding which had been put in place by the government itself (see chapter 22). The final step in Koop's strategy was the conclusion by the Consensus Development Conference that liver transplantation was not experimental.

At the last minute, the executive branch took a stance that undercut its own original purpose. Margaret Heckler, the secretary of HEW, announced at Gore's congressional hearing that liver transplantation would be classified by Medicare as a service for those under the age of eighteen but, incongruously, that it remained experimental for anyone older. Although the ruling shielded Medicare from fiscal responsibility, it sent a message to insurance companies that restored for adults the very situation from which we had just rescued ourselves with Koop's assistance. This attempt to reach a Solomon-type decision meant that sick children with liver disease could be cared for, but not their parents.

» «

Heckler's attempt to conciliate both points of view did nothing to slow the legislative momentum. When Congress passed the Gore Bill and sent it to President Reagan, he signed it into law. The tug of war between his executive branch and Congress was over the broader political question of how large, pervasive, and powerful the government bureaucracy should be in the affairs of daily life. Restriction of government intervention was the Republican party line, and expansionism was the battle cry of the Democrats.

Reagan himself was anything but callous. From 1983 onward, he threw himself into the campaign to increase public awareness of the organ shortage. He talked of it often on his weekly Saturday morning radio broadcast and offered airforce planes to children who otherwise were unable to find emergency transportation to Pittsburgh in time to receive their new livers. Four of the children came from the Washington area. All recovered and are still well.

President Reagan's personal attention to the problem had a greater positive impact on organ donation than any other single factor in the mid 1980s. Before June 1983, the supply of donors was a trickle. During the next twelve months, this changed to a torrent, and fifty-one infants and children were treated at Children's Hospital in Pittsburgh. The liver recipients became known as the "Reagan children," to the delight of Reagan's supporters and the chagrin of his detractors, who accused him of hypocrisy.

Sometime later, I was invited with several of these small patients to a private meeting with Mr. Reagan. This had been arranged by Mike Batten, a liaison officer appointed to sort out and do something about the anguished appeals from desperate patients or their despairing relatives that were flooding the White House. Mr.

Reagan was preceded into the room by a wildly excited but friendly spaniel who was reputed to be refractory to house training. Reagan looked more physically powerful than I had imagined and much younger than the seventy-five years he carried. He spent a long time with the children. It was not a photo opportunity with the children as a prop. He genuinely cared.

Although this was not my last trip to the White House, I understood from that time onward why he was called a "teflon president." Mud could not stick to someone like this. Years later, during the first days of the war in the Persian Gulf, I turned on the television one night to see Reagan facing a large crowd after he had given a speech in Utah. A hostile member of the audience asked him why the government during his administration had tilted to Saddam Hussein and contributed to the present situation. Instead of an evasive half-truth, he blurted out without hesitation, "I guess I pulled a boner," and went on to the next question. There was something about him that repelled defilement.

One of the so-called Reagan children was a three-year-old boy named Austin Szegda from Iowa. On January 20, 1984, I was visiting with John Fordtran at the Baylor University Hospital in Dallas, to assess with him the possibility of setting up a much-needed liver transplant program for that part of the country. While I was in his office, a call came from Paul Taylor, who had stayed in Colorado when I moved to Pittsburgh. There was a brain-dead donor at the Porter Hospital in Denver.

The twenty-one-month-old donor had been abandoned by (or taken from) his parents and placed by a court order with foster parents. In his new home, he had been abused to death, the fatal blow being to the head. The government, which had declared itself his guardian and placed him in his lethal environment, now had to decide what to do. I flew to Denver and went to the court. Judge Orrelle Weeks, a gray-haired woman, heard the story first and then my testimony about the dying Szegda child in Pittsburgh. Herself a mother, Judge Weeks could not hide her grief over the tragedy. At last, she gave permission to remove the organs.

By the time we reached the hospital, the wretched little donor was in the operating room on a breathing machine. Photographers from the coroner's office and police were there to record the cigarette burns on his arms and legs and the bruises all over. I do not believe that a word was spoken until we finished and left for the airport. Flying east through the night, the Lear jet crossed two time zones and arrived in Pittsburgh as dawn broke.

Austin recovered uneventfully after his liver transplantation and several years later made his own trip to the White House. His mother wrote me often about these adventures and about small problems of the kind seen in all children. Because it was public knowledge, she knew the circumstances of the donor's death. The knowledge stalked her with a lingering sadness. I wrote back and explained that circumstances had permitted a part of the unwanted donor child to finally find a cherished home in her son and added, "I still have terrible nightmares about Austin's little donor who was tortured to death in Denver. I doubt if I will ever really be able to get the sight of that tormented little body out of my mind. I am so glad that you love Austin. Please do not worry too much about the teeth since the real ones will be coming along soon." In the summer of 1991, Austin came back to Pittsburgh. He was eleven years old now and bore no resemblance to the moribund invalid I first saw so long ago when his life was ebbing away. His mother and I embraced silently and watched her fair-haired son play in the corridor.

A month or so later, I sat alone in a restaurant in the Sheraton Hotel in London, Ontario. Up on a platform, concealed by the piano he was playing, a black man sang a love song in tones so sad and beautiful that I wondered if he would ever be able to sing it so well again. As far as I could tell, no one was listening except me. The words came, "You're always on my mind," and with them a flashback to the awful scene in the operating room in Denver. I left without eating and went to my room.

» «

By the time the Gore Bill finally passed in 1984, no one knew what to do with it. A task force was convened to recommend how to distribute organs equitably and effectively. It was chaired by a distinguished surgeon named Olga Jonasson who later became chair of the Department of Surgery at Ohio State University. After holding its own public hearings for almost a year, the group established broad, written guidelines for organ distribution. The task force categorically rejected discrimination on the basis of sex, race, national origin, or economic class. It urged caution in giving any weight to such criteria as age, life style, the presence of a social network, or other factors that might only be judgments of social worth.

Although Denny had bitterly fought passage of the Gore Bill, he was nominated to serve on this committee by the University of Pittsburgh transplantation team. What better way was there to create unity in our program and nationally than to acknowledge and honor the minority contingent and its spokesman? It was an unwise decision.

The Pittsburgh turf war over who would perform kidney transplantations and for what patients now was transferred to a national stage where charges and innuendos of commercialism and use of slogans like "selling the gift" could be promulgated on a grander scale. Documents were fed in confidence to gullible reporters from one of the Pittsburgh newspapers, complete with interpretations implying that the transplant surgeons, the general surgical service, or members of the hospital administration had been involved in payoffs and other irregularities. These innuendos later were found by a community oversight committee and federal investigators to be unfounded. This was long after they were published as news.

Two days before Christmas 1985, a copy of a letter to Mr. Denny appeared in my office. It was written by Dr. Charles B. Carter, the director of an organ procurement agency in Indiana and a friend of Denny's whom I did not know. It read:

Dear Don:
This letter concerns copies of the recent Pittsburgh Press articles which were sent to our institution by you. As I understand it, these copies were sent unsolicited to our program and many others around the country. . . .

These articles are very harmful to the organ procurement process and the transplant field in general. In my opinion, they are unfair and factually in error in many places. By choosing to distribute these widely, you have done a major disservice to the field. Since the vast majority of newspapers in the country did not choose to carry these, I do not understand your action in distributing them. . . .

I feel it is not your role to distribute these articles especially in view of your position on the Transplantation Task Force and in NATCO, an organization which is dedicated to improving organ procurement.

There was nothing here we did not already know, but the letter itself created a crisis. A copy had been sent to Dr. Jonasson, the chair of the federal task force on which Denny sat, and to others. Soon, its accusation of subversion of the commission's purpose would be seen by many people. At noon on December 20, 1985, Bahnson met with Denny to discuss the letter. Bahnson never told me what was said and I never asked him.

Denny resigned that afternoon as director of the Transplant Organ Procurement Foundation (TOPF). I agreed with Bahnson that the circumstances would not be disclosed. The promise was studiously kept even though a final news story on Denny's career portrayed him as a disillusioned man whose departure had been precipitated by his defense of lofty principle. The rhetoric of administrative turf war is camouflage by which all reasons for an action are given except the correct ones.

Nine months later, in early October 1986, the truth emerged during a program on public television. A series for national syndication about advances in medicine called "Managing Our Miracles" had been produced by Fred Friendly, the man responsible for the Edward R. Murrow news shows of the 1950s. It was his program that had exposed Senator Joe McCarthy's abuse of power during the postwar witch hunt for communists. Now in academia, Friendly was professor of journalism at Columbia University. The program on transplantation was filmed in Philadelphia in April 1986, with Denny and me as panelists along with seven or eight physicians from other major centers as well as legislators and medical media specialists. To promote its release in early October, Friendly and the local Pittsburgh station (WQED) planned a similar round table, but this would be aired live and use only Pittsburgh panelists. With me would be Angus McEachran (editor of the Pittsburgh *Press*), Don Denny, and four or five others. In the dressing room prior to the session, McEachran and Denny gave every appearance of meeting each other for the first time and even of not knowing what the other looked like.

The one-hour Pittsburgh program was dull for the first thirty minutes until Friendly asked McEachran what was meant by the accusation in his newspaper, as it had been reported to him, that we had transplanted organs "for valuable consideration." Mr. McEachran's explanation was evasive. Friendly then asked Denny why he had resigned from TOPF. Because his explanation was the same falsified one as had been reported in McEachran's newspaper, I was obligated to tell the truth and did. Two days later, on October 10, 1986, I sent Friendly a brief note which read: "Dear Fred: "Thank you for what you made possible. Senator McCarthy revisited!!""

The morning after the television program, I gave medical rounds at Mercy Hospital where Denny had taken an administrative job following his resignation. After parking, I came face to face with him and asked directions to the auditorium. Unsmiling but courteous, he obliged me. I have never seen him since, but I often have thought of him and inquired about how he is doing. He left Pittsburgh a year or so later and returned to university graduate studies. Soon he will have a Ph.D.

There was a period of potential greatness in his life which he cast away. Perhaps there can be one again. I keep looking for people like Denny because they have the fire and determination to change the world. They have it in them to be great men or women. If only I had not arrived in his life already labeled as the enemy whom he had not yet even met, it might have been different.

» «

The recommendations of the Jonasson committee report were incorporated into a contract which was let in 1986 by the federal agency empowered to establish a national organ procurement and distribution system. The contract was given to the United Network for Organ Sharing (UNOS), a previously private and nonprofit organization which already had been carrying out these functions unofficially. Denny's nemesis, Gene Pierce, was named the executive director of UNOS and became the subject of a scathing investigative report by a Pittsburgh newspaper. An English surgeon provided some of the most damning quotations against Pierce; he himself was soon to be suspended because of misconduct from transplant activities in his own country and from membership in professional transplantation societies. Investigations cleared Pierce of any wrongdoing.

UNOS committees that attempted to develop an organ distribution plan were unable to reach a consensus as the deadline of May 1987 approached for submission of the plan to the government. Failure to have a plan would put UNOS in default. In April 1987, they requested me to develop two proposals, one for the national distribution of cadaver kidneys and one for the fair deployment of other organs, principally the liver and heart.

The request to me was prompted by the fact that we had devised in Pittsburgh a system for kidney distribution that gave credit points to potential recipients. The plan that we had put in place in 1985 had taken the decision about who would be given a cadaver kidney out of the hands of Denny's procurement agency employees. Instead of vague criteria for such decisions, the Pittsburgh plan allowed credits to be acquired for time waiting, quality of tissue match, medical need, and other technical factors. *This was the only such system in the United States.* The results of its use were described in an article to be published in the medical literature. A slightly different plan also was in use in Pittsburgh for liver and heart distribution.[1]

I cut up these two articles with scissors and reassembled the pieces in slightly different order to comply with the format to be used for the national distribution plans. The proposals were accepted by the UNOS board of directors, found by the government to fulfill the contract obligations, and put into effect on October 1, 1987. All this was the maturation and politization of a technology. There were no magic moments. To accomplish it, the clock of progress froze in patient care. It did not thaw again until 1989.

» «

The turf war in Pittsburgh came as a delayed reaction to the transplant revolution of the early 1980s. It could have ended in administrative murders, but it did not. Instead, those who wanted to work stayed and the others left. The Pittsburgh organ distribution system became the national standard. The organ procurement agency was reorganized in 1985 along the lines mandated by the Gore Bill and was shaped thereafter by its own high aims. Now, it belonged to the community and to the nation.

The anonymous allegations, investigative reporters, selected leaks of uninterpretable information, and political agendas had created a public relations hurricane in the spring and early summer of 1985. While it was going on, my hidden allegiance was with the reporters, their numerous factual errors notwithstanding. They were doing something that I thought was needed but could not do alone. While searching for villains with their spotlights, two reporters for the Pittsburgh *Press*, Andrew Schneider and Mary Pat Flaherty, unwittingly had illuminated the whole scene and thus became the instruments of reform, some of it contrary to what they had advocated editorially. Seasoned by their earlier experience, they wrote in the autumn a seven-part study of worldwide issues in transplantation which was crowned in 1986 with a Pulitzer Prize for specialized reporting.

These were not the only laurels for Pittsburgh. In the same year, the television station KDKA, and the Westinghouse Broadcasting Group with which it is affiliated, won the highest professional distinction in their medium, the George Foster Peabody Award for community service. It was one of the four journalistic honors earned by a television series, introduced by President Reagan, that promoted organ donation. I was named overall Pittsburgh Man of the Year (a 1981 award had been in science and medicine), was given keys to the cities of Milan and Venice, and received other honors including elevation to a distinguished service chair at my own university.

To understand how all of this could have happened without a systematic administrative plan, it is necessary to understand Hank Bahnson, chair of the surgical department, who already had passed his sixtieth year by the time Iwatsuki and I arrived in Pittsburgh. Bahnson's greatest assets and human qualities were fairness and integrity. When he was a child, he was an innocent bystander in an accident which became a linchpin of his character. While he was nearby, his mother fell down a steep flight of stairs in a church near their home in Winston-Salem, North Carolina. To his horror, he realized that she thought that she had been pushed—by him. He told me this in June 1985, while we walked down a quiet street in Vienna. We were there for his induction as an honorary member of the Austrian Surgical Society. The week before, one of the Pittsburgh newspapers had published a sensational report about alleged improprieties in the transplant program. I heard in his voice the pain that the unfair childhood accusation and now the recent ones had caused.

Who was responsible for the distorted information that had been leaked as ammunition in the intramural turf war? There would be no rush to judgment in Bahnson's life. This trait paralyzed him in his executive functions, but it created a protective buffer for those who were in the fusion of the old and new in the transplant world. No complaint, however minor, went unattended by him personally. The paper trail—notes of meetings, letters sent and unsent, answers to complaints, summaries of testimony—showed without intending to the purity and purpose of the new program and destroyed the web woven over it by those intent upon its destruction or fractionation.

This was the old-fashioned way of management. When Bahnson retired from surgery in 1987, the turf wars were over. If they were to recur, it would have to be through the councils and oversight committees that were designed to prevent them. Transplantation had been institutionalized in Pittsburgh, setting the stage for the next harvest of ideas and new technologies. These already were simmering on the back burner.

At a national level, a law had been passed and put into effect. Transplantation was being woven into the fabric of American society and of conventional medical care. The problem was that no one knew how to pay for it.

24

Understanding Governor Lamm

Richard Lamm, governor of the State of Colorado from 1978 to 1986, was not the first person to question the cost efficiency of transplantation, but he became the most celebrated. Because I admired him so much, I was sorry to be chosen as his debating adversary. Few men or women in public life will speak their convictions so honestly as Lamm did routinely. This kind and courteous man already had provoked a fire storm by criticizing the wisdom of more than supportive medical care for the aged, and by suggesting that the old had an obligation to wither and die as leaves must fall from trees to make way for new ones.[1]

Lamm was discussing more than money when he poetically described the duty of the obsolete generation to leave the scene. His point was that senile leaves (or people) can inhibit or destroy the next generation or generations as yet unborn. Lamm knew ecology, and his political career had begun as a conservationist. He was stating his understanding of the continuum between the past and future.

Lamm occupied the Colorado governor's office during many of the important developments in transplantation at the University of Colorado. The developmental work brought more than $50 million in outside revenue to his state over a period of nineteen years. When the time came for its more general application, transplantation became for Mr. Lamm the symbol for fiscal inefficiency and irresponsibility in health care. This was unfortunate because Lamm's important overall message was thereby lost. In the summer of 1987, he wrote an article entitled "Health Care as Economic Cancer" for the journal *Dialysis and Transplantation*, saying:

> Health care is clearly entering into a new era: Infinite health needs have run into finite resources. The miracles of medicine have outstripped our ability to pay, and some thoughtful and equitable thinking has to be done to ensure that America gets the most health care for its limited dollars.
>
> It is a very serious mistake to deny that a major change is in the wings. No sector of the economy, no matter how important, can continue to grow at two-and-a half times the rate of inflation. We are heading rapidly toward an America that has rusting plants, closed factories, staggering trade deficits. Health care cannot continue to operate under the illusion that it can continue with business as usual.
>
> Once we accept the fact that there are limits to what the nation can afford (and, increasingly, people are recognizing this truth), then we will begin a process of asking how to get the most health benefits for the most Americans for our money. We should have asked this question years ago. It is outrageous that this country spends five to eight times what other countries spend, and yet has no better health outcome. America is going to demand more accountability for the more than one billion dollars a day it now spends on health care. Many countries give a high level of health care to all their citizens for a fraction of what we spend, and yet keep them healthier. We are no longer rich enough to give a blank check to an inefficient health care industry.
>
> Once we start to apply even minimum management standards to the health care industry, we will see some substantial changes. If we ask how to get the most health benefits for the greatest number of Americans for our tax dollars, many of today's practices will not meet the test. If we zero-budget all that we now do in health care, we shall inevitably close unnecessary hospitals, close excess ICU units, and look much more closely at utilization factors and outcomes. We shall have to develop a concept of cost-effective medicine. Virtually every health care provider will agree that much of what we do today in medicine has "marginal utility." When a society faces fiscal reality and seeks to optimize its dollars, it not only starts on the road to financial sanity, but it also brings dramatic change to existing medical practices. Dialysis and transplantation will undoubtedly undergo major change. The "opportunity costs" in other areas of medicine are clearly greater than much of what is being done today. The bottom line is that we can save more lives and bring better health care to more Americans for many of the dollars we are spending today.

Economist Lester Thurow suggests that, to impress upon health providers what they are doing when they order marginal services, we should require them to imagine an American worker sentenced to a period of slavery long enough to pay the medical bill for that procedure. Dr. Thomas Starzl recently gave a liver transplant to a 76-year-old woman. It cost $240,000. Dr. Starzl should understand that with the average U.S. family making $24,000 a year, he has sentenced 100 U.S. families to work all year so that he could transplant a 76-year-old woman.

Such actions are cheating our children of resources that they desperately need to build a better life and to revitalize the United States economically. If all of us, or even a significant percentage of us, take $240,000 in high-tech medicine as we are on our way out the door, we are stealing resources that our children and our grandchildren desperately need. Health care is important, but it cannot be the only value of our society. It cannot continue on its growth curve without bankrupting America.

Health providers are not used to thinking this way. Many of you will cry foul and think this heresy. But alas—it is true. A nation that runs $200 billion deficits and borrows 20 cents from its children out of every dollar it spends must one day demand more accountability from its politicians, from its industries, and from its health providers. That day is near at hand, and we should welcome it—for our children's sakes.[2]

The journal editors asked me for a response. I complied because Mr. Lamm had specifically criticized the use of liver transplantation for a seventy-six-year-old woman who was my patient and still is. As it has turned out, this patient recently passed the five-year post-transplant mark and lives a full life at home. A teenaged Colorado girl whose care also was opposed by Mr. Lamm in his capacity as governor remains well, now seven years after liver transplantation. Thus, my reply to Mr. Lamm in 1987 has seemed more sustainable with each new year:

It would be unjust to describe a public servant of Richard Lamm's distinction and courage in any but the most flattering terms. Mr. Lamm has contended for a number of years that health care costs must be contained. He has pointed out that too much of the high-intensity care provided for aged or hopelessly ill patients is not only costly, but may also be inhumane when all that is achieved is prolongation of painful dying. These messages are so important that they deserve the kind of thoughtful examination that depends upon accuracy more than rhetoric.

Two cases can illustrate the point. The first came to my attention and to Governor Lamm's in October, 1984. A 13-year-old girl was admitted to the Colorado General Hospital in Denver with acute liver failure from previously undiagnosed Wilson's disease. She required ventilatory support [breathing with a machine] because of unconsciousness, hemodialysis [artificial kidney] because of the hepatorenal syndrome [combined liver and kidney failure], and repeated closed cardiac massage. Her physicians realized that liver transplantation was the only treatment that would be more than symbolic and that would allow real recovery.

Governor Lamm was reported, perhaps incorrectly, to have disallowed public assistance for this purpose on grounds that this would be a costly exercise in futility [see article by S. Burling in *The Rocky Mountain News*, October 17, 1984, p. 16]. Support mechanisms in Denver, Houston, and Pittsburgh were quickly developed, whereby the child was transferred to the Presbyterian University Hospital of Pittsburgh. Liver transplantation was carried out on October 17, 1984. The girl returned home to Colorado on December 1, 1984. The cost of her care was $87,322, of which $54,000 was paid eventually by Colorado State Medical Assistance. Today, she leads a normal life on the farm where she was reared.

The second example concerns the 76-year-old lady mentioned by Mr. Lamm in his editorial. The extent to which the ethical and societal issues in this case were examined by a broad consortium of interested parties has been exceptionally well-documented [e.g., *The Wall Street Journal*, October 14, 1986, p. 1]. The fact that advanced age alone does not preclude liver transplant candidacy or significantly degrade postoperative survival also has been reported [T. E. Starzl et al., "Liver Transplantation in Older Patients," *New England Journal of Medicine* 316 (1987):484-85]. The seventy-six-year-old patient whose treatment was decried is coming up to the one-year follow-up mark in excellent condition at home. The enslavement of 100 families, working for one year to pay a $240,000 medical bill, was not required. Surgical fees were written off. The hospital cost of $68,000 has not been paid and may never be. The willingness of the Presbyterian University Hospital and its University of Pittsburgh faculty to take responsibility for this case without assurance of payment was an expression of a moral position like that of the Colorado physicians in Case One.

It has been said that society and its institutions are judged by the way they treat those who cannot defend themselves, as exemplified by its very young and very old. It would have been members of these extreme age groups who would have been deprived of effective care by their exclusion from transplantation in late 1984 and more recently. In the process, Mr. Lamm, a decent and compassionate man, had no objection to the expensive care provided to the child and to the old lady who had become invalided and hospital-bound by their diseases. Incongruously, the objection was to transplantation which was the only treatment that was capable of liberating them from hospital life, restoring them to society, and putting an end to a continuous accrual of expenses down a therapeutic cul-de-sac.

It is conceivable, but highly unlikely, that society someday will decide that no patient with liver disease, or diseases of certain other organ systems, such as the heart or kidney, will be treated. If so, Mr. Lamm's arguments will have great force, and physicians (those who are left) will want to determine the cheapest way to exercise what will have become a priestly, not therapeutic, function. Until then, the proper first decision by those serving society will be whether treatment should be carried out. If the answer is yes, the appropriate second question will be, what is the best way. Then, what will be purchased per health care dollar will be real, not symbolic.

Developments in transplantation and artificial organ technology have changed forever the philosophy by which organ-defined specialties such as nephrology [kidney], hepatology [liver], and cardiology [heart] are practiced. Until recently, what could be offered victims of vital-organ failure was a rear guard approach designed with diet, medicines, or surgical procedures to extract the last moment of life-supporting function from the failing organ. Now, and for the first time in human history, the breathtaking possibility has emerged of starting over when all else fails, with an organ graft or with a manufactured organ.

Much of the groundwork for this revolution was laid at the University of Colorado during Mr. Lamm's enlightened gubernatorial administration and during that of his predecessor, Governor John Love. The failure of Mr. Lamm to take advantage of what has happened under his own sponsorship is like giving birth to a beautiful child and then trying to starve it so that it will not threaten the food supply.[3]

Closing comments were allowed for Mr. Lamm after he had seen my arguments. What he said was persuasive but it was not published after I was given the privilege of a further comment. In Mr. Lamm's view, the exchanges were degenerating into a never-ending spiral. His unpublished parting remarks were:

Dr. Starzl continues to miss the point. He is so busy dedicatedly saving specific individuals that he cannot see the larger societal dilemma. A compassionate society has the duty to use its limited resources to save the maximum number of its citizens. The American health care system already denies care to millions of people—some of whom die every day for lack of treatment. A compassionate society should first give everyone basic health care—then, as resources allow—move to more complicated procedures. I know of no health official who claims transplants are a cost-effective way to bring a society good health. There are a myriad of ways we can and should be spending our limited health care dollars that would save more lives than do transplants.

It was a pity to terminate the discussion. Mr. Lamm's was a description and defense of statistical morality, and mine was the same justification of the doctor-patient relationship which I had used as my lifetime ethical standard as outlined twenty years earlier (see chapter 16). Only the circumstances were different. My unpublished riposte was:

I understood perfectly the arguments in Mr. Lamm's editorial, and I explained in mine why I disagreed with them. When the state is seen as the agent and protector of the good of the public, notions of utilitarian balance can be invoked with the result that the interests of the state can always be placed ahead of the needs or claims of the very individuals whom the state supposedly serves. Those who believe that an individual human life is above bartering also believe that the preeminent and transcendent status of the human personality is the bedrock of our secular, pluralistic society. The taking or debasing of life by withholding effective treatment ought not to be justifiable no matter how great the offsetting "benefit" to the public good.

I often have wondered about the efforts by physicians or non-physician planners to find a dollar and cents figure for health care per unit population as if all people (here called units) are the same. Most of the patients whom I see have never been seriously ill until the arrival of the one great problem that brings them to special hospitals like those at the University of Pittsburgh Health Sciences Center. What the patient seeks at that moment is "tertiary care," a kind of treatment requiring unusual knowledge or skills, cooperation among specialists, and hospital resources that are not routinely available. Such care often enables the patient to evade death or prevents permanent invalidism in what may seem to be heroic rescue.

Tertiary care is expensive, and its misuse and abuse were the targets of Governor Lamm's remarks. Who should be allowed to have it? To put it differently, who decides who is to be rescued and who is to be left behind?

25

The Drug with No Name

Forty-five miles from Tokyo, the University of Tsukuba is located at the foot of the mountain from which the school and the village in which it is located take their name. Although the university is only two decades old, 10 to 15 percent of all the scientists in Japan are on its faculty. One reason is that more than 40 government institutes plus an additional 100 private institutes endowed and run by major corporations contribute to its campus. When I visited it in 1977, the village of Tsukuba was largely farmland. A decade later, it was an intellectual hotbed—and one of the fastest growing cities in the country.

The founding chairman in 1975 of the Department of Surgery of the new Tsukuba medical school was Yoji Iwasaki, the former University of Colorado transplant fellow whose studies of antilymphocyte globulin (ALG) in 1964 and 1965 enriched the field of transplantation (see chapter 13). In 1986, Iwasaki was appointed chair of the Institute of Clinical Medicine—a unique position in Japan—in addition to his surgical chair. Now he is in charge of education in all clinical medical specialties in this astonishing school.

Sometime in the spring of 1986, I heard about a drug with the code name FR900506 that was discovered by scientists at the institute established on the Tsukuba University campus by the Fujisawa Pharmaceutical Corporation. Their project was to systematically screen natural substances in the soil for their anticancer or antirejection properties. One product of the search was a fungus (a special kind of germ) found in the soil at the foot of Tsukuba Mountain, not far from Yoji Iwasaki's office. The fungus produced a substance that interrupted or prevented immune reactions in their test systems. The substance had not yet been described in the scientific literature, and it was not available for investigation outside the Fujisawa laboratories.

The drug receded into the background until August 1986 when I went to Helsinki for the biannual meeting of the Transplantation Society. Scheduled on the program in one of the smaller sessions with no more than forty or fifty people in the audience was a paper with the mystery code number FR900506 in the title. It was to be given by a young Japanese surgeon named Takenori Ochiai of Chiba University near Tokyo.

Nearby, in an amphitheater overflowing with most of the congress participants, progress and problems in kidney transplantation under cyclosporine were being discussed. In the larger meeting, the marvelous qualities of cyclosporine were being extolled, but its limitations also were receiving attention. The most serious side effect, which had been well known since 1980, was the kidney injury which cyclosporine could cause at the same time as it protected kidney transplants from the damage of rejection. The same kidney injury also was being reported in recipients of other kinds of organs, including the liver and heart. In addition, cyclosporine in high doses caused high blood pressure, excessive growth of hair, an annoying heaping up of the gums, and a tremor. When the cyclosporine doses were reduced to relieve these side effects, the risk of rejection increased.

Transplant surgeons with an obsession for perfection wondered if FR900506 might have a better margin of safety. Roy Calne of Cambridge was one of those waiting for Ochiai's presentation. I was another, and sitting with me was a Japanese surgeon named Satoru Todo whom I had met in October 1980, in the city of Fukuoka on Kyushu Island at the southern tip of Japan. Kyushu was Todo's ancestral home and the location of the university where he was trained in surgery. Then thirty-three years old, Todo was a surgeon in search of a mission. When he spoke, I had the eerie sensation that I was listening to myself in a time warp from October 1960. He was determined to master liver transplantation, an operation that he knew only from books and journals—it could not be performed in Japan. Because brain death was not accepted in Japan and would not be for many years, there could be no cadaver liver donors. Todo was the right man but he lived in the wrong time and place. He had decided to try to come to Colorado to pursue his dream, not yet knowing that the program would be in Pittsburgh instead.

On that day in 1980, Joy and I walked with Todo on the sand beaches of Kyushu Island and drove along the coastline, which was deserted because of a typhoon which had struck the day before and was playing out its final fury. That night we ate with a large group of surgeons and physicians from the University of Kyushu. Todo towered over most of them. He is a very large Japanese, five feet eleven inches tall and weighing 210 pounds. With his strong moon face and powerful body, he looked more like a Buddha God than a native son.

I had no position for him in Pittsburgh and told him so. From the way he talked, I suspected that he would come anyway. He finally made it in January 1984, prepared to work with no salary which he did for the first 12 months. After arriving, he spent every day for two and a half years learning and perfecting the liver transplant procedures in dogs and rats that would enable him to efficiently test new drugs or answer other questions that bore on patient care. Then, almost every night he worked in the human operating room, assisting more experienced surgeons. By the summer of 1986 he too was ready for the next challenges. Many of these would stem from Ochiai's paper about FR900506 which we had come to Finland to hear.

Ochiai began his talk with a summary of the properties and mechanisms of action of FR900506. In addition, he reported the results of heart transplantation in a small number of rats. Rejection had been prevented with remarkable reliability and safety. During the discussion that followed, Calne said that he recently had tested the drug, which had been supplied to him by the Fison Corporation, an English pharmaceutical company which had obtained the drug through a trade agreement with Fujisawa. Calne was concerned about the drug's toxicity, and especially the violent vomiting which it caused in dogs. In the months to come, Calne became increasingly convinced of the drug's deficiencies. However, to me the properties of the drug, including the fact that it was one hundred times more potent per weight unit than cyclosporine, looked too promising to abandon. It was the beginning of a disagreement that lasted for more than three years.

The trade arrangement between the Fujisawa and Fison corporations precluded our obtaining a supply for testing through normal channels. A few weeks later, Todo and I left Pittsburgh for Japan. On the first day, we met in Nagoya with Fujisawa executives and discussed with them our plan for laboratory research. In response to our meeting, Hiroshi Imanaka, the executive manager of the FR900506 development, flew to London for a meeting with Fison officials.

After they had gone, I was gently reminded of my age. Reaching sixty years is discretely ignored in many American institutions, but it is a major cultural event (called *kanreki*) in Japan. That evening, nearly a hundred former Japanese students held a belated *kanreki* ceremony organized by Shun Iwatsuki and Hiro Takagi (chair of surgery, Nagoya University) to mark my passage into antiquity, which had actually occurred the previous March 11. Joy was with me. After reminiscences, the climax of the evening was bestowal of a brilliant red velvet waistcoat with half-length sleeves and a matching flat hat similar to those used at graduation exercises. After this moment, the burden of constant striving that is traditional in this remarkable country is lifted, and a new life begins.

The timing of the rite of passage seemed particularly appropriate because of the physical and emotional cost of the preceding ten years. Fatigue had become my seductive and constant partner, preaching expediency and caution instead of boldness. Perhaps it would be a blessing *not* to obtain the drug and not begin a new cycle of anxiety and controversy. While the days passed, Todo and I with our wives (Noriko and Joy) waited in Japan for the outcome of the Fujisawa negotiations in London. Carried by the gentle current of Japanese society, we moved from Nagoya to Tokyo and then south to Todo's home in Fukuoka.

After a week, Dr. Imanaka returned from England. The outcome of the discussions with the Fison officials was announced to us at a meeting in the lobby of a Fukuoka hotel. The conversation was polite and painfully slow, almost ceremonial. For those of us who were not bilingual, Todo translated. At the end, we were given approximately one one-hundredth of an ounce of FR900506. There was enough to fill the bottom of a very small thimble.

The race was on again. With the tiny prize, Adriana Zeevi and the other cellular immunologists in Pittsburgh could test the drug, using minute and carefully rationed quantities in tissue culture experiments. Within a month, more drug arrived for testing. Thousands of transplantation experiments followed with rats and subsequently in dogs, monkeys, and baboons. Every Monday night a research conference was held. At first, eight or ten people came. By the end of 1986, the conference room could not contain the growing number which eventually was nearly one hundred, all waiting eagerly for weekly reports on the tissue culture experiments, an account of transplant experiments in rats performed by a pediatric surgeon named Noriko Murase, and the results from dog transplant experiments carried out by Todo. Each piece of new information added to the excitement. The drug was more potent than cyclosporine and did not seem prohibitively toxic.

» «

If this was to be the last great scientific journey, it would not be an easy one. On Christmas Eve, 1986, an accident occurred during a liver transplantation in the operating room of Children's Hospital. The recipient was an infant whose blood would not clot. As the night wore on, I used an instrument known as a ruby light to dry up the tissues that were oozing blood in the deepest recesses of the wound. Forgotten were the instructions to avoid looking at the brilliant light at the tip of an instrument which cauterized the bleeding targets. I cannot remember any pain when the ruby light burned the back of the eye, but when Christmas morning came, the child had died and I was partially blind.

At first there was the vague sense of not knowing precisely where my hands were. On the way home, I found out why. When I closed my right eye, the vision in my left eye was restricted to an outer rim. In the middle, where a stop sign should have been on a familiar street corner, was a dark gray hole with nothing in it. Back at the emergency room, the eye specialist found a telltale blister in the back of the left eye where the ruby light had left its mark. The right eye was spared by some protective reflex which had caused me to close it. When I came home and told Joy, she cried at first and then said, "Thank you, Jesus."

"What do you mean, 'Thank you, Jesus?'" I asked. "I am blind."

"This means you won't have to work so hard," she answered.

It was true, but only temporarily. During the rest of the week, I watched video movies out of one eye with Joy and my grandson, Ravi, who had come to Pittsburgh for the holidays with my oldest son, Tim, and his wife, Bimla. Before our houseguests returned to Colorado, a possible alternative explanation for the blindness rose. Throughout their visit, I had daily fevers and night sweats. These continued throughout January 1987, and in February I was admitted to the Presbyterian University Hospital emergency room with pneumonia of the right middle lung lobe.

I had lost weight and suspected that I was having symptoms of AIDS. The magnitude of this threat to transplant patients and those who cared for them had become obvious after the development of screening tests for the HIV virus and the widespread use of these tests beginning in the spring of 1985. By studying the stored sera of patients treated in earlier times, we discovered that between 2 and 3 percent of the liver recipients and a smaller number of heart and kidney recipients had been unknown HIV carriers at the time of their transplantation.[1]

In these cases I had been the surgeon most commonly, but there were others with multiple exposure to the virus including Byers (Bud) Shaw, who had moved to Omaha in 1985, Andreas Tzakis, Satoru Todo, Shun Iwatsuki, Rob Gordon, and Leonard Makowka. It seemed possible that some of these surgeons, and perhaps all, had been infected. Shaw had gone through an unexplained illness similar to mine lasting three months in the autumn of 1984; the diagnosis at the time was viral encephalitis. Makowka, the Canadian, had been prostrated with an unexplained ailment which was attributed to overwork. In addition to heavy patient care duties, Makowka was founding the research laboratory that later became the basis for the Pittsburgh Transplantation Institute and the fountain from which would come the next wave of advances. It seemed that he never slept.

All the surgeons at risk were notified and urged to have HIV tests. To provide an example for the others, Makowka and I did this publicly every three months for one year. Those who were exposed had spent hundreds of hours in the operating room—sometimes in direct contact with infected blood after their hands or fingers were stuck with needles or cut with surgical instruments as had occurred in the hepatitis epidemics of the mid 1960s. To my surprise, everyone was negative. The virus had not infiltrated the staff. That this could have happened was illustrated tragically several years later in another part of the country when seven patients were infected with HIV from a single cadaveric donor of tissues and organs.

» «

The eye healed in six months. Although I was able to return to the operating room, the purpose no longer could be the mere compilation of cases. The *kanreki* of 1986 had in fact marked the beginning of a new cycle of activities, most of which involved FR900506. A few days after the blinding accident, our optimism was dampened by information from Calne's English laboratory that FR900506 was intolerably toxic, not only in dogs as Calne had mentioned the previous summer in Helsinki, but also in rats and baboons. Abstracts describing these observations had been submitted to the program committee for the June 1987 meeting of the European Society of Organ Transplantation (ESOT) which was to be in Gothenburg, Sweden.

Fearing that these reports would kill the development of this promising drug, I arranged through the transplant surgeons Carl Groth (Stockholm), Hans Brynger (Gothenburg), and Walter Land (Munich) to have an afternoon symposium on the day before the official congress at which all the available information on FR900506 could be exchanged. No articles about the drug had yet been published. Essentially all the research had taken place at four centers: the Fujisawa laboratories (Tsukuba and Osaka), Chiba University (in Tokyo), Cambridge University (England), and the University of Pittsburgh. The Gothenburg symposium was published in *Transplantation Proceedings* as a separate volume of 104 pages, of which 46 were contributed by Pittsburgh authors.[2]

Anyone reading the articles, and especially someone who was in the audience at the Gothenburg conference, might have wondered if the different investigators were discussing the same drug. The reports from Cambridge were gloomy, those from Pittsburgh were optimistic, and those from Chiba were noncommittal. The burial ground for controversial drugs beckoned. If this was to be its fate, the headstone would be easier to read because the name of FR900506 had been simplified to FK 506.

Before the Gothenburg symposium, all the same work from the Pittsburgh laboratories was presented by six members of our team to a smaller and more critical audience, consisting of about a dozen scientists from the Oncology and Pulmonary Disease section of the FDA in Rockville, Maryland. The preliminary meeting was convened in May 1987, at my initiative in order to alert the FDA to the impending conference in Sweden that was certain to generate media interest and controversy.

We summarized our own results as well as the adverse reports from Cambridge, explaining that we were not agents of the Fujisawa Corporation with which we had neither financial ties nor contracts. Our objectives were to provide an early account of an experimental drug which someday might be considered for clinical trial, to obtain scientific input and advice from the FDA scientists, and to be sure that what we were doing was in compliance with FDA regulations.

The stereotyping of government agencies could be exemplified by the FDA. No week goes by without a newspaper or television story about overregulation by the FDA that has prevented the orderly development of a drug or device, or about underregulation and release of an unsafe product. We were astonished at what we found. Each of the FDA scientists was an expert in his or her own right and understood perfectly what we had to report. When we finished, they pointed out the gaps in our research (mostly toxicology), what safeguards they thought would be necessary if clinical trials ever were to be considered, and how our work so far did or did not fulfill FDA requirements. They invited us to return when we had more results to report.

Not long afterward, we learned that Gregory Burke, one of the FDA team members, a physician and oncologist (cancer specialist), had been placed in charge of the FK 506 project and would be our contact person for further inquiries and discussions. I knew exactly who Burke was. For me, he had been the single most memorable figure in our conference even though his appearance may have been the most forgettable. Slight of build and with short sandy hair, he seemed almost lost in the crowd until a second startled look detected the faint luminescence with which nature paints unusual people. Throughout the meeting, he sat at one end of the long table, alertly listening while the others talked. Occasionally, he jotted down one or two words on a note pad.

I reflect from time to time on how important it is for government to attract people like Burke to its service. When he said something, it was as cryptic as his notes. Shy but friendly, this hardworking man rose during his stewardship of the FK 506 development to be the director of his FDA division. His suggestions about FK 506 always were creative, and his last one almost two years later prevented a tragedy when the drug was first given to a human being.

» «

In the pharmaceutical industry, there is a little-known process by which new compounds are given for the first time to professional risk-takers. Studies of these healthy young men and women, who are carefully examined medically to rule out diseases of all the organ systems, provides preliminary information on how the human body disposes of the new drugs, and in turn how the drugs affect the body. Scattered in large cities around the world, these subjects must be people without self-destructive behavior patterns such as alcohol or other substance abuse. These vices could alter the function tests of the liver or other organs, which are carefully monitored during and after the test doses of the new drugs. The human guinea pigs are handsomely paid and are enrolled with meticulous attention to informed consent. For many of them, this is their only work. To qualify for the job, the first condition is that they must be completely normal.

This preliminary step of drug development may be omitted with hazardous drugs such as those used for cancer chemotherapy. The steps had not been taken when Burke issued to us an investigational new drug number for FK 506. How to proceed was left up to me and my associates subject to the Institutional Review Board (IRB) of the University of Pittsburgh. What followed illustrated the maturation of the IRB system from the time of the cyclosporine trials eight years earlier (see chapter 21). The IRB decisions were even more difficult than those made prior to the cyclosporine trials in 1981. As in the earlier period, the mixed background of members precluded a uniform understanding of transplantation. Moreover, opinions about FK 506 from outside reviewers were not helpful because most of the available information came from our own research group.

Richard Cohen, professor of child psychiatry, was chair of the IRB throughout the FK 506 development. Later he remarked that dealing with the drug quickly became a full-time job. Cohen, a slender and almost pathologically handsome sixty-eight-year-old man, looked one or two decades younger than his stated age in spite of a full head of snow-white hair. His energy, grasp of the complex issues in transplantation, and air of dignity inspired the confidence of the IRB members and of the investigators in spite of their disagreements with him. His first decision about FK 506 was so shrewd that a quandary was created from which there was no escape later: we were able to demonstrate the therapeutic superiority of FK 506 almost from the outset.

Because the preliminary testing of FK 506 had not been done in healthy volunteers, Cohen wanted to give it for the first time to liver recipients who were losing their transplanted organ in spite of the best and strongest antirejection treatment available, including cyclosporine. Such patients faced death or retransplantation and had nothing to lose.

Burke was willing to follow this strategy, but when the first patient finally was selected for rescue therapy, he called back urgently. The starting intravenous dose, he said, was too large, based on the information we had given him from laboratory experiments. We reduced the dose according to his recommendation. From what we learned later, we came to believe that without Burke's input our first patient might have died of an overdose.

The human being whose life was spared by the telephone call of a man whom she would never meet was a twenty-eight-year-old woman named Robin Ford who was slowly rejecting her third liver graft eight months after its transplantation. Rescue treatment with FK 506 was started on February 28, 1989. She recovered. The next patient, a thirty-eight-year-old man who had received five livers during the preceding four years, was an even more severe test. He was now rejecting the fifth liver only three months after the last transplantation. As in the Ford case, rejection was controlled. More cases followed. In the first ten liver recipients switched from cyclosporine to FK 506 from February to July 1989, seven of the grafts were saved and still function today, more than two years later.

The surgeon who managed these trials was another of a new breed whose talents allowed fresh ideas and technologies to force their way into the light as flowers do through cracks in concrete. John Fung was a halfway surgeon and a complete immunologist when he came to Pittsburgh in June 1984, a few months after Todo arrived. Armed with a Ph.D. from the University of Chicago in addition to his M.D. degree, Fung was midway in his residency training in general surgery at the University of Rochester when he took two years off for laboratory research. He had helped develop tissue culture systems henceforth called "mini transplant" models which had allowed Adriana Zeevi and René Duquesnoy to learn as much in a few days about the effectiveness and mechanisms of action of FK 506 as had required months or years in the past. Now, a fully trained surgeon as well as a professional investigator, he sat at the bedside, equipped with unique knowledge and skills. He had not yet reached his thirty-second birthday.

I later met Fung's father when he was admitted to Presbyterian University Hospital because of heart disease. Many years before, Mr. Fung had emigrated from China in order to make a better life for his family. In May 1986, John, who was born in California, took his father home to see the village where he himself might have lived but for his father's youthful courage. The village had not changed in a thousand years. When I ate dinner with the two of them one night, I caught John looking at his father with wonder. There was a tear in the corner of his eye and I realized that whatever he did in his life was going to be for both of them. For the time being at least, this would involve FK 506.

» «

The fact that FK 506 could rescue grafts that were being rejected despite all previously available therapy was known only to a handful of people at the beginning of the autumn of 1989. Two of the insiders were Henry Pierce, a science reporter for the Pittsburgh *Post-Gazette*, and an assistant managing editor, Mark Roth. Both men had closely watched the development of FK 506 from the time the drug was merely interesting and promising. Although they knew that clinical trials had begun, they had promised not to publish the information until it was reported in a medical journal.

The promise was strained when Larry Altman, a reporter from the New York *Times*, came to Pittsburgh in late September, a few days after a telephone interview about some new and controversial operative procedures involving transplantation of multiple abdominal organs. Altman originally called me because he had wind of criticism directed at these advanced surgical techniques, which we had stopped using temporarily earlier in the year. Now, he had heard that we were resuming the operations and his question was why. After all attempts to evade his telephone cross-examination had failed, I reluctantly told him that the justification was our ability to give better antirejection treatment. Altman, an academic physician as well as the science editor of his newspaper, realized that FK 506 was the real story, not the operations which initially had interested him. He spent the next two weeks in Pittsburgh where he developed a report on FK 506 which could compete in the quality of science with medical reports, aside from the fact that it was more skillfully written than most.

Altman insisted on seeing every patient and pored over the records with the meticulousness of a born researcher. He also agreed to hold off his New York *Times* account, knowing that the Pittsburgh *Post-Gazette* was doing the same. Both papers knew that a description of the first ten cases was scheduled for publication in the British journal *The Lancet* on October 28, 1989.

The voluntary news embargo was important to us because we feared that a premature news release would jeopardize our impending publication with *The Lancet*. While we held our breath, the embargo held until the late afternoon of October 18, 1989, several days before the curtain would be lifted by the advance copies of *The Lancet* routinely issued to the media. Late that afternoon, Pierce called to tell me that the *Post-Gazette* could wait no longer and that the story which they had been sitting on for six months would be broken in their evening edition. With his permission, I notified Altman in New York, who said that they would follow suit in the morning *Times* edition which was just going to press.

Chaos followed. The FK 506 reports competed with the San Francisco earthquake on the front pages of both newspapers on the morning of October 19. By the time I called London, *The Lancet*'s editor, Robin Fox, had a copy of the New York *Times* front page in his hands. I explained exactly what had happened, confirming what Fox already had heard from Larry Altman a few minutes before. *The Lancet* publication proceeded on schedule[3] and a week later, a ten-hour symposium on FK 506 was held in Barcelona at the annual meeting of the European Society of Organ Transplantation.

Overnight, FK 506 became the court of last appeal for liver recipients and for recipients of other organs in whom transplant rejection could not be controlled with conventional treatment. As the news became known, patients with failing grafts migrated to Pittsburgh from other centers. In the meanwhile, trials in Pittsburgh were started with FK 506 from the time of transplantation rather than for rescue purposes. By the end of October, experience using FK 506 as first line treatment had been acquired with liver, kidney, heart, and lung transplantation.

Those caring for all of these different kinds of organ recipients were quickly convinced that FK 506 was superior to previously available drugs. The incidence of rejection was reduced, the amount of prednisone required was lessened, and the time and expense of hospitalization were lowered. Although the side effects, including kidney damage, were similar to those caused by cyclosporine, they were not worse. The new treatment had a better margin of safety than the old one, or so it seemed to the care givers.

Would the lottery known as a randomized trial (see chapter 21) be required? The University of Pittsburgh IRB which governs the

Presbyterian University Hospital said yes and overrode the University Ethics Committee which said no. The IRBs for Children's Hospital and the VA hospitals said no. Here the patients, their families, and the surgeons could have a voice.

This would not be the end of discussions about patients' rights versus obligatory randomized trials of FK 506. Nor would these discussions be confined to transplantation. The same kinds of immune cells that cause rejection are known or thought to be responsible for many human diseases which are called autoimmune disorders. The ability of FK 506 to stop and reverse rejection of transplants when all other antirejection measures had failed was predictive of the drug's potential value for the autoimmune afflictions that can involve the skin (psoriasis, for example); liver, kidney, and heart (many leading to organ failure and the need for transplantation); eyes (causing certain kinds of blindness); endocrine system (sugar diabetes); bowel (such as ulcerative colitis and Crohn's disease); blood vessels and joints (including rheumatoid arthritis); and the nervous system (probably including multiple sclerosis).

Should an experiment on the lottery principle be imposed on each of these groups of patients, knowing that half are apt to be benefited in a randomized trial and half are not? The question quickly became urgent when six of the autoimmune diseases were shown to respond to FK 506 therapy.

Greg Burke had made clear to us the position of his FDA Division of Oncology and Pulmonary Disease. In his opinion, a lottery involving transplant or non-transplant patients must be ordered by the IRB supervising a new drug trial and the physicians conducting it, not by scientists at the FDA. If he had made a randomized trial a condition for issuance of an investigational new drug number (IND), Burke would have become the de facto instigator of a human experiment and a partner in the silent collusion of a government agency with the IRB, the investigating physicians, or both. To him, this was morally abhorrent even though he would welcome randomized trials decided on in good faith independent of the FDA.

We came to realize that not everyone at the FDA was of one mind concerning this division of responsibility and authority. At first, a randomized trial was made a condition for issuance of an IND in some of the other FDA divisions that were responsible for drug trials for autoimmune diseases. In a few of these autoimmune diseases, patients whose luck of the draw was not to receive FK 506 would be consigned without knowing it during the course of the trial to *no therapy* (placebo) or to treatment which already was known to be worthless or in some instances dangerous. The ethical dilemma delayed the exploration of the effectiveness of FK 506 in treating many important diseases such as multiple sclerosis.

» «

Even as the merits of randomized trials and protection of patients' rights were being debated, other developments in transplantation were evolving to which FK 506 contributed. However, more important than the drug was the presence of a third surgeon named Andreas Tzakis who had come to Pittsburgh in July 1983, preceding Todo and Fung by a few months. Tzakis, a Greek native who had trained in New York with the transplant pioneer, Felix Rapaport, also had developed a passion for liver transplantation, an operation he had never seen and did not understand. Because Rapaport sincerely liked Tzakis he advised him not to come to Pittsburgh and he advised me not to take him. His opinion was that Andy was too clumsy and too slow to ever perform such a difficult operation as liver transplantation. When he received my letter of rejection, Tzakis refused to accept the decision and took the next plane from New York in order to defend his candidacy face to face. I lost the battle of wills, and he began his two-year transplant fellowship on July 1, 1983. No one ever worked so hard and accomplished so little. Rapaport had been right.

More than a year later, I met with Tzakis and told him that I could never permit him to attempt a human liver transplantation. It would not be safe or justified. I apologized for allowing him to waste his time and assigned him to the kidney service where the less difficult kidney transplant operations would be within his capabilities. He thanked me, accepted the assignment, and told me that he would remain a fellow for however long was required to be qualified to perform liver transplantation—even to the extent of relearning layer by layer the basic movements and coordination of surgical technique. This is what he did. Every place he went, he carried instruments with him, fondling them and flipping them like a gunfighter practicing his draw until these pieces of steel called hemostats and scissors were like natural extensions of his hands and fingers. No string or thread was spared the indignity of being a tangled mass of surgical square knots, tied to a chair or bed post.

Now, glimpses of precious metal could be seen within the crude ore. Tzakis *could* do liver transplantation and did. One night at 4 A.M., I was awakened by an anesthesiologist who asked me to come to the operating room and order Andy Tzakis to pronounce dead a recipient whose heart had quit beating while the liver was being sewed in. Against the advice of the more senior surgeon assisting him and the anesthesiologist, Andy had refused to give up trying to restart the heart. When I arrived, I told the person who called that I would not give the order she wanted. I went upstairs to the observation dome and watched the activities below. It was a scene in pantomime because those on neither side of the glass could hear the others.

Using their hands as a makeshift pump, members of the surgical team performed heart massage and propelled the life-giving blood through the inert heart to the waiting body. Periodically, the heart was shocked and would jump, only to fall motionless once again. Finally, it shuddered like a dog awakening from a long slumber, and began to beat. The patient lived. Every Christmas since then, he has written to me, always giving the date of his transplant as the anniversary of his second life. It also was the day when Tzakis completed his training. The process had been slower than with many others but it may have been the most complete. He had become one of the best surgeons in the world.

Now Tzakis learned that reaching a cherished goal can be a cruel illusion. After he had learned to use them so well, his hands began to lose their sensation and their strength because of a condition that is a professional hazard of surgeons. He was slowly being paralyzed by a large herniated disc which pressed on the nerves to his arms and hands. He could abandon his surgical career or have the disc removed with an operation in the neck. No one was surprised at his choice. A few days after having the disc taken out, Tzakis was on a plane to Greece, a rubber ball in each hand for squeezing exercises; two months later, he was back in the Pittsburgh operating rooms.

Now, I realized that Tzakis too would take a step beyond where anyone had been before. No one in more than twenty years of trying had been able to transplant pancreatic islets in humans. These islets are the tiny bits of tissue in the pancreas which are the source of insulin, the hormone that controls blood sugar and prevents the development of diabetes. If the islets could be made to function as free pieces, it would not be necessary to transplant the entire pancreas in order to treat sugar diabetes.

Successful islet tranplantation was accomplished on January 6, 1990, at Children's Hospital. A fifteen-year-old girl with an otherwise hopelessly advanced malignant tumor of the liver that had spread to the pancreas was treated by taking out the liver, pancreas, stomach, and all of the other organs in the upper abdomen of the child, followed by liver transplantation under FK 506. While Tzakis was doing this, another team headed by Camillo Ricordi, a surgeon from Milan, and Dan Mintz, a physician from Miami, removed and purified a third of a million of the insulin-producing islets from the pancreas of the liver donor. These islets were infused into the portal vein of the newly transplanted liver. The islets distributed themselves throughout the liver, took up residence in their unnatural new location, began producing insulin, and spared the child from the development of diabetes. Antirejection therapy was with FK 506. It was the first successful pancreatic islet transplantation in history.[4]

News of this success spread rapidly by word of mouth. A report by Tzakis in *The Lancet* on this first case and subsequent successes evoked a fiery letter to the editor from a physician in Hereford, England, who commented: "I read . . . the report . . . with mounting horror. . . . I thought that this sort of mutilating surgery . . . had ceased long ago. How many more cruel and inhumane operations will be done in the name of advancement of science? . . . this practice . . . is unethical and immoral and disregards man's spirituality and ineffectually tries to deny his mortality. . . . It is time that rampant scientific endeavor was brought under some humane and ethical control. . . . Death is not a failure, it is a natural process."[5]

It is best not to answer letters like this in kind. The first child and several others in the controversial series still are alive and well. However, in our response, we pointed out that the purpose of our report was not to describe the treatment of cancer but rather "to describe islet cell transplantation. . . . The technology developed for this objective and demonstration of its efficacy have ramifications for the treatment of patients with diabetes mellitus."[6] This is what had happened. The first patient still is insulin-free twenty months later.

The port city of Piraeus had been Tzakis's childhood home. No more than one hundred yards from the seawater and the docks, his mother and father lived there in a small apartment far from the controlled comfort and splendor of the central Athens hotels where medical conferences are held to which Andy is now often invited as a distinguished guest. He always stays at the apartment where I also have been a houseguest.

The seaman's life of Mr. Tzakis had been a hard one until his retirement — often far from home and on the open seas — but his last days were content until his death in March 1990. Toward the end, he sat in the center of the modest apartment in front of his television set. He listened and watched intently on Cable Network News (CNN) for reports about the activities of his famous son who stood surrounded by reporters, five thousand miles away in Pittsburgh, calmly answering questions about his operations. To those in the apartment in Piraeus it looked as if their son was not being properly fed, or so they said. It was the ageless tactic by which parents conceal their pride.

Another mystery being dispelled was that of the transplanted intestine. Experimental bowel transplantation was first described in 1958 by Richard Lillehei, a surgeon at the University of Minnesota who died in 1981 without seeing his operation used successfully in humans.[7] In 1959 I had described a different operation in which the entire intestine was included as part of a complex transplant that also included the other principal abdominal organs — the liver, pancreas, and stomach (see chapter 7).[8] No means of preventing rejection were available then, but even after antirejection treatment was developed for other organs, progress was not made with the intestine. The bowel was unusually susceptible to rejection, which in turn led to the leakage through its damaged wall of the germs (bacteria and fungi) that normally are confined inside the intestine and contribute to the digestion of food.

Entering the surrounding tissue and the blood stream, these germs spread quickly throughout the body, causing uncontrolled total body infections. Also, lymphocytes and other immune cells normally present in the intestine were found capable of mounting a lethal counterattack on the recipient in what is called "graft versus host disease" (GVHD). Between 1967 and 1987, about a dozen attempts at intestinal transplantation were made in humans in Europe, South America, Canada, and the United States. All failed.

A three-and-a-half-year-old child named Tabatha Foster reawakened hope that the human intestine could be transplanted when on November 1, 1987, she underwent the same multivisceral transplantation developed in dogs nearly three decades before. Her medical problems began when her intestines were lost shortly after birth. Although she was kept alive by intravenous feeding, she developed liver failure, for which she was brought to Children's Hospital of Pittsburgh.

Tabatha recovered promptly from the difficult multivisceral operation. Under cyclosporine treatment, her organs were not rejected and she had no evidence of the dreaded graft versus host disease. She was able to eat for the first time in her life. It was the first demonstration that transplantation of a complete intestine from a cadaver donor might be feasible. Then, three months after the operation, at the moment of greatest hope, she developed a white blood cell cancer (lymphoma) in both the new liver and intestine.[9] When she died after six months, she was mourned worldwide. Before long, the criticisms and ethical debates began, similar to those after each of the previous steps in transplantation of the other organs.

On the morning of her death, a twenty-seven-year-old nurse named Marianne Stewart, who had cared for Tabatha, left the hospital to drive home. A few blocks away, she was killed instantly when her car ran off the road into a telephone pole. Whether her vision was blocked with eyelids closed by exhaustion or by a veil of tears will never be known.

The next day I tried to answer the questions of a crowd of news reporters whose demand for explanations about Tabatha's course and cause of death I could not satisfy. My sorrow was deepened by what they did not know and never learned—that a vital young woman had entered the shadows hand in hand with her tiny patient. I was unable to continue the interview. The picture of the nurse and child together still hangs on the wall of the ninth floor ward of Children's Hospital of Pittsburgh.

The matter was not finished. Throughout 1988, Tabatha's multivisceral operation or modifications of it were performed in Chicago (James Williams); Innsbruck, (Raimund Margreiter); Madison, Wisconsin (Munci Kalayoglu); and London, Ontario.[10] Life was prolonged in each instance but only to a maximum of nine months, except in the Canadian case. On November 23, 1988, a team from London, Ontario, led by David Grant, William Wall, and Calvin Stiller succeeded in transplanting a multivisceral graft which was pared down to the liver and intestine before its insertion. This patient has lived (and eaten) for nearly three years.[11] A second patient named Faith Ann Larson with this operation (by the same team) has survived for almost two years. I met Ms. Larson during the first week of October 1991. She gave me a prayer that she had composed during her recovery: "I never stopped believing, not really, and I never gave up hope! . . . You were there all along, even when I despaired and You have given me the courage . . . we are never alone!"

By the time I met Ms. Larson, a third patient in the Canadian series was well nine months after the same complete multivisceral operation that was used in Tabatha Foster. The intestinal barrier had been shattered, at least in those patients whose new set of bowels came with the liver of the same cadaver organ. The next step of transplanting the intestine as a single organ was not yet practical. However, beginning in 1989, it was shown by Noriko Murase, Todo, and other surgeons in the Pittsburgh laboratories that it was easier in animals to control intestinal rejection and graft versus host disease using FK 506 than with any previously used drug. Beginning in May 1990, five consecutive patients in Pittsburgh were given successful complete small intestinal transplants under FK

506. Four received new livers at the same time, as in the first two Canadian cases. The fifth had received only the intestine.

More than a year later, at the annual meeting of the American Society of Transplant Surgeons (June 1, 1991), Satoru Todo, Andreas Tzakis, and John Fung showed pictures of these five recipients, two adults and three children.[12] All five were eating—no longer slaves to the fluid pumps and intravenous feeding tubes which had kept them alive. With the Canadian and American successes, the intestine was a forbidden organ no longer. Todo, who delivered the lecture, was given a standing ovation. A person from a nondemonstrative culture, he did not know how to respond.

» «

For John Fung also, 1990 was a vintage year. In August, he won a cash prize and medal at the Transplantation Society meeting in San Francisco for his award-winning investigations of FK 506 in patients. He had no time to spend it. By year's end, he was in the uniform of his country as the Army Medical Corps braced for Desert Storm. Out of the army by June 1991, Fung sat with Tzakis in the audience while Todo talked in Chicago about successful intestinal transplantation.

Immobilized by pain, he did not yet know that his blinding headache was due to a tumor at the base of his brain. Within a few days, he would go to the operating room, but on the other end of the scalpel. It was his turn to be a patient.

26

The Day the String Broke

I also would have a turn as a patient. Just after midday on May 29, 1981, I had realized that an unseen figure was waiting for me in the shadows. The day before, I had flown to Norfolk, Virginia, to remove a liver for a child from the state of Washington named Heidi Armeijo who had biliary atresia and was extremely ill in the intensive care unit of Children's Hospital of Pittsburgh. Her swollen abdomen was crisscrossed with multiple scars from previous operations in the midst of which were two "rose buds"—the open ends of intestine that had been brought to the skin surface during these procedures. Because the liver transplant program in Pittsburgh still was recovering from its disastrous beginning, I was counseled not to attempt the case, which was seen as a predictable disaster. As it turned out, it was a triumph, but one that required twenty-four hours of continuous and intense effort in the operating room. More than ten years later, Heidi remains well.

While Shun Iwatsuki and I were closing the abdomen after completing the marathon procedure, a nurse held the telephone to my ear with a call from a surgeon named Nicholas Terezis who himself was in an operating room at St. John's Hospital in Steubenville, Ohio. I had met him in Pittsburgh at a surgical grand rounds three months earlier where I described for the audience some techniques of partial liver removal which we were using to treat liver cancer and for other purposes including liver rupture. The development of the methods had been stimulated by the referral through the years of patients for transplantation whose cancers we were able to remove short of transplantation with these improved or new operations.[1] They had been done with consistent success only in Denver and now in Pittsburgh. Terezis was standing over a patient who could be saved only with such an operation, and only if it was performed immediately. He asked me to leave my patient in Pittsburgh and come to his hospital in Steubenville.

We pled with each other. I begged him to understand that I was too exhausted to help him. He explained that his nurse was holding the phone to his ear, that he had his finger in a hole in the great vein (vena cava) at the back of the shattered liver of an eighteen-year-old boy who had been in a motorcycle accident, and that the blood bank supply of western Pennsylvania had been exhausted by the case. He said that he could have a Pittsburgh life-flight helicopter at Trees Field, an athletic playing field two blocks from Children's Hospital, in five minutes.

I wrapped fifteen or twenty of the unwashed special blood vessel instruments from the back table and left with the transplant fellow Carlos Fernandez-Bueno, arriving in a squad car at Trees Field simultaneously with the chopper; twenty minutes later it set us down fifty feet from the front entrance of St. John's Hospital. Dr. Terezis had not been exaggerating. Both his hands were in the abdomen, and like the Dutch boy at the dike, one of his fingers was inserted into the lethal hole while his free hand tried to compress the bleeding raw surface of the ruptured liver. He was pale, but looked flushed in comparison to his patient, whose skin was like white marble.

The boy was dying. There was not time even to wash the bloody instruments from Pittsburgh or to wash my hands. Within about ninety minutes, we removed the portion of the ruptured liver that overhung the hole in the vein, exposed Terezis's finger, liberated it, closed the blood vessel defect, and dried up the wound. Not only a life, but a lifetime was the reward for the patient. After a brief lunch with the Sisters, it was time to collect the instruments and return.

As the chopper flew back, I lay on the floor, peering over the side at the hills and forests of western Pennsylvania. It was the most beautiful green I had ever seen. Was it to be the last time? Something was wrong inside. There was a curious feeling in my chest, beneath the breast bone, not really painful but like something trying to eat its way out. After we landed, I went to the clinic for an electrocardiogram. It was normal. The strange presence in my chest came and went over the next nine years, eluding detection by heart tests and the examinations of consultant physicians. But I always knew that this cunning thing was waiting, ready to spring.

Finally, it identified itself on July 11, 1990, the day after my first vacation in seven years. The vacation began with ten leisurely days at the end of June which we spent in Kauai, one of the smaller and less densely populated of the Hawaiian Islands. Because Joy was with me, it was disappointing to be so tired. I yearned for the night and sleeping to the tune of breakers just outside the window. I dreamed of floating away on a flower-filled barge.

After Kauai we flew to Japan, hotbed of industry and high technology where social and legal inertia had frozen the conditions of organ donation into the mold that the Western world had shattered two decades before. Brain death was not accepted, and public debate over what defined this condition remained at the same level as when I visited Japan for the first time in 1968. Consequently, there were still no cadaver donors. In the meanwhile, an army of incredibly talented Japanese surgeons waited in all the major cities for the signal that would allow a network of cadaver organ transplantation to materialize overnight from one end of their country to the other. After my lectures in Osaka and Tokyo, I felt too weak to have a discussion period. We flew home immediately.

This strange fatigue had reached the peaceful lassitude where help is neither sought nor accepted. I didn't mention it to Joy, but it was as if the central string to a puppet had frayed to a single strand and stretched. Early the first morning back in Pittsburgh, I drove to my office over the Pizza Hut on Fifth Avenue where, halfway between the first and second floors, the string broke. The slightest movement caused a cylinder of fire beneath my breast bone that erupted like a volcano into my neck. Crawling up the stairs inch by inch to the second floor landing, I lay there sweating and panting for an hour, before trying the next flight.

My office is on the third floor of this ancient building where the faint smell of pizza sauce substitutes for the odor of cedar or other wood that normally gives character to such old structures. After creeping to the office, my resting place for the next hour was a rug on the floor. I could look up and see three weeks of correspondence neatly organized in stacks by my secretary. Nearby were two dictating machines. The sight was energizing.

Finally reaching a sitting position and immobile as a statue except for my arms, I worked through the piles of mail for twelve hours, answering and disposing of everything in front of me. It was Saturday, and no one came throughout the day or evening. At midnight, I was able to walk down the steps and drive the six blocks back to our house. Stair steps had to be climbed and then there was fitful sleep in the familiar bed.

When morning came, I drove to the emergency room and arranged for an electrocardiogram to measure the electrical activity of the heart and for some chemical tests that can detect heart damage. Both were normal. By the time the cardiologist, Bruce Wilson, arrived, Andy Tzakis and I had left the emergency room and were on the way to our cars, convinced that the episodes of chest pain had been indigestion. Wilson was irate and explained that these were classic symptoms of angina pectoris. We agreed to a compromise. We would walk together down the steep two-block hill to a milk shake parlor, and if I could make it back, I could go home.

It was easy to walk down, but when we started back, I could go only a few feet before the suffocating pain returned. Tzakis, circling close by in his car, picked us up and raced back to the hospital, defying the reverse traffic of the one-way street. A few minutes later, I was rolled on a stretcher into the cardiac catheterization suite of the operating room.

Anxious faces surrounded the cart. Someone mentioned that my blood pressure was 60. It was much too low, but I noted the observation with impersonal interest rather than alarm. White-faced, an old friend, Father Logue, arrived and offered to give me last rites, which I declined. I had not been a practicing Catholic since my mother died. If there was to be a judgment day, it would have to be on the whole record, not the last moment of it.

When a tube (a cardiac catheter) was inserted from a leg artery and advanced upward through the main blood vessel (aorta) toward the heart, I could watch its tip in my chest on the X-ray screen. It looked like a snake's head probing for the origin of the main heart arteries. Into these, it discharged its benign brand of venom, a dye that allowed the structure of the vessels to be seen down to the last detail. I felt no pain. Lying on my back with the screen overhead, I watched the movement of the catheter with the detachment of a third-party observer while Wilson explained the maneuvers as he might have done for a student.

A surgical team crept unnoticed into a corner of the room, hooded and cloaked like monks or Ninja warriors. Their anonymity was betrayed when one of them spoke. It was John Armitage, the thoracic surgeon who was in charge of the trials with FK 506 for heart transplantation. If my heart stopped beating, the operating room was a few feet away where my chest could be opened.

As soon as the catheter tip found the opening of the two arteries supplying the heart and dye was injected, the diagnosis was made. The right main heart artery had a tight waist near its origin, so extreme that it was more than 99 percent closed off. Through the tiny pinhole that remained, a jet stream passed to its intended destination in the heart muscles. Beyond the nearly complete blockage, the main heart vessel returned to normal. However, it was starved for blood and looked like a tree trunk that had been divested of its branches and leaves by a wind storm. The other (left) main heart artery was open but it was very small. This was single-vessel coronary artery disease, so limited that no symptoms would have been caused if the rest of the blood vessel anatomy of the heart was normal. The problem was that it was not. The involved right coronary artery carried almost all the heart's blood supply.

The objective now was to open up the waist by dilating it with an inflatable balloon at the catheter tip (balloon angioplasty). When the tip was pushed through the pinhole, the blockage was made complete. The chest fire was reignited, and far worse than it ever had been before. In a reflex, my arms and legs came up in a furious effort to resist. When I woke up, I was in a different place. It was the intensive care unit. The first thing I realized was that Joy's hand was in mine. The second was that the exhaustion of the previous weeks was gone. I wanted to go home.

It would have been a grand success if this could have been the end of it. Before long, Wilson came to the bedside and explained that the diseased artery had been opened by the procedure, restoring the heart's blood supply. However, the offending plug in the vessel had cracked as it was stretched open, creating two blood channels, one inside the other and separated by a circular shell. In medical terms, this was called a "dissecting aneurysm." The practical implication was that the vessel might close off again.

The following day, I went to work. It was easy to climb the stairs to the third floor of the Pizza Hut. When I opened the office door, I saw that my radio and CD player had been stolen. News of my illness had traveled fast.

» «

My three days in the hospital gave me an unplanned chance to see a serious disease from the inside instead of through the minds and words of others. Throughout it all, the possibility of death was an interesting statistic but not a cause for fear. Calculating the odds as for a baseball game, I was a spectator in the stands, while down below I also came to bat. In this team exercise of skill and chance, Wilson devised a strategy that I admired from afar and also was involved in as a player on the field. The player half and the spectator half wanted me to be cleanly out or to make it home. Neither half could accept a disabling injury on the base paths. I would rather lose. As it turned out, the great scorekeeper awarded my time at bat with a standing triple. But when the inning ended, I was stranded on third base. The dramatic restoration of energy that followed the emergency dilation of the heart artery was only temporary.

When the original symptoms began to recur about two weeks later, it was obvious that the double channel left by the first procedure was closing off. An open chest operation would be necessary, and preferably soon. It would have been hard to find a worse time to have a health problem. In five weeks, on August 21–24, the biennial meeting of the Transplantation Society was scheduled in San Francisco. I was the incoming president.

The congress was special in another way. This was the first international meeting at which our experience with FK 506 for human organ transplantation and other purposes was to be presented. Nearly forty lectures or displays from the University of Pittsburgh were on the scientific program, and the majority concerned this new drug, including the first reports on intestinal and pancreas islet transplantation. The manuscripts I had to write or supervise had not been prepared, and a heart operation would make this impossible.

The first week of August 1990 now had come and gone. If I underwent a coronary artery bypass now, it was doubtful if I would be able to go to the meeting at all, much less prepare for it. After discussing the risk of delay with Wilson, the Pittsburgh heart surgeons, and Michael DeBakey of Houston, I decided to go to San Francisco first and to undergo the coronary bypass operation the day after the convention.

If this was to be a calculated risk, why not in San Francisco, the city that gave dreams substance? This was where in 1960 I had decided to chance everything by abandoning a conventional career in surgery and by changing universities to pursue the mirage of transplantation. It was where I returned seven years later to debate the ethics of the new field of organ replacement and to announce that our program of human liver transplantation, which had failed earlier, was soon to be reopened. In those earlier days, I could climb mountains. This time, I knew that I would have trouble walking to the stage. I told Joy not to come. Any extra effort caused by a temptation to go to the society's social functions would be disastrous.

I moved through the five days in San Francisco in a state resembling suspended animation. The center of my world was a large room on the twenty-fourth floor of the Fairmont Hotel to which Bob Starzel, my Uncle Frank's son, who was practicing law in San Francisco, anxiously came each day. Every excursion to a conference hall was planned for economy of movement. On the last afternoon, Roy Calne, immersed by now in his avocation as an artist, asked me to sit for him in a quiet garden court of the majestic cathedral at the top of Nob Hill. The next time I saw his painting it was in an exhibition of his art in England. His gifts with the brush and palette had captured in the portrait an air of hopelessness.

At midnight of the fifth day, after discharging my duties as president, I took the nonstop flight back to Pittsburgh for the coronary artery bypass the next day. The operation, by Gary Marrone and Scott Stuart, was performed without a blood transfusion while a heart-lung machine provided for my circulation and breathing. I left Presbyterian University Hospital three days later and returned to work four days after that.

» «

The same illness from which I had just recovered would have led to invalidism or possibly death twenty years earlier—and still does even today in medically underserved communities. Fortune had placed me in a time and place where my care was not even challenging. Yet it was hard to forget that the quality of all the rest of my life, and presumably much of its duration, would be a gift. My life curve was altered by tertiary care.

I was not alone. Of the four surgeons who began the FK 506 trials together, only Todo remained intact throughout. In another time and place, Andy Tzakis's dreams would have turned to ashes as paralysis set in. When I was a medical student, John Fung's pituitary gland tumor would have required an operation so dangerous and mutilating that it probably would not have been advised at all. Yet after a surgical procedure at Presbyterian University Hospital in 1991 carried out by the same neurosurgeon who operated on Tzakis, Fung left the hospital in four days and returned to work in a week.

All three of us had become part of a new population. It is one that could be a liability if made up predominantly of wretched and diminished people whose fundamental purpose is survival—avoidance of the last great experience of dying. In that case, the human product of man's ingenuity would be an expensive collection of the leaves described by Governor Lamm whose obstinate refusal to let go could strangle and prevent the new harvest. On the other hand, the salvaged group of people could be an asset to humanity by its collective wisdom and experience. Who could deny that crossing over and coming back imparts an understanding or imbues a quality that was not there before, or lay dormant? Whether this intervention is justified or wise was the fundamental question asked by Governor Lamm (see chapter 24). Every transplant patient is an example. I was not their brother but now I would claim to be their cousin.

It was all so safe. My gratitude was boundless to the cardiologist Wilson and the surgeons Marrone and Stuart for their competence. But the debt was deeper by far. It went back to those surgeons who first thought of salvaging hearts by restoring their blood supply. What sacrifices did they make and what opposition did they face? This is the fabric of recorded history—accessible to scholars. But who were the patients who endured the coronary artery operations when they were not yet perfected? Ultimately, they were the ones who made my operation safe. It seemed shameful not to know their names.

It was the same in transplantation. All triumphs in medicine are the forgotten sorrows of past days. Mourning of the losses was what drove progress more by far than the vain exaltation of success. Success came later.

27

The Little Drummer Girls

Stormie Jones lost her anonymity and gained her life when she received a combined liver-heart transplantation on St. Valentine's Day (February 14), 1984. Movie starlets might have envied her creative name and a smile that once seen was never forgotten. Notwithstanding these advantages, she had become a prisoner of intensive care units just after her sixth birthday because of a fast-forward version of a kind of heart disease usually reserved for older people.

Stormie had been brought to the precipice by an inherited disorder of cholesterol metabolism which kills before or during the teenage years. What it is that snuffs out small and vulnerable girls was held at bay with Stormie's heart-liver transplantation. Then, study of her case proved how the human liver regulates cholesterol, a fat in the blood stream that can plug the arteries supplying the heart and cause heart attacks in patients of all ages.

Although hers was the first heart-liver transplantation, it was by no means the first example of multiple organ transplantation, which usually included the kidney or liver. These complex operations went beyond the previously conceived technical limitations of surgery, but they usually failed primarily because of the inability to safely control rejection. When the more powerful antirejection treatment based on cyclosporine became available, multiple organ transplantation was reassessed. In the new era that began in 1980, long survival of multiple organ recipients became the rule.

» «

Stormie Jones became a puzzle child from a base of information and experience laid down long before. It was known that certain proteins and other products secreted by the liver varied from person to person and could be identified by laboratory tests that determined their chemical "fingerprints." In the 1960s, it was demonstrated in recipients that such substances produced by the liver promptly became those of the original donor after liver replacement. Ken Porter, the London pathologist, showed why by studying the transplanted livers of patients whose donors had been of the opposite sex. Because cells have sex markers, he was able to see under the microscope whether any given cell in the new liver was female or male.

Porter's findings were astonishing. The specialized liver cells that are responsible for the complicated function of this organ retained their original sex. However, in less than one hundred days, other cells (Kuppfer cells and macrophages), past which recipient blood flows to nourish the aristocratic liver cells, changed sex to that of the recipient. It was as if the rich vegetation in a cultivated farm permanently maintained its special character while the walls lining the terminal irrigation ditches changed to that of the fluid and debris flowing through them.

These discoveries had major implications for the potential treatment of numerous diseases called "inherited inborn errors of metabolism" in which the patient begins life with faulty chemistry. If the fundamental defect was exclusively or primarily in the liver, as often is the case, it was conceptually possible to correct the problem by replacing the liver—with assurance that the correction would be permanent.

Attacking the problem from a different perspective, the biochemists had started a revolution that gave focus to such dreams. Beginning in 1956, they had probed for missing or malfunctioning gears in the total chemical machinery of patients suspected of having these inherited disorders. In the blood and tissues of such patients they examined the proteins, fats, carbohydrates, and minerals—looking for structural abnormalities and especially for the presence or absence of the small proteins (enzymes) that regulate the production or elimination of the end products. This line of research created a framework within which it could be predicted if a faulty liver was responsible for a number of previously mysterious disorders.

Armed with information from these dual lines of inquiry, more than a half dozen such inborn errors were "cured" metabolically between 1969 and 1983 by liver transplantation in Denver and Pittsburgh. Since then, the list has grown to nearly two dozen.[1] In about half the diseases found by actual trial to be correctable with a new liver, success was almost certain because the chemistry of the inborn error was so well understood and so clearly caused by a missing liver enzyme. In the other half, the expectation of benefit was from circumstantial evidence, and the transplantation itself became the means by which the liver's role in the disease was verified or clarified. The high blood cholesterol from which Stormie Jones suffered was an example of the latter, and because of this she became an instrument of discovery.

» «

Where blood cholesterol came from and what regulated it were questions viewed from different vantage points by the Pittsburgh and Dallas groups that eventually joined for the treatment of Stormie Jones. The interest of the University of Colorado surgeons (who later moved to Pittsburgh) was initially aroused by an incidental observation in dogs, and later in patients, with a different inborn error called "glycogen storage disease." In both the animal experiments and in the human, the blood cholesterol was sharply reduced when the portal venous blood that normally nourishes the liver was rerouted around it by the operation known as portacaval shunt, portal diversion, or Eck's fistula (see chapters 5 and 17).

The finding seemed immediately applicable to the care of a twelve-year-old girl named Jody Plute who was admitted to the Colorado General Hospital in the autumn of 1972. Her diagnosis was *familial hypercholesterolemia*, the same lethal metabolic disease as would be faced by the yet unborn Stormie Jones, and with very similar consequences. The high blood cholesterol was layering out on her heart valves and in her arteries, including those supplying her heart muscle. She grew steadily worse, and after having a serious heart attack in early February 1973 she was transferred to the intensive care unit for the treatment of heart failure.

The same kind of cholesterol deposits that were plugging her blood vessels could be seen easily in the bulging sacks covered with reddish skin beneath her eyes. Similar lumps protruded from her elbows, buttocks, and the back and front of her knees. Even larger ones dangled from her heels. She had scars where an unwise surgeon had attempted to whittle these away.

In spite of these cosmetic deformities, she was a beautiful girl. Although she knew that she was nearing death, her manner was cheerful and philosophic. She was an honor student at a junior high school in Golden, Colorado, and her only expressed regret was that there would be a vacant seat when her class graduated. She had been promised this remembrance.

I cannot remember being more determined to help someone, because I was convinced by now that the portal diversion procedure would reduce her blood cholesterol and possibly even allow absorption of the widespread cholesterol deposits in her blood vessels and tissues. When I recommended that the portal operation be carried out, the opinion precipitated a crisis conference with the pediatric staff. Their resistance persisted, even at the eleventh hour when it appeared that the opportunity to intervene was being lost to procrastination. If the matter had been handled by consensus, only two votes would have been cast to go forward.

Fortunately, the other yes ballot would have come from Jody's doctor, a very able pediatrician named Peter Chase. He had seen her deteriorate in spite of the most stringent dietary restrictions imaginable and the closely supervised administration of all the drugs known to lower cholesterol. Chase agreed, and so did the patient and her mother. The operation was performed without incident on the morning of March 1, 1973.

Afterward, we were scarcely able to believe what was happening. The tense and unsightly red excrescences, which also were found between the bases of and on the knuckles of her fingers, looked smaller and lighter in color. The resorption of the tissue cholesterol was understandable because the cholesterol in the blood, which had been five times the normal level, was reduced by more than half. The masses were slowly melting back into the blood stream where the cholesterol belonged. It took more than a year for all traces of the larger ones to disappear.

Now, our hope was that the cholesterol incrustations inside the arteries and on the heart valves were disappearing too. There was evidence for this. Heart pain (angina pectoris), which had been continuous before the operation, disappeared. After two weeks Jody Plute returned to school to a heroine's welcome.

In reporting the case in *The Lancet*, our explanation of the astonishing effect was simple.[2] We believed that cholesterol production had been reduced to a crawl by depriving the liver of the portal blood that had special qualities (particularly a high insulin content) necessary for normal liver function. This was the essence of the so-called hepatotrophic concept which for other reasons was under intense study in our research laboratory at the time, and ultimately accepted universally (see chapter 17). By means of this operation we had created a subtle kind of liver disease that inhibited the manufacture of many substances, not just cholesterol. The significant consequences of portal diversion varied in different species. In the dog and baboon they were lethal (including brain injury); in rats and humans the effects were much milder. Thus, the penalty of portal diversion for this disease was acceptable in humans because of the gain achieved by lowering the blood cholesterol. However, this information, including the species difference, was known in 1973 only to us and contradicted prevailing dogma.

In addition, the hepatotrophic hypothesis that explained the liver changes was heretical at the time and would continue to be for several more years. Finally, acceptance of our explanation would involve a derivative heresy. If we were correct in the hepatotrophic hypothesis, the corollary was that the liver was central to regulation of body cholesterol. This also proved to be true, but it remained a contentious issue until the next decade.

The divergence of our views from those held by most leading liver and cholesterol experts of that era was unnerving. On August 1–2, 1974, a special task force was convened at the Center for Lipid Research of the National Institutes of Health in Bethesda, Maryland, to discuss our use of the portal diversion operation for hypercholesterolemia, and especially why it seemed to work. Robert I.

Levy, director of the center, was particularly interested in the disease. Five years earlier, he had shown that the body's failure to eliminate cholesterol rather than its overproduction was the principal explanation for its accumulation.

I gave a poor account of myself. The language of those with detailed knowledge of the cholesterol field was so specialized that I had difficulty understanding their conversation, much less comment on it. The meeting was summarized by Bob Levy in a November 1974 issue of *The Lancet* with the announcement of an international registry of patients treated with portal diversion, sponsored by the National Heart and Lung Institute of the National Institutes of Health and run by Dr. Sheila Mitchell.

Although my explanation for the cholesterol lowering caused by portacaval shunt was rejected, there was no need to give ground. In dog experiments, we already had shown an 80 percent reduction in liver cholesterol production after this operation.[3] Because these were normal animals, it seemed obvious that the liver was the ruler of cholesterol in healthy subjects as well as in those with hypercholesterolemia. David Bilheimer of Dallas subsequently published studies from one of his patients named Mary Cheatham on whom I performed a portal diversion procedure in October 1974. Accompanying the patient was a young scientist named Michael Brown who came to the operating room in Denver and collected samples. Their findings of reduced cholesterol production after the portal diversion in the patient were similar in principle to those in our dog experiments.[4]

By this time, I listed familial hypercholesterolemia as one of the potential indications for liver transplantation. Its inclusion came to be criticized bitterly because of a discovery by Mike Brown and Joseph Goldstein of Dallas in 1974, the first of a series of scholarly contributions leading to the Nobel prize in 1985.[5] At the time and for several years afterward, the interpretation of their results pointed away from the liver instead of to it, thus undermining my advocacy of liver transplantation for this disease. They demonstrated a fundamental defect in *all* cells of patients like Jody Plute (and Stormie Jones). There was a deficiency of attachment sites to which circulating cholesterol-rich particles are bound in the process of normal cholesterol elimination. Even with a normal rate of cholesterol production it would inexorably accumulate because there was no means of disposal. Like cars in a junk yard, the cholesterol stacked up in the tissues and arteries.

It was hard to see how liver transplantation could correct the problem when the binding site defect was everywhere. The answer came later in a series of reports from Brown and Goldstein and workers elsewhere between 1977 and 1981. They showed that a high proportion of the binding of cholesterol-complex occurred in the liver, which became again a candidate to be kingpin of cholesterol metabolism.

Interest in liver transplantation to treat familial hypercholesterolemia promptly revived, this time with the support of the cholesterol establishment. Three of its key members had referred and collaborated in the care of two or more patients treated in Denver with portal diversion. One was Bilheimer (with Goldstein and Brown) in Dallas. Another was Ernest Schaefer, Levy's successor as director of the Center for Lipid Research. The third was E. J. (Pete) Ahrens of Rockefeller University in New York City. I proposed liver transplantation to all three.

Before going farther with such a drastic step, it was crucial to make a final assessment of what could and could not be expected with the safer portal diversion operation. By the end of 1981, I had treated twelve patients with this operation during the preceding eight and a half years and knew of twenty-six additional cases reported from other centers with similar results. All our patients had a 20 to 55 percent decrease in blood cholesterol, but to a level that still was far too high. Nine of the twelve were alive, and most seemingly were well. However, the three losses were from heart attacks, and all the survivors had heart disease which either failed to regress after early improvement or was slowly worsening. The heart remained the limiting factor. In the race against time fueled by the high cholesterol, the portal diversion only slowed the clock.

Our princess, Jody Plute, was one of the missing three. Sixteen months after her operation, when all the skin lesions were gone, her heart was restudied by inserting catheters into it and injecting dye (as would be done to me sixteen years later). The valve in the main outflow vessel of the heart had improved markedly, but there remained three tightly constricting waists in the principal arteries supplying the heart muscle itself. After deluding ourselves that these might regress with the lowered blood cholesterol, like the skin and heart valve deposits, a fatal mistake was made by deciding against a coronary artery bypass operation.

Two and a half months later, as she was skipping down the street in Golden on the way home from school, she dropped dead. When I came to the morgue to see her, I stopped at the door—gagging at the thought of what was inside. She lay on her back on the white table, with her long hair spread out like a black star imprinted on the snow beneath. The room felt colder than I ever remembered before. Her sightless eyes stared at the checkered ceiling. I prayed that she had died so fast that she was never afraid. This disease was worth hating.

» «

In early 1982 after the move to Pittsburgh, we finished a manuscript describing our twelve patients as well as the world experience with portal diversion. Its review and rejection by the *New England Journal of Medicine* and *The Lancet* caused a delay in publication for more than a year. Eventually, the work was presented to the American Surgical Association in May 1983 and published in the *Annals of Surgery* the following September. In the final paragraph of the discussion, we recommended liver transplantation for definitive therapy. Ernie Schaefer, Pete Ahrens, and Dave Bilheimer were among the co-authors.[6]

Of the three, Pete Ahrens was the most determined to move forward with transplantation. With his concurrence, I approached the Institutional Review Board of Children's Hospital about establishing a collaboration with Rockefeller University where it was proposed to study a French boy named Florent Vinay in the metabolic unit before and after liver transplantation, which would be carried out in Pittsburgh.

Six years previously, in August 1975, I had performed a portal diversion operation on Florent, who was eight years old at the time and almost too handsome to be a boy. As if atoning for poor chemical workmanship, nature seemed to endow these children with an ethereal beauty that shone through the yellow or red lumps in the skin. In the mind's eye, the children were luminescent because we knew so well what was going on inside. By X-ray studies, it was learned that the outflow valve of Florent's heart was nearly closed down and that a huge sausage-shaped mass of cholesterol occupied most of the large vessel (thoracic aorta) that carries blood to the entire body.

During the six years since Florent's portal operation, these findings stayed much the same, but the heart chambers had begun to dilate when the family visited Pittsburgh in 1981. I spoke to them about liver transplantation and sent both parents to Ahrens. In turn, Ahrens drafted a formal proposal to the boy's mother and to professors Jean Rey and Jacques Schmitz, the physicians at the Université René Descartes in Paris who were caring for Florent. A letter dated December 30, 1982, was particularly elaborate and humane and included provision for uninterrupted education by special tutors during Florent's confinement.

It was a very difficult decision for the family. Because the deposits of cholesterol in the skin had long since disappeared, Florent did not have a mark on him. He was an immensely popular teenager now. He had learned to ski and was jogging and playing soccer. After months of thought, the plan was turned down. Seven years later, in 1988, I was saddened to learn from his mother that Florent had died suddenly while dancing.

Because the mother expressed guilt in her letter about what might have been, I wrote back: "Even though Florent died, you were able to enjoy his company and share his life with him for another 13 years after 1975. If you had gone forward with the liver transplantation in 1982, we might have lost that opportunity since there was a risk associated with this option. Thus, I think that your decision at the time when it was made was a correct one. I once saw an inscription in a book, written by one grieving parent to another, which I hope might give you some comfort. It read, 'In memory of your son and mine who by the wisdom of God will remain young throughout eternity.' Please write me again some day and tell me how things are going for you."

A second candidate, a sixteen-year-old patient of Ernie Schaefer's and Jeff Hoeg's at the National Institutes of Health, came close to a combined heart-liver transplantation thirty months after undergoing a portal diversion procedure in Denver. The boy arrived in Pittsburgh in heart failure in December 1981 and was found dead in his hospital bed one day later. The autopsy revealed a large blister from one of the heart chambers such as one sees in a blown-out tire.

There was a different kind of communication with Mike Brown in Dallas. In Kyoto, a Japanese scientist named Yoshio Watanabe had been able to breed a rabbit strain which, insofar as could be determined, had exactly the same disease as humans with familial hypercholesterolemia. A few of these animals, all males, had been sent to the United States, where they were as precious as gold. I contacted workers at Rockefeller University and the National Institutes of Health about collaborating in liver transplantation experiments, but they did not have a continuous or reliable supply of animals. Mike Brown, who contacted me about the same kind of research, had also obtained some Watanabe rabbits and had established his own breeding colony. In Pittsburgh, the surgeon Munci Kalayoglu was assigned two tasks: first, to perfect the operation in healthy rabbits, and second, to apply the procedure to the frail Watanabe variety.

In spite of his great skill and a time investment of nearly a year, Kalayoglu was not able to succeed with the first step. When he completed his two-year fellowship in July 1983, the project was discontinued. Although we had been thwarted, the experiment no longer seemed essential. With the evidence we now had, the question was not if liver transplantation should be done if it was needed, but why the trial had been delayed so long.

As so often happens, patient need forced our hand. In November 1983 I heard the name Stormie Jones for the first time when Dave Bilheimer telephoned me from Dallas, described her case, and asked me to accept her for an emergency portal diversion operation. In September and October, Stormie had undergone exhaustive metabolic examinations which established the diagnosis of hypercholesterolemia. These studies were of the highest sophistication in preparation for the testing of an experimental cholesterol-lowering drug. During their performance, Stormie's heart function rapidly deteriorated, necessitating two double coronary artery bypass operations in quick succession and replacement of one of her heart valves. She remained in heart failure in the intensive care unit of a Fort Worth hospital.

By coincidence, I was scheduled to address the Dallas County Medical Society a few days later (November 22) at the invitation of John Fordtran, with whom I sat at the head table. Bilheimer joined us from the crowd and gave further details about his patient. When he was finished, I told him that we were discussing the wrong operation and that we should consider liver transplantation instead of portal diversion. I also pointed out that as in Schaefer's earlier case, we should plan to replace her heart, which had been irreparably damaged. Bilheimer's first reaction was amazement, but he expressed interest and promised to discuss the proposal with his colleagues and with the child's mother. Eventually, all parties agreed. By the Christmas season, Stormie had recovered from her chest operations enough to be transferred to Pittsburgh.

» «

In Pittsburgh, an army quickly gathered of surgeons, pediatricians, nurses, social workers, and others with a direct or peripheral role in Stormie's care. Outnumbering all the others were kibitzers, well-wishers, and spectators. We attempted a blackout, but this was futile because the Dallas media were aware of the case and watched every development closely.

Like so many others with this disease who had preceded her, Stormie was utterly fearless. Transferring from one intensive care unit to another two-thousand miles away was a high adventure. For us, there was an air of urgency. I had seen one too many sudden deaths to be beguiled by appearances. Those who did not understand familial hypercholesterolemia asked why we were planning such draconian treatment for this child with the honey-colored hair and sweet disposition. At a distance, she seemed more physically perfect than the idealized dolls she cradled in her arms. A debate raged within the Children's Hospital IRB about the rationale for transplanting the two organs and the odds that the liver would rectify the cholesterol problem.

After seven weeks of waiting, a donor was found in Buffalo, New York. Robert Hardesty, a heart surgeon, and I brought the organs back. The heart portion of Stormie's transplantation was performed by the oldest member of the team, Hank Bahnson, who at sixty-three was nearing retirement. The liver was sewed in by Bud Shaw with the aid of Shun Iwatsuki, the unflappable and enormously experienced Japanese-American surgeon who had come with me from Colorado three years before. Thirty-three years old, Shaw was just beginning his career and had been on the university faculty for less than eight months, but before that, he had participated as a fellow in almost every case of liver transplantation from 1981 forward. The operation was perfect.

The media attention was beyond description. At times, the atmosphere resembled a war theater with its hordes of correspondents. When the gunsmoke lifted, the little drummer girl whose life or death was the heart of the story miraculously stood unscathed in the middle of the battlefield. Oblivious to the scientific strategy and the stakes involved, she was surrounded by an aura in which many would bask. No matter how cynical a reporter might be, there was no way to distort the innocence which was her armor. Little did she realize that she would never leave this battlefield or escape the attention of those who fed vicariously on the triumphs and sorrows of her life. She had become one of the most celebrated children in the world.

Within one day of the operation, her blood cholesterol fell from 1000 to 300, drifting down to the 200–250 range by the time she left Pittsburgh four weeks later. This was only slightly above normal for her age. A report of the outcome was sent to *The Lancet*, drawing attention to the pathfinding role of Jody Plute which had been recorded eleven years earlier in the same journal. The authors were from Pittsburgh except for Dave Bilheimer.[7]

Because of the exhaustive earlier investigations of Stormie obtained in Dallas for the drug trial, it also was possible to say exactly how the transplanted liver had made the cholesterol correction. After she returned to Texas, these baseline studies were repeated by Bilheimer. The results were as predicted during the soul-searching that had preceded the operation and confirmed the view of the body's cholesterol world painstakingly constructed by the experiments of Brown and Goldstein. The manuscript from Texas had

Dallas authors except for me. It was accepted by the *New England Journal of Medicine*[8] but with a faintly disapproving comment in the editor's letter to Bilheimer that the earlier *Lancet* report had "taken the bloom off the rose."

These two reports actually were reinforcing. After years of wandering, the Pittsburgh and Dallas workers had arrived at the same destination by different routes. Following the original Jody Plute report, Pete Ahrens had written a survey of the cholesterol field in *The Lancet* of August 1974 entitled "Homozygous [familial] Hypercholesterolemia and the Portacaval Shunt: The Need for a Concerted Attack by Surgeons and Clinical Researchers."[9] This is exactly what had happened.

Vindication was a commonly used word at Children's Hospital in Pittsburgh, and undoubtedly in Texas also. But what of Stormie's dreams? The life of the small town child whose favorite sport before her illness was climbing trees would not be the same again. There were visits to the doctors in Dallas, tests to be endured, medicines to be taken, and precautions to be observed. The thrill of being a celebrity wore off quickly as she learned the price of fame.

When she came back to Pittsburgh, which was not often, the television crews and reporters would be waiting at the gate for her and her mother, Suzie. She knew that what she said would be quoted; therefore, she learned to say nothing. Some complained that she had changed, but when talking to her privately, this was not true. She grew normally until she almost was a woman. What changed was the size of the jeans and sweat shirts that made up her uniform. Always, at least one lace of her tennis shoes was loose, and usually both.

In keeping with her celebrity status, the demands on her mounted. Usually, these involved fund-raising for research. She did what was asked, but it was not easy for her and her mother to be part of history on special occasions and to worry about next month's rent the rest of the time.

In October 1987, Stormie uneventfully went through a small operation to correct a partial block of the channel (bile duct) draining the transplanted liver. After this, she did well until late 1989 when the liver showed signs of failing. A small piece of it examined under the microscope showed hepatitis. Although it could not be proved, we suspected that she had been infected by a virus in one of the blood transfusions given at the time of the transplantation nearly six years earlier. Her main antirejection drug was changed from cyclosporine to FK 506. Her condition improved, but this was temporary. On February 20, 1990, she underwent a second liver transplantation in Pittsburgh, performed by Andy Tzakis.

She left the hospital after four weeks, but soon it was discovered that the virus had infected the second liver transplant. The damage was occurring far more quickly than the first time. She was back on the tight rope. An antiviral drug called interferon was begun, and to allow it to be effective, the amount of antirejection treatment was slowly reduced. The liver was watched closely for signs of rejection, which under the FK 506 treatment did not occur. She was able to return to Texas. During my own hospitalization in the summer and early autumn, Stormie's medical reports were satisfactory, but I knew that the odds for the long future were against her.

» «

In the first week of November 1990, nine weeks after undergoing my coronary artery bypass, I began a journey halfway around the world which would have been unthinkable except that it was to honor two old friends whom I considered to be great men. The first leg was three thousand miles west to Los Angeles. Paul Terasaki, the father of clinical tissue matching, was host of a meeting that reunited pioneers in his field, many of whom reflected on their achievements. Although an outsider, I also was invited, and I reminisced about how Paul's courage and integrity twenty years earlier had shaped his specialty (see chapter 11).

The next day, I flew from Los Angeles to Athens to contribute to a conference honoring Sir Roy Calne and to attend the ceremony awarding him an honorary doctorate from the University of Athens. It was my first excursion from Pittsburgh since my heart operation. Andy Tzakis, also attending the meeting, met me at the Athens airport. He would accompany me home.

On the way back via Paris, we made an unplanned detour to Nice to visit Jacques Poisson, the man who had kept for twenty-seven years the memorandums written by Will Goodwin about the surprise visit to Colorado on the night of the first technically successful liver transplantation (see chapter 9). We registered at a motel and spent the next two days studying the documents. No one knew where we were until Tzakis notified his office. Five minutes later, the phone rang in my room. My wife, Joy, was at the other end, sobbing with the news that Stormie had died, a few hours after being rushed to Pittsburgh from Dallas with the diagnosis of "flu." Because Joy could not speak easily, the conversation was mostly silence.

I was glad that there was a good friend in the next room. When I told Andy, he asked what had caused her death. My answer was, "I think we forgot the heart," hoping that it was not true. When we arrived in Pittsburgh, we learned that my suspicion was correct. At her autopsy, the liver was damaged by hepatitis but it contained little evidence of rejection. The heart transplant from the original donor was filled with the cells (lymphocytes) that cause rejection. Most of the findings were of recent origin. If someone had thought of this possibility, she might have been treated and potentially saved with high doses of steroid drugs, even during the desperate last hours of her life. The knowledge was more cruel than a stake through the heart.

» «

I never operated again. I had planned to stop performing surgery at the end of the year, and it was a comfort to know that the surgeons whom I had trained were more capable than I was, or perhaps had ever been. It would be important to make them believe this.

The winter came and when it had passed, I reached the age of sixty-five. It was a landmark that no responsible bookie would have predicted or bet on. Having passed the hurdle, there would be time to write this book, to truly be with Joy for the first time in the ten years of our marriage, and to think about research that might ease the way of the next generation scrambling up behind or forging ahead. What had been learned in transplantation was sure to change the practice in all of medicine, in ways that already had begun and in ways that were not yet obvious. Who could guide the ripples better than one who dropped the stone?

After ten years in Pittsburgh, I did not know where the parks were. The closest one is just beyond the campus, eight or ten blocks from my office and across a concrete bridge. By then turning left, the bottom of a huge grassy amphitheater is reached, lined with trees on each side and capped at the top by a small forest. During the day, students and lovers stroll there, but late at night, the park is deserted. It is the favorite place of our two dogs, who race up and down the green hillside in a frenzy of delight.

Late one day, ten months after leaving Nice, I went there just before sunset. Far up the slope, half hidden in shadows, were two young girls, one with honey-colored hair, clad in jeans and a sweat shirt. She wore tennis shoes, and as she walked the laces trailed behind. The other had dark hair to her shoulders. She was dressed in pleated slacks and an impeccably pressed blouse that seemed slightly out of style in the casual teenage world of 1991. I guessed their age as thirteen years.

The girls moved aimlessly to and fro, slowly advancing from the trees toward the slope, laughing, reaching out to touch each other as they came, and talking with gestures as they made fine circles and designs in the air. I wondered what they could be discussing that made them so happy. They looked like Stormie Jones and Jody Plute. I had wanted so much to have these girls grow up, but God froze them in time instead. Embarrassed by my sentimental thoughts, I turned away. When the distraction had passed and I looked up again, the distant figures were gone.

There is a strange thing about the dimming vision of aging eyes. What cannot be seen clearly, the mind fills in more vividly than reality. It was almost dark. The time had come to collect the dogs and go home.

28

Afterthought

When recognition comes to young men, it nourishes them like drops of gentle rain. With the burden of memories toward the end, honors can be like hailstones. In June 1991 in New Orleans, there were more prizes, beginning with a reception Saturday night. Remnants of the past moved in from the shadows, alive and well. Messages came from the first wave of kidney recipients—who had now entered their thirtieth year—and from the happy young wife who had been four years old when she received her liver more than twenty years before in January 1970.

A Dallas contingent already was there. Behind me, I heard the soft drawl of John Fordtran, the medical specialist who had been our best man when Joy and I were married in 1981. His son, Billy, who received a cadaver kidney in Denver in 1971, had returned to school after his recovery, became a pharmacist, and after that a husband.

Much later, the other two Fordtran children who had inherited the same disease also underwent kidney transplantation, both from cadaver donors. They too are well. Their need came at a better time, when cyclosporine was available and cadaver transplantation was no longer the uncertain gamble which it still was in 1971. One of these girls, now fully grown and beautiful, escorted her father to the reception. Her transplantation in 1990 was performed in Dallas by Goran Klintmalm, a Swedish surgeon and protégé of Carl Groth's. We had trained Klintmalm at our Colorado-Pittsburgh program in 1979–81.

Thus, instead of dying away, the ripples from the earlier days of transplantation had became stronger and more complex. As medical director at the Baylor University Hospital in Dallas, Fordtran decided in 1984 to establish a liver transplant program, and it was primarily for this purpose rather than to create another kidney center that he recruited Klintmalm from Stockholm. The objective was met.

The beginning of the Dallas liver program came earlier than planned. In early December 1984, a four-year-old child named Amy Garrison was flown from her home in Kentucky to place an ornamental star at the top of the White House Christmas tree. This was a traditional event for those occupying these grand quarters, and it marked the unofficial opening of the Washington holiday season. It was expected to be Amy's last Christmas. She was dying of biliary atresia, the disease for which liver transplantation was first attempted on Bennie Solis almost twenty-two years earlier. In the days after the ceremony, her condition rapidly deteriorated.

No organ donor could be found until the evening of December 22 when a response came from Hamilton, Ontario. While Amy's family packed in preparation to come to Pittsburgh, it was found that there was no room at the inn called the Children's Hospital. The intensive care unit was jammed with mortally ill children on breathing machines. A manger had to be found. The only possibility was Dallas. Klintmalm had barely arrived from Stockholm and had not had time to obtain a Texas state medical license, assemble a team, or even collect the required special equipment.

Back in the White House, Nancy Reagan had not forgotten the child. With the assistance of her staff and the administration of Baylor University Hospital, an executive order from the governor of Texas was obtained granting me permission to operate there. The plane carrying Amy headed south. Loaded with equipment and with experts who knew about every phase of liver transplantation, our plane flew north to the Canadian hospital.

Several hours later, after bringing on board the precious liver in a refrigerated lunch cooler, we took off from Hamilton in pursuit of Amy's plane, picking up the Mississippi river on our southern course before veering southwest to our destination more than two-thousand miles away. In Dallas, we met Amy in the operating room for her second nativity. The operation was successful.

Later that day, we returned to Pittsburgh. Every year, Hank Bahnson had a Christmas party at his home, on or just before Christmas eve. The University of Pittsburgh surgeons provided the entertainment by dressing in costumes and singing carols for the benefit of the gathered children, accompanied by Bahnson's harmonica. Since joining him after leaving Colorado, I had never missed the party. Without changing clothes, I drove from the airport to his house and slipped in through the garage door. The first thing I heard was the harmonica and the dissonant sounds of "We Three Kings of Orient Are." Still unnoticed, I joined the chorus line.

Amy Garrison is still well. The Dallas liver transplantation program was born. In the long run, Fordtran had overcome adversity, engineered the salvation of his children, and become the architect of one of the largest liver transplantation centers in the world. When in June 1991 he was given a Distinguished Educator Award by his gastroenterology association two days after my Saturday night reception, the citation was for his public accomplishments. As the wiry balding Texan wended his way to the rostrum, I was warmed by my knowledge of the more complete story. His was a puzzle family. Although he was not himself an organ recipient, transplantation had reshaped him. His life had been shattered by the siege of a terrible familial disease—and then reassembled piece by piece, stronger than ever. He too was a puzzle person.

Back at the Saturday reception, the crowd was swollen by arriving recipients. One waited in a corner, too shy to join the others in the receiving line and unnoticed until the speeches began. Even then, his words were few. Talking into the microphone, he expressed his appreciation for the second chance at life given to him by his new liver in Pittsburgh seven years earlier. Then, he gave me a copper plaque that he had made himself. It was inscribed: "Dr. Starzl: No one understands your achievements better than your recipients. Thank you. Tom Blanford, 'Grocer'." Few who were there knew what this meant, or the reason for the tears that welled into the eyes of Sandee Staschak, the leader of the nurse coordinators who had helped take care of him. Like John Fordtran, there was much more to know about Blanford.

After he was born in 1958, Blanford's eighteen-year-old mother was unable to care for him and placed him for adoption. His life was ordinary until his mid twenties when he developed liver disease. The question that had haunted him all his life now assumed new importance. Who was his natural mother? It was suspected that he had an inherited disorder of the liver, but this could not be proved without examining his biologic parents and doing special studies on them. A hunt for the parents was organized, and before long, Blanford got a phone number where his mother could be reached.

When he called, he realized that this was someone he knew. It was a woman who had moved recently from eastern Iowa to Coal Valley, Illinois, where he lived and managed a grocery store. For reasons neither could understand, they had been drawn to each other and had exchanged many kindnesses. Providence, which separated them at the time of his birth, had arranged a mother-and-child reunion in time for Blanford's death. Touched by the sight, fate stayed its hand on May 5, 1984, with a new liver in the Presbyterian University Hospital operating room. The stars that had found each other in the vast universe were permitted to remain together.

The reception wore on. Paul Taylor, the black man and jack-of-all-trades, who two decades earlier was the first full-time organ procurement coordinator in the world, could be seen moving confidently through the New Orleans crowd, snapping photographs of old friends who were embracing and reminiscing. In his youth, he would not have been welcome in this room except as a servant. Graying now, he still carried in his head the names and fate of the earlier patients saved by the cadaver organs he had obtained. He also stayed in touch with the donor families long after the world had forgotten them. It was like a personal religion.

One after the other, those who were there spoke, each with their own memories and feelings. Once they had known each other as doctors, nurses, patients, parents, and technicians. Through a mystical fusion, each had absorbed a part of the others and had become a puzzle person. They were friends now with no professional or cultural barriers. It was a happy time. At the end, a message was read from President and Mrs. Bush, a congratulatory video taped earlier by Governor Robert Casey of Pennsylvania was played, and it was time to adjourn.

» «

On the following day, Sunday, I was told to go to the lobby of my hotel to meet with Michael Field, a distinguished professor of medicine and a specialist in diseases of the gut and liver at Columbia University. I knew him only by his reputation in science. His mission this morning was to explain the meaning and background of two prizes that I would receive the following morning. In response, I was expected to deliver a twenty-five-minute lecture on transplantation with particular emphasis on liver replacement.

As Field and I talked, he revealed that he himself had undergone a liver transplantation performed more than a year previously by Bud Shaw at the University of Nebraska. Shaw, the surgeon who sewed in Stormie Jones's first liver, had transformed Field's decaying life and health back to normal, as if he were a magician whose trick was performed with a touch of a wand. There were many surgeons now who were capable of this, and almost all had been trained in Pittsburgh or Colorado.

Field continued to explain. He described his struggle for many years with liver disease and his determination to contribute as much as he could to medicine and science in spite of his handicap and before it overcame him. He spoke of his long belief that liver transplantation was only a fantasy and could not be a practical solution for his problem. He had watched the pieces of liver transplantation fall into place as the years went by, and now he wanted to thank me for what eventually had happened.

Field's language was even, with no hint of sentimentality. His detachment was that of a soldier who needed help to come back from no man's land after performance of a hard duty, but who had not expected at first to receive it. Or of a mountain climber who was too exhausted to make it back down after scaling a peak and was satisfied that he had done his best, no matter the outcome.

Much as I appreciated Field's kind words, I knew that the real tribute was to him and to other patients who like him found the will to strive and survive. It is true that transplant surgeons saved patients, but the patients rescued us in turn and gave meaning to what we did, or tried to. This thought was going to be in my first sentence the next day when I gave the Beaumont Lecture.

The audience the following morning contained more people than the town in Iowa where I was born and raised. Stunned by the size of the crowd, I remember regretting that my dead mother and father could not be with me at that moment, and then reflecting, who was to say that they were not. Either way, I felt certain that I had not shamed them. This might be as close as I could come to the riddle of my own jigsaw puzzle. If so, it would be close enough.

Notes
Index

Notes

Preface
1. Thomas E. Starzl, "My Thirty-five-Year View of Organ Transplantation," in *History of Transplantation: Thirty-Five Recollections*, ed. P. I. Terasaki (Los Angeles: UCLA Tissue Typing Laboratory, 1991), pp. 144–82.

Chapter 2. Printer's Ink
1. *The American Heritage Dictionary*, 2d College Edition.

2. Dr. Friedrich Katscher, a Viennese medical journalist who writes for the *Wiener Zeitung*, made an effort to find the meaning of the name Starzl, which he correctly identified as Austrian in origin. His primary source was J. Andreas Schmeller, *Bayerisches Wörterbuch, Sammlung von Wortern und Ausdrucken* [Bavarian Dictionary, Collection of Words and Expressions] (Stuttgart und Tübingen: Verlag der J. G. Cotta'schen Buchhandlung, 1836), pp. 659–60.

> Der Starz (diminutive *das Starzl*): 1. stock of cabbage plants 2. a piece of bone, stone, wood etc. that is put upright at the Plattel game to overthrow it 3. tail of animals, in high German *Sterz* 4. the piece of the long wooden pole that stands out behind a rack-wagon 5. the rear-end of a thing opposite to the head-end.
> *Der Sterz, das Sterzlein*: 1. same meaning as *Starz*, to stand upright like a *Sterzlein* (*l* or *lein* at the end of a word mean a diminutive like *y* in English), the grip of a plow 2. the end-piece of a round loaf of bread that is cut first or remains at the end 3. a kind of thick mush of flour, potatoes and the like.

Dr. Katscher, who provided the English translation, added, "Now you must select which your name means. . . . Sterzl in Viennese dialect means little man, shortie and that could be the origin, pronounced Starzl in other parts of the Austro-Hungarian monarchy."

3. "John Starzl Trial Is Postponed Again," *Sioux City Tribune*, January 9, 1918, p. 9.

4. John C. Miller, *Crisis in Freedom: The Alien and Sedition Acts* (Boston: Little, Brown, 1951).

5. M. McStay, *Colin* (Dublin: Poolbeg Press, June 1986).

Chapter 3. Medical School (1947–52)
1. T. E. Starzl and H. W. Magoun, "Organization of the Diffuse Thalamic Projection System," *Journal of Neurophysiology* 14 (1951):133–46; T. E. Starzl, C. W. Taylor, and H. W. Magoun, "Ascending Conduction in the Reticular Activating System, with Special Reference to the Diencephalon," ibid., 461–77; T. E. Starzl, C. W. Taylor, and H. W. Magoun, "Collateral Afferent Excitation of the Reticular Formation of Brain Stem," ibid., 479–96; T. E. Starzl and D. G. Whitlock, "Diffuse Thalamic Projection System in Monkey," ibid. 15 1952):449–68.

Chapter 4. The Johns Hopkins Hospital
1. T. E. Starzl, R. A. Gaertner, and R. C. Webb, Jr., "The Effects of Repetitive Electric Cardiac Stimulation in Dogs with Normal Hearts, Complete Heart Block and Experimental Cardiac Arrest," *Circulation* 11 (1955):952–62; T. E. Starzl, R. A. Gaertner, and R. R. Baker, "Acute Complete Heart Block in Dogs," ibid. 12 (1955):82–89; T. E. Starzl and R. A. Gaertner, "Chronic Heart Block in Dogs: A Method for Producing Experimental Heart Failure," ibid. 12 (1955):259–70.

Chapter 5. A Trip South
1. T. E. Starzl, R. K. Broadaway, R. C. Dever, and G. B. Reams, "The Management of Penetrating Wounds of the Inferior Vena Cava," *American Surgeon* 23 (1957):455–61.

2. F. N. Cooke, F. T. Kurzweg, and T. E. Starzl, "Blood Vessel Bank: Organization and Function," *Bulletin of the University of Miami School of Medicine and Jackson Memorial Hospital* 2 (1957):26–31.

3. A. E. Walker, J. P. Dawson, and R. Lattes, "Faculty-Administration Relationships: The School of Medicine at the University of Miami (Florida)," *AAUP Bulletin*, Spring 1961, pp. 24–39.

4. W. H. Meyer, Jr., and T. E. Starzl, "The Effect of Eck and Reverse Eck Fistula in Dogs with Experimental Diabetes Mellitus," *Surgery* 45 (1959):760–64.

5. N. V. Eck, "K voprosu o perevyazkie vorotnois veni: Predvaritelnoye soobschjenye," *Voen Med J* 130 (1877):1–2 (translated by C. G. Child III in *Surgery, Gynecology, and Obstetrics* 96 [1953]:375–76).

6. M. Hahn, O. Massen, M. Nencki, and J. Pavlow, "Die Eck'sche Fistel zwischen der unteren Hohlvene und der Pfortader und ihre Folgen für den Organismus," *Archives of Experimental Pathology and Pharmacology* 32 (1893):161–210.

7. T. E. Starzl, V. M. Bernhard, R. Benvenuto, and N. Cortes, "A New Method for One-Stage Hepatectomy in Dogs," *Surgery* 46 (1959):880–86.

8. C. S. Welch, "A Note on Transplantation of the Whole Liver in Dogs," *Transplantation Bulletin* 2 (1955):54.

Chapter 6. A Fertile Vacuum
1. T. E. Starzl, H. A. Kaupp, Jr., D. R. Brock, R. E. Lazarus, and R. V. Johnson, "Reconstructive Problems in Canine Liver Homotransplantation with Special Reference to the Postoperative Role of Hepatic Venous Flow," *Surgery, Gynecology, and Obstetrics* 111 (1960):733–43.

2. T. E. Starzl and O. H. Trippel, "Reno-Mesentero-Aortic-Iliac Thromboendarterectomy in Patients with Malignant Hypertension," *Surgery* 46 (1959):556–64.

Chapter 7. Substance or Stunts?
1. F. D. Moore, H. B. Wheeler, H. V. Demissianos, L. L. Smith, O. Balankura, K. Abel, J. B. Greenberg, and G. J. Dammin, "Experimental Whole-Organ Transplantation of the Liver and of the Spleen," *Annals of Surgery* 152 (1960):374–87 (T. E. Starzl's discussion of Moore's presentation is on p. 386); T. E. Starzl, H. A. Kaupp, Jr., D. R. Brock, R. E. Lazarus, and R. V. Johnson, "Reconstructive Problems in Canine Liver Homotransplantation with Special Reference to the Postoperative Role of Hepatic Venous Flow," *Surgery, Gynecology, and Obstetrics* 111 (1960):733–43.

2. D. M. Hume, T. Benjamin, C. F. Zukoski, H. M. Lee, H. M. Kauffman, and R. H. Egdahl, "The Homotransplantation of Kidneys and of Fetal Liver and Spleen After Total Body Irradiation," *Annals of Surgery* 152 (1960):354–73.

3. T. E. Starzl, G. W. Butz, Jr., D. R. Brock, J. T. Linman, and W. T. Moss, "Canine Liver Homotransplants: The Effect of Host and Graft Irradiation," *Archives of Surgery* 85 (1962):460–64.

4. F. D. Moore, "Life and Contributions of David Hume," *Transplantation Proceedings* 6 (1974):153–56.

5. The eulogies appear in *Transplantation Proceedings* 6 (1974):141–45 (Harrison); 156–59 (Merrill); 159–62 (Murray).

6. T. E. Starzl and H. A. Kaupp, Jr., "Mass Homotransplantation of Abdominal Organs in Dogs," *Surgical Forum* 11 (1960):28–30.

7. C. F. Zukoski, H. M. Lee, and D. M. Hume, "The Prolongation of Functional Survival of Canine Renal Homografts by 6-mercaptopurine," *Surgical Forum* 11 (1960):470–72.

8. R. Y. Calne, "Rejection of Renal Homografts: Inhibition in Dogs by 6-mercaptopurine," *The Lancet* 1 (1960):417.

Chapter 9. The Failed Liver Transplant Trials
1. T. E. Starzl, T. L. Marchioro, K. N. Von Kaulla, G. Hermann, R. S. Brittain, and W. R. Waddell, "Homotransplantation of the Liver in Humans," *Surgery, Gynecology, and Obstetrics* 117 (1963):659–76.

Chapter 10. Time
1. *Surgery, Gynecology, and Obstetrics* 117 (1963):385–95.

2. T. E. Starzl, *Experience in Renal Transplantation* (Philadelphia: W. B. Saunders, 1964).

3. J. E. Murray, R. Gleason, and A. Bartholomay, "Second Report of Registry in Human Kidney Transplantation," *Transplantation* 2 (1964):660–67.

4. T. E. Starzl, G.P.J. Schroter, N. J. Hartmann, N. Barfield, P. Taylor, and T. L. Mangan, "Long Term (25 Year) Survival After Renal Homotransplantation: The World Experience," *Transplantation Proceedings* 22 (1990):2361–65.

Chapter 11. Tissue Matching
1. J. Hamburger, J. Vaysse, J. Crosnier, J. Auvert, C. M. Lalanne, and J. Hopper, "Renal Homotransplantation in Man After Radiation of the Recipient," *American Journal of Medicine* 32 (1962):854–71.

2. P. I. Terasaki, T. L. Marchioro, and T. E. Starzl, "Sero-typing of Human Lymphocyte Antigens: Preliminary Trials on Long-term Kidney Homograft Survivors," in *Histocompatibility Testing 1965*, ed. P. S. Russell, H. J. Winn, D. B. Amos (Washington D.C.: National Academy of Sciences, 1965) pp. 83–96.

3. T. E. Starzl, K. A. Porter, G. Andres, C. G. Halgrimson, R. Hurwitz, G. Giles, P. I. Terasaki, I. Penn, G. T. Schroter, J. Lilly, S. G. Starkie, and C. W. Putnam, "Long-term Survival After Renal Transplantation in Humans: With Special Reference to Histocompatibility Matching, Thymectomy, Homograft Glomerulonephritis, Heterologous ALG, and Recipient Malignancy," *Annals of Surgery* 172 (1970):437–72.

4. See P. I. Terasaki, T. L. Marchioro, and T. E. Starzl, "Sero-typing of Human Lymphocyte Antigens."

Chapter 12. Why Not Two Livers?
1. C. S. Welch, "A Note on Transplantation of the Whole Liver in Dogs," *Transplantation Bulletin* 2 (1955):54.

2. T. E. Starzl, T. L. Marchioro, D. T. Rowlands, Jr., C. H. Kirkpatrick, W.E.C. Wilson, D. Rifkind, and W. R. Waddell, "Immunosuppression After Experimental and Clinical Homotransplantation of the Liver," *Annals of Surgery* 160 (1964): 411–39.

3. T. L. Marchioro, K. A. Porter, T. C. Dickinson, T. D. Faris, and T. E. Starzl, "Physiologic Requirements for Auxiliary Liver Homotransplantation," *Surgery, Gynecology, and Obstetrics* 121 (1965):17–31.

4. T. L. Marchioro, K. A. Porter, B. I. Brown, J. B. Otte, and T. E. Starzl, "The Effect of Partial Portacaval Transposition on the Canine Liver," *Surgery* 61 (1967):723–32.

Chapter 13. A Counterattack on Rejection
1. T. E. Starzl, T. L. Marchioro, K. A. Porter, P. D. Taylor, T. D. Faris, T. J. Herrmann, C. J. Hlad, and W. R. Waddell, "Factors Determining Short- and Long-term Survival After Orthotopic Liver Homotransplantation in the Dog," *Surgery* 58 (1965):131–55.

2. T. E. Starzl, "Inaugural: Presidential Address, American Society of Transplant Surgeons," *Surgery* 79 (1976):129–131; T. S. Kuhn, *The Structure of Scientific Revolutions* (Chicago: University of Chicago Press, 1962).

3. I. I. Metchnikov, "Etudes sur la résorption des cellules," *Annales de l'Institut Pasteur* (Paris) 13 (1899):737–69.

4. T. E. Starzl, T. L. Marchioro, K. A. Porter, Y. Iwasaki, and C. J. Cerilli, "The Use of Heterologous Antilymphoid Agents in Canine Renal and Liver Homo-transplantation, and in Human Renal Homotransplantation," *Surgery, Gynecology, and Obstetrics* 124 (1967):301–18.

Chapter 14. The Donors and the Organs
1. The proceedings were published in G. E W. Wolstenholme and M. O'Connor, eds., *Ethics in Medical Progress: With Special Reference to Transplantation* (Boston: Little, Brown, 1966).

2. "Definition of Irreversible Coma: Report of the Ad Hoc Committee of the Harvard Medical School to Examine the Definition of Brain Death," *Journal of the American Medical Association* 205 (1968):337–40.

3. W. E. Burger, "The Law and Medical Advances," in *The Changing Mores of Biomedical Research: A Colloquium on Ethical Dilemmas from Medical Advances*, ed. J. R. Elkinton, *Annals of Internal Medicine* 67 suppl. 7 (1967):15–18.

4. J.R.W. Ackermann and C. N. Barnard, "Successful Storage of Kidneys," *British Journal of Surgery* 53 (1966):525–32.

5. L. Brettschneider, P. M. Daloze, C. Huguet, K. A. Porter, C. G. Groth, N. Kashiwagi, D. E. Hutchison, and T. E. Starzl, "The Use of Combined Preserva-tion Techniques for Extended Storage of Orthotopic Liver Homografts," *Surgery, Gynecology, and Obstetrics* 126 (1968):263–74.

Chapter 15. A Liver Summit Team
1. T. L. Marchioro, C. Hougie, H. Ragde, R. B. Epstein, and E. D. Thomas, "Hemophilia: Role of Organ Homografts," *Science* 163 (1969):163–88.

2. J. H. Lewis, F. A. Bontempo, J. A. Spero, M. V. Ragni, and T. E. Starzl, "Liver Transplantation in a Hemophiliac," *New England Journal of Medicine* 312 (1985):1189–90.

3. Rheology is a science dealing with the deformation and flow of matter (*Webster's Ninth New Collegiate Dictionary*).

Chapter 16. A Pyrrhic Victory
1. The proceedings were published in J. R. Elkinton, ed., *The Changing Mores of Biomedical Research: A Colloquium on Ethical Dilemmas from Medical Advances*, Annals of Internal Medicine 67 suppl. 7 (1967):1–83.

2. T. E. Starzl, "Ethical Problems in Organ Transplantation," ibid., pp. 32–36.

3. Ibid.

4. T. E. Starzl, C. G. Groth, L. Brettschneider, I. Penn, V. A. Fulginiti, J. B. Moon, H. Blanchard, A. J. Martin, Jr., and K. A. Porter, "Orthotopic Homotransplantation of the Human Liver," *Annals of Surgery* 168 (1968):392–415.

5. T. E. Starzl and C. W. Putnam, *Experience in Hepatic Transplantation* (Philadelphia: W. B. Saunders, 1969).

Chapter 17. Icebergs and Hammer Blows
1. T. E. Starzl, C. W. Putnam, C. G. Halgrimson, G. T. Schroter, G. Martineau, B. Launois, J. L. Corman, I. Penn, A. S. Booth, Jr., C. G. Groth, and K. A. Porter, "Cyclophosphamide and Whole Organ Transplantation in Human Beings," *Surgery, Gynecology, and Obstetrics* 133 (1971):981–91.

2. C. Clifford, *Counsel to the President* (New York: Random House, 1991).

3. T. E. Starzl, A. Francavilla, C. G. Halgrimson, F. R. Francavilla, K. A. Porter, T. H. Brown, and C. W. Putnam, "The Origin, Hormonal Nature, and Action of Hepatotrophic Substances in Portal Venous Blood," *Surgery, Gynecology, and Obstetrics* 137 (1973):179–99.

4. The funeral of this child is described in T. E. Starzl, "In a Small Iowa Town," *Transplantation Proceedings* 20 suppl. 1 (1988):12–17.

5. T. E. Starzl, K. Watanabe, K. A. Porter, and C. W. Putnam, "Effect of Insulin, Glucagon, and Insulin/Glucagon Infusion on Liver Morphology and Cell Division After Complete Portacaval Shunt in Dogs," *The Lancet* 1 (1976):821–25.

6. J. L. Bollman, "The Animal with an Eck Fistula," *Physiological Reviews* 41 (1961):607–21.

7. L. Thomas, *The Lives of a Cell* (New York: Viking Press, 1974).

8. T. E. Starzl, K. A. Porter, C. W. Putnam, G. P. J. Schroter, C. G. Halgrimson, R. Weil III, M. Hoelscher, and H. A. S. Reid, "Orthotopic Liver Transplantation in Ninety-Three Patients," *Surgery, Gynecology, and Obstetrics* 142 (1976):487–505.

9. Written by Forrest J. Ackerman of the Science Fiction Institute, Los Angeles.

Chapter 19. The Kidney Wars
1. J. F. Borel, C. Feurer, H. U. Gubler, and H. Stahelin, "Biological Effects of Cyclosporin A: A New Antilymphocytic Agent," *Agents and Actions* 6 (1976): 468–75.

2. R. Y. Calne, K. Rolles, S. Thiru, P. McMaster, G. N. Craddock, S. Azis, D. J. G. White, D. B. Evans, D. C. Dunn, R. G. Henderson, and P. Lewis, "Cyclosporin A Initially as the Only Immunosuppressant in 34 Patients of Cadaveric Organs: 32 Kidneys, 2 Pancreas, and 2 Livers," *The Lancet* II (1979): 1033–36.

3. T. E. Starzl, R. Weil III, S. Iwatsuki, G. Klintmalm, G. P. J. Schroter, L. J. Koep, Y. Iwaki, P. I. Terasaki, and K. A. Porter, "The Use of Cyclosporin A and Prednisone in Cadaver Kidney Transplantation," *Surgery, Gynecology, and Obstetrics* 151 (1980):17–26.

Chapter 20. A Tale of Four Cities
1. T. E. Starzl, S. Iwatsuki, G. Klintmalm, G. P. J. Schroter, R. Weil III, L. J. Koep, and K. A. Porter, "Liver Transplantation, 1980, with Particular Reference to Cyclosporin A," *Transplantation Proceedings* 13 (1981):281–85; T. E. Starzl, G. B. G. Klintmalm, K. A. Porter, S. Iwatsuki, and G. P. J. Schroter, "Liver Transplantation with Use of Cyclosporin A and Prednisone," *New England Journal of Medicine* 305 (1981):266–69.

Chapter 21. Letter in a Birmingham Jail
1. *Webster's Ninth New Collegiate Dictionary.*

2. M. L. King, "Letter from Birmingham Jail," in *Black Writers of America: A Comprehensive Anthology*, ed. R. Barksdale and K. Kinnamon (New York: Mac-Millan, 1972), pp. 865, 866.

3. F. D. Moore, "Discussion of T. E. Starzl, C. G. Groth, L. Brettschneider, I. Penn, V. A. Fulginiti, J. B. Moon, H. Blanchard, A. J. Martin, and K. A. Porter, 'Orthotopic Homotransplantation of the Human Liver,'" *Annals of Surgery* 168 (1968):414–15.

4. *The Belmont Report: Ethical Principles and Guidelines for the Protection of Human Subjects of Research*, Report of the National Commission for the Protection of Human Subjects of Biomedical and Behavioral Research (Washington, D.C.: Department of Health, Education and Welfare, April 18, 1979; GPO publication 887-809), p. 2.

5. *Federal Register* 46 (January 26, 1981):8366–92: ibid. (January 27, 1981):8942–80.

6. M. M. Ravitch, "Colleagues Suborned," *Perspectives in Biology and Medicine* 25 (1982):404–05.

7. J. T. Rosenthal, T. R. Hakala, S. Iwatsuki, B. W. Shaw, Jr., and T. E. Starzl, "Cadaveric Renal Transplantation Under Cyclosporine-Steroid Therapy," *Surgery, Gynecology, and Obstetrics* 157 (1983):309–15.

8. T. E. Starzl, T. R. Hakala, S. Iwatsuki, T. J. Rosenthal, B. W. Shaw, Jr., G.B.G. Klintmalm, and K. A. Porter, "Cyclosporin A and Steroid Treatment in 104 Cadaveric Renal Transplantations," in *Cyclosporin A*, ed. D.J.G. White (Amsterdam: Elsevier Biomedical Press, 1982), pp. 365–77.

9. T. E. Starzl, "Protecting the Patient's Interest," *Kidney International* 28 suppl 17 (1985):31–33.

10. M. Angell, "The Nazi Hypothermia Experiments and Unethical Research Today," *New England Journal of Medicine* 322 (1990):1462–64.

Chapter 22. The Liver Wars
1. P. Yomtoob and T. Schwarz, *The Gift of Life* (New York: St. Martin's Press, 1986).

2. R. Schmid, "Issues in Liver Transplantation," *Hepatology* suppl (1984):1–104.

3. Her pictures appeared in T. E. Starzl, T. R. Hakala, B. W. Shaw, Jr., R. L. Hardesty, T. J. Rosenthal, B. P. Griffith, S. Iwatsuki, and H. T. Bahnson, "A Flexible Procedure for Multiple Cadaveric Organ Procurement," *Surgery, Gynecology, and Obstetrics* 158 (1984):223–30.

4. Today, all three men are professors of surgery and directors of liver transplant programs. Makowka is at UCLA (Cedars Sinai); Mosimann at the University of Lausanne, Switzerland; and Henderson at Emory University, Atlanta.

5. N. V. Jamieson, R. Sundberg, S. Lindell, R. Laravuso, M. Kalayoglu, J. F. Southard, and F. O. Belzer, "Successful 24- to 30-hour Preservation of the Canine Liver: A Preliminary Report," *Transplantation Proceedings* 20 suppl. 1 (1988): 945–47.

Chapter 23. Politics
1. T. E. Starzl, T. Hakala, A. Tzakis, R. Gordon, A. Stieber, L. Makowka, J. Klimoski, and H. Bahnson, "A Multifactorial System for Equitable Selection of Cadaveric Kidney Recipients," *Journal of the American Medical Association* 257 (1987):3073–75; T. E. Starzl, R. D. Gordon, A. Tzakis, S. Staschak, V. Fioravanti, B. Broznick, L. Makowka, and H. T. Bahnson, "Equitable Allocation of Extrarenal Organs: With Special Reference to the Liver," *Transplantation Proceedings* 20 (1988):131–38.

Chapter 24. Understanding Governor Lamm
1. R. Lamm, "The Coming Era of Hard Choices" (interview by Emily Friedman), *Hospitals* 59 (1985):96–100.

2. R. D. Lamm, "Health Care as Economic Cancer," *Dialysis and Transplantation* 16 (1987):432–33.

3. T. E. Starzl, "New Options" (editorial), ibid., pp. 432–33.

Chapter 25. The Drug With No Name
1. A. Tzakis, M. H. Cooper, J. S. Dummer, M. Ragni, J. W. Ward, and T. E. Starzl, "Transplantation in HIV + Patients," *Transplantation* 49 (1990):354–58.

2. T. E. Starzl, L. Makowka, and S. Todo, eds., "FK 506: A Potential Breakthrough in Immunosuppression," *Transplantation Proceedings* 19 suppl. 6 (1987):1–103.

3. T. E. Starzl, S. Todo, J. Fung, A. J. Demetris, R. Venkataramanan, and A. Jain, "FK 506 for Human Liver, Kidney, and Pancreas Transplantation," *The Lancet* 2 (1989):1000–04.

4. A. G. Tzakis, C. Ricordi, R. Alejandro, Y. Zeng, J. J. Fung, S. Todo, A. J. Demetris, D. H. Mintz, and T. E. Starzl, "Pancreatic Islet Transplantation After Upper Abdominal Exenteration and Liver Replacement," *The Lancet* 2 no. 336 (1990):402–05.

5. M. Barker, "Pancreatic Islet Transplantation" (letter to editor), *The Lancet* 2 no. 336 (1990):1323.

6. T. E. Starzl and A. Tzakis (letter to editor, response to Barker), *The Lancet* 2 no. 336 (1990):1323.

7. R. C. Lillehei, B. Goott, and F. A. Miller, "The Physiologic Response of the Small Bowel of the Dog to Ischemia Including Prolonged In Vitro Preservation of the Bowel with Successful Replacement and Survival," *Annals of Surgery* 150 (1959):543–60.

8. T. E. Starzl and H. A. Kaupp, Jr., "Mass Homotransplantation of Abdominal Organs in Dogs," *Surgical Forum* 11 (1960):28–30.

9. T. E. Starzl, M. I. Rowe, S. Todo, R. Jaffe, A. Tzakis, A. L. Hoffman, C. Esquivel, K. A. Porter, R. Venkataramanan, L. Makowka, and R. Duquesnoy, "Transplantation of Multiple Abdominal Viscera," *Journal of the American Medical Association* 261 (1989):1449–57.

10. T. E. Starzl, S. Todo, A. Tzakis, M. Alessiani, A. Casavilla, K. Abu-Elmagd, and J. J. Fung, "The Many Faces of Multivisceral Transplantation," *Surgery, Gynecology, and Obstetrics* 172 (1991):335–44.

11. D. Grant, W. Wall, R. Mimeault, R. Zhong, C. Ghent, B. Garcia, C. Stiller, and J. Duff, "Successful Small-Bowel/Liver Transplantation," *The Lancet* 2 no. 335 (1990):181–84.

12. S. Todo, A. G. Tzakis, K. Abu-Elmagd, J. Reyes, J. J. Fung, K. Nakamura, A. Yagihashi, A. Jain, N. Murase, Y. Iwaki, A. F. Demetris, D. H. Van Thiel, and T. E. Starzl, "Cadaveric Small Bowel and Small Bowel–Liver Transplantation in Humans," *Transplantation* 53 (1992):369–76.

Chapter 26. The Day the String Broke
1. T. E. Starzl, R. H. Bell, R. W. Beart, and C. W. Putnam, "Hepatic Trisegmentectomy and Other Liver Resections," *Surgery, Gynecology, and Obstetrics* 141 (1975):429–37; T. E. Starzl, S. Iwatsuki, B. W. Shaw, Jr., P. M. Waterman, D. Van Thiel, H. S. Diliz-P, A. Dekker, and K. M. Bron, "Left Hepatic Trisegmentectomy," *Surgery, Gynecology, and Obstetrics* 155 (1982):21–7.

Chapter 27. The Little Drummer Girls
1. T. E. Starzl, A. J. Demetris, and D. H. Van Thiel, "Medical Progress: Liver Transplantation," part I, *New England Journal of Medicine* 321 (1989):1014–22.

2. T. E. Starzl, H. P. Chase, C. W. Putnam, and K. A. Porter, "Portacaval Shunt in Hyperlipoproteinemia," *The Lancet* 2 (1973):940–44.

3. T. E. Starzl, I. Y. Lee, K. A. Porter, and C. W. Putnam, "The Influence of Portal Blood Upon Lipid Metabolism in Normal and Diabetic Dogs and Baboons," *Surgery, Gynecology, and Obstetrics* 140 (1975):381–96.

4. D. W. Bilheimer, J. L. Goldstein, S. M. Grundy, and M. S. Brown, "Reduction in Cholesterol and Low-Density-Lipoprotein Synthesis After Portacaval Shunt Surgery in a Patient with Homozygous Familial Hypercholesterolemia," *Journal of Clinical Investigation* 56 (1975):1420–30.

5. J. Goldstein and M. S. Brown, "Binding and Degradation of Low Density Lipoproteins in Cultured Human Fibroblasts: Comparison of Cells from a Normal

Subject and from a Patient with Homozygous Familial Hypercholesterolemia," *Journal of Biological Chemistry* 249 (1974):5153–62.

6. T. E. Starzl, P. Chase, E. H. Ahrens, Jr., D. J. McNamara, D. W. Bilheimer, E. J. Schaefer, J. Rey, K. A. Porter, E. Stein, A. Francavilla, and L. N. Benson, "Portacaval Shunt in Patients with Familial Hypercholesterolemia," *Annals of Surgery* 198 (1983):273–83.

7. T. E. Starzl, D. W. Bilheimer, H. T. Bahnson, B. W. Shaw, Jr., R. L. Hardesty, B. P. Griffith, S. Iwatsuki, B. J. Zitelli, J. C. Gartner, Jr., J. J. Malatack, and A. H. Urbach, "Heart-Liver Transplantation in a Patient with Familial Hypercholesterolemia," *The Lancet* 1 (1984):1382–83.

8. D. W. Bilheimer, J. L. Goldstein, S. M. Grundy, T. E. Starzl, and M. S. Brown, "Liver Transplantation to Provide Low-Density-Lipoprotein Receptors and Lower Plasma Cholesterol in a Child with Homozygous Familial Hypercholesterolemia," *New England Journal of Medicine* 311 (1984):1658–64.

9. *The Lancet* 2 (1974):449–51.

Index